PARENTING FOR PEACE

PARENTING *for* PEACE

*Raising the Next
Generation of Peacemakers*

Marcy Axness, PhD

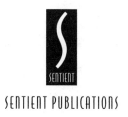

SENTIENT PUBLICATIONS

First Sentient Publications edition 2012
Copyright © 2012 by Marcy Axness, PhD

A Caress, 1891, Mary Stevenson Cassatt, 1845-1926, pastel on paper, 29 1/4 x 23 3/4 in., is included with permission from New Britain Museum of American Art and Harriet Russell Stanley Fund, 1948.14.

A paperback original

Cover design by Kim Johansen, Black Dog Design (www.blackdogdesign.com)
Book design by Timm Bryson

The information in this book is not intended as a protocol for the treatment of individual patients and is not a substitute for professional medical help. The author, publisher, and all others associated with this book cannot be held liable for any consequences of undertaking ideas or suggestions in this book whether or not under the care of a licensed professional.

Library of Congress Cataloging-in-Publication Data
Axness, Marcy, 1956-
  Parenting for peace : raising the next generation of peacemakers / Marcy Axness.
    p. cm.
  Includes bibliographical references.
  ISBN 978-1-59181-176-3
  1. Child rearing. 2. Parenting. 3. Peace--Psychological aspects. I. Title.
  HQ769.A93 2012
  649'.1—dc23
                           2011047141

Printed in the United States of America
10 9 8 7 6 5 4 3 2 1

SENTIENTPUBLICATIONS
A Limited Liability Company
1113 Spruce Street
Boulder, CO 80302
www.sentientpublications.com

You are the bows from which your children
as living arrows are sent forth.
The archer sees the mark upon the path of the infinite,
and He bends you with His might
that His arrows may go swift and far.

—KAHLIL GIBRAN

To Eve and Ian, our wondrous arrows…

CONTENTS

STEP TWO

ATTUNED CONCEPTION—A QUANTUM COLLABORATION 55

STEP FIVE
NATURE'S PEACE PLAN—INSTALLING PEACEMAKER HARDWARE IN YEAR ONE   169

EPILOGUE   395

ACKNOWLEDGMENTS

This book is a love letter to the researchers, clinicians, authors, and educators named in these pages, threads of whose landmark work I have woven through emerging perspectives on early human development to stake out new territory on behalf of coming generations. Curt Sandman consistently encouraged my talents as a popular translator of scientific concepts. Bruce Lipton patiently tutored me in the basics of such frontier fare as genomic imprinting and (the now mainstream) epigenetics. William Emerson has gentled me along through almost twenty years of prenatal psychology ah-hahs. In addition to his extraordinary ideas I have cited, I must also thank Joseph Chilton Pearce for his championship, his counsel, and for introducing me to my guardian agent, Barbara Neighbors Deal. Without Barbara's guidance you wouldn't have this book in your hands. Her vision was unwavering about whom she wanted to publish it, and how lucky we were that Connie Shaw at Sentient welcomed and honed it with such a keen eye.

While only a handful of their stories are included, the heroic spirit of all my counseling clients permeates these pages: my gratitude to the parents-in-progress who shared their struggles and triumphs with open-hearted, courageous generosity. My heartfelt appreciation to early readers of the manuscript, for their discerning input—the meticulous Winifred Fleet, the rarified Michael Shea, the playful Howard Moody, the enthusiastic Patrick Houser, the thoughtful Jan Bowman. My thanks to Lynn Franklin for her encouragement and guidance in the early conceptual years. And no words can adequately capture her consummate devotion and pivotal importance to *Parenting for Peace:* my soul sister, my Sanchi—Laura Uplinger. In my mind, your name hovers there on the cover with mine, so imbued is this book with your wisdom, precision, and expansiveness.

This book is the result of more than research, writing, and editing; it grows out of a lot of lived life. Thanks are due to my dear late mentor Annette Baran, who, along with many other Jewish-mothery acts of love, urged me to get my doctorate so I could be heard. Before that, Randolph Severson helped me find my voice, and Jim Gritter invited me to use it out loud. Mary Anne Cohen coaxed semi-poetry out of me. Elizabeth Memel opened a new world of perception and permission that was seminal for me, through two years of weekly RIE classes with each of our two children.

I am filled with gratitude for the countless healing practitioners of all stripes over the years whose collective treatment helped me back into my skin, my heart, my life, abundantly—too many to list, so I'll trust you to know who you are.

For his unflagging support both financial and moral, for his invaluable brainstorming and troubleshooting, for his great sense of humor and mad skills on computer, and for being an extraordinary father to our children, my enduring thanks to John Axness. Ian and Eve, thank you for your enthusiastic participation in the process of creating this book. I am unspeakably proud of what thoughtful, engaged, loving people you are, and the unwavering integrity you bring to the art of living your lives. Being your mother has brought me everything.

Introduction

Do You Know How Powerful You Really Are?

A towering question lives today in the minds and hearts of young people, perhaps more strongly than ever before in human history, as they feel the growing shadow of our global human and environmental crises: "Is there *anything* I can do to change the world?"

A few years from now, these same young folks may ask another question: "Do I really want to bring a child into today's world?" Each generation's challenges seem more daunting than anything that has come before, but indeed, any thoughtful person contemplating parenthood in the twenty-first century has many stark and vivid reasons to ask this question. Our world presents complex challenges, with imbalance and complications seeming to grow at an exponential speed. The real question on the minds of future parents is, "Will my child survive in today's world? And in tomorrow's?"

What if there were a handful of uncomplicated—and amazingly little known—principles that would assure you that the answer to all of these questions can be a resounding *Yes?* What if you could feel confident that with these principles at work in your life and in your parenting, you and your child will not only survive but *thrive* in a world of ever changing complexities and challenges? And that a generation living with these principles will have what it takes to make sure our world also survives and thrives?

Today's culture exerts tremendous pressure on well-meaning parents to make choices that simply aren't good for kids, or for our future as a human family. But knowledge is empowering: heartened by the promise of simple principles backed by leading-edge research, parents can feel confident in their ability to raise children who are "hardwired for peace."

I have a proposition for you: If you're deeply concerned about today's world and where it's going...if you feel like something more is needed to heal our social and environmental issues...if you feel like you want to participate in a "solution revolution" but don't quite know how...then as Gandhi so famously urged, be the change you want to see in the world, and raise children whose very beings are woven from that change. Raise the generation who has what it takes to turn this world around. The principles in this book will help you do just that. (To be honest, it's more about *not*-doing—entering into a potent collaboration with Nature, learning how to finally stop impeding her rather perfect plan for the kind of evolutionary leap we're talking about.)

How can I claim to offer you such empowerment? And why would such revolutionary information be contained in a book but not on the front pages of every newspaper on Earth? That's a great question, and indeed why I wrote this book! These principles are sometimes written about, one at a time, here and there. But they have never been put together in quite this way to empower a new generation. Even though you have flour, eggs, sugar, and chocolate in your kitchen, years or decades could pass before you put them together and make a cake. Think of this book as a cake—or better, a lasagna—made largely from ingredients available to everyone: I've combined the latest scientific research in such fields as brain science, cell biology, epigenetics, psychology and mind-body science, folded in some perennial philosophy, layered it with timeless spiritual principles, and seasoned it with understandings gleaned from my own experiences.

I grew up the daughter of five parents, and have mothered a son and daughter to the cusp of adulthood. I share the parenting journey with a husband of twenty-seven years. I have studied meditation with devoted masters, and early development with renowned researchers. I've delved deeply into personal psychology and honor its strengths and its limitations, together with the fundamental importance of a transpersonal ("beyond the personal") perspective. I am an early development specialist who teaches graduate students and counsels parents, and am an active research junkie. I am, above all, a student and lover of Life.

The result of this recipe, which you hold in your hands, offers us one kind of chance—perhaps the best kind of chance—to heal our global family. This is an invitation to a new way of thinking about children and ourselves, about how we develop to be the people we are, and how we choose daily to become who we will be tomorrow. This book can be read at any point in your parenting journey, even long before you embark upon parenthood, since it is intended to seed your mind with ideas that over time will take root and grow within your own relationship with Life.

The idea for this book came from a column I wrote during my three-year stint with the *Wet Set Gazette*, a small Los Angeles parenting publication. I titled it "From Presence to Simplicity: Cliff Notes for P-A-R-E-N-T-S," and in it I explained that in my twenty years of being a parent, a student of human development, a human *in* constant development, an impassioned researcher of the human sciences, and a parent counselor engaged with the challenges and triumphs of real moms and dads, I have gathered a superabundance of excellent information. But I had come to recognize that one of the greatest gifts in this era of information overload is to arrive at the *other* side of a gazillion helpful facts to essential nuggets that are simplified without being simplistic. So I distilled seven solid-gold nuggets, informed by research in fields ranging from neurodevelopment to theology—foundational principles for effective, healthy and joyful parenting.

Wary of systems, techniques, or even instructions for parents, I realized that a handful of *principles* was something I could get behind. Unlike rigid rules, principles encompass individual differences in temperament, sensibilities, pacing, and cultural orientation. While rules are static, principles give room to breathe, to discover, to inhabit. Where rules constrain, principles offer an endless palette of application. Principles are timeless yet practical, like a handy, pocket-sized toolkit—at the ready anytime, anywhere. Equally wary of gimmicks—and a big fan of Boggle—I found myself whimsically realizing that the seven enduring principles I wanted to convey were considerate enough to begin with letters that spelled out PARENTS: Presence, Awareness, Rhythm, Example, Nurturance, Trust and Simplicity. My readers may not need the mnemonic assist, but I do! At the end of each step are examples—Principles

Presence — *Being fully engaged right here, right now with your body, your thoughts, your feelings*

Awareness — *The knowledge needed to be effective*

Rhythm — *A fundamental human pacing need, often forgotten in our technoautomated world*

Example — *The ultimate mode of teaching, and learning*

Nurturance — *The practical demonstration of love*

Trust — *Calm reliance upon processes outside of your immediate perception and control; cousin to humility*

Simplicity — *The absence of complication and excess*

to Practice—of ways you might apply the principles during that step; these are not meant as a definitive list, nor as a prescription, but are offered as ideas for you to try out, experience and improvise upon.

If my Cliff Notes column was the seed of this book, its seminal agent was a segment I saw on a network morning show entitled How to Raise A CEO. It featured a mother sharing insights into how she had raised three children who all had the qualities needed to become successful corporate executives. It occurred to me that people might be interested in what capacities a person needs to be a successful agent of peace and innovation, and how *those* are fostered. Since I know that such a process optimally begins before other parenting books begin—prior to conception—the idea of a timeline came to me. Thus was conceived the idea of a book featuring seven steps—from pre-conception through adolescence—and seven principles to be applied at each of the seven steps in a fluid, friendly, yet revolutionary way. A book about parenting as social action. A book about parenting for peace.

Everything in existence first begins as an idea—this book, the chair you sit in, the utensils you use to eat your food. Before moving to where you live now, you most likely gave a lot of thought to it, developing an increasingly vivid idea of *home*. We often do weeks of research before buying a particular car, envisioning ourselves driving various models, imagining how each would feel. Of all the things we might ever pursue, bringing children to life is undoubtedly the most monumental in its impact—upon us, certainly upon our children, and ultimately upon the world. It merits devoting time and care to envision the model of parenting we choose to embrace. Hopefully the model you choose is equipped to channel the awesome power—and responsibility—that comes with raising children.

Why We Must Rethink Our Parenting—and Our World

Most of us would subscribe to the goal of a peaceful, ecologically sustainable world where our great-grandchildren can thrive, but that goal seems far out of reach. Staggering evidence of human and planetary strife is scattered across the globe. U.S. foreign policy ostensibly seeks to export America's high quality of enlightened democratic life, but just how high is that quality of life? Depression is our leading cause of disability![1] A joint 2004 study by Harvard and the World Health Organization found that the U.S. suffers the highest rate of depression (9.6 percent, meaning more than nine out of every one hundred people) of the fourteen surveyed countries, including war-torn Lebanon (6.6 percent) and poverty-stricken Nigeria (0.8 percent).[2] While the truth is not quite as straightforward—in countries where mental illness is still shrouded in shame and secrecy, depression is bound to be under-reported—the troubling fact remains that many people are suffering in a country with the world's greatest material wealth.

Much of our advanced technology and scientific muscle is geared toward finding more effective drugs to *treat* depression, rather than ways to understand it more meaningfully and thus have more success at preventing it. The use of antidepressants and other psychotropic drugs for school-aged children (and even preschoolers!) has risen steadily over the past decades.[3] Youth suicide has become the third leading cause of death in American 15-24-year-olds,[4] and has doubled in the 5-14-year-old age group over the last twenty years.[5] Along with our late-model cars and flat-screen TVs, the U.S. also has more violence and higher murder rates than any Western European country, and by far the highest incarceration rate in the world.[6] As Princeton's Daniel Kahneman points out, "Standard of living has increased dramatically and happiness has increased not at all, and in some cases has diminished slightly."[7] And, for the first time in recorded history, children in the U.S. today are the first generation to have a shorter life expectancy than their parents![8]

What happened to the shining vision held dear to your great-grandparents and their kin that through hard work they could get ahead, make good money, and have a better life than their parents? Well, ironically, it seems that perhaps a good deal of our everyday suffering—represented in those bleak statistics above—is because, as Melissa Etheridge sings, we "never woke up from the American Dream." Keeping up with the Joneses has led to anxiety disorders at home, military bullying abroad and environmental crises everywhere. What if we were to conceive a new dream, suited to today's world? A dream we can embrace with confidence that it will bring riches in the moment and dividends in the future, of the deeply human sort that money cannot buy, and yet abundance tends to pursue?

Many countries are asking just such questions, as they have come to realize that Gross Domestic Product—the historical yardstick for progress—is grossly insufficient for measuring a society's wellbeing. Economist Ronald Colman points out, "Our growth statistics were never meant to be used as a measure of progress as they are today, when activities that degrade our quality of life, like crime, pollution, and addictive gambling, all make the economy grow. The more fish we sell and the more trees we cut down, the more the economy grows. Working longer hours makes the economy grow. And the economy can grow even if inequality and poverty increase. For decades, we have made a tragic error—confusing economic growth with wellbeing."[9]

In an attempt to remedy this limited view, many nations now participate in the Global Project on "Measuring the Progress of Societies"; for example, the Canadian Index of Wellbeing (CIW) calculates data from a rich array of criteria to assess its country's overall health and progress. Standard of living, health, quality of the environment, education and skill levels, how people use their time, the vitality of their communities and cultural pursuits, their participation in the democratic process—these measures as well as the interactions among them paint a picture of a richer kind of national dream.

It's great news that countries around the world are moving away from the strictly industrial context within which they assess their success and wellbeing. Unfortunately, individuals and families—at least here in the U.S.—continue to slog their way through the mire of the industrialist worldview. You might not be aware of even having a *worldview*—it sounds so pretentious—but we all do. We've all been raised in the context of a particular worldview, an overarching context for life that is made up of a largely unquestioned, inherited, subliminal set of beliefs, attitudes, perceptions, and assumptions through which we filter our understanding of the world and our place in it. I'll discuss more about the process of the kind of invisible learning that shapes a worldview in Step One.

Several basic assumptions inherent in the industrialist worldview—that economic wealth is the truest sign of progress; that more is better and we live in a world of scarcity; that successful achievement requires competition—work like an invisible pumice to erode the potential for confidence, ease, and joy in the experience of parenting and family life. When we judge ourselves according to the values of this linear, predictable worldview, while pursuing the mysterious, ever changing, sometimes chaotic process of parenting, we're doomed to disappointment. We become so busy *doing* and *going* and *acquiring* and *achieving*—and also evaluating—that we miss out on the supposed greatest experience ever that parenting is romantically cracked up to be. To add ironic salt to that wound, we then add our missing enjoyment to the long list of perceived daily failures that accrue within the industrialist worldview from which most of us operate.

As the cofounder of Families for Conscious Living, Lisa Reagan has worked for almost fifteen years with hundreds of families faced with the challenge of making wellness choices in a culture whose worldview doesn't value wellness. As a facilitator of the Worldview Literacy Project through the Institute of Noetic Sciences (IONS), Reagan highlights the importance of becoming aware of your personal lenses, "which can be as tricky as fish becoming aware of the water they swim in." Becoming aware of your worldview involves mindfulness practices that question whether the stories we live by are true, in an effort to rewire our brains to see other story possibilities and take action to consciously make choices according to the values of the new story. These seemingly small and personal actions toward wellness are actually profound steps for the individual and the planet. As Reagan says, "Worldviews create worlds." This process of consciously revising the lenses that make up your worldview is popularly referred to as *paradigm shifting*.

Reagan believes the need for Worldview Literacy is especially imperative for thoughtful parents earnestly trying to "do it better." She explains, "As the internet has helped foster awareness of and interest in healthy lifestyles, parents trying to do the best for their children decide they're going to be 'holistic' or 'natural.' If you make this choice without being aware of your personal lens on life—and the fact that you most likely need to begin to adjust that lens—you end up with an even longer yardstick to beat yourself up with: 'Did I buy all organic food? Unbleached diapers? The right sling?' The joy of parenting for peace can get squashed by the whirl of production and evaluation."[10]

So before we can change the world (or even just how we parent in the world), it is helpful to begin noticing our worldview. Reagan suggests that paradigm shifting, like parenting for peace, asks us to embark on a hero's journey—that mythic process in which seekers heed a call to adventure, a call that asks them to leave their familiar world behind, perhaps gradually, to venture into new, unfamiliar territory. Unlike our sanitized image of the Teflon hero who doesn't flinch at danger, the true hero has mixed feelings or is even down-right scared. But with the help of wise mentors and magical guides, they navigate the many challenges and their fears—and return matured, transformed and possessed of a radiant new body of knowledge. In all cases, the hero's task is to bring renewed life to an ailing culture—oneself, one's family, one's kingdom, one's world.

But embracing that new worldview requires a leap of faith—or rather, many small hops of faith, on an hourly basis! As Richard Rohr points out, we don't *think* our way into new ways of living, but instead, we *live* our way into new ways of thinking. Like letting go of your plan of what was supposed to happen later this afternoon, in favor of giving in to the tug of now—the delight of your three-year-old's fascination with finger paints…leaping for process over product—which may feel so unfamiliar as to be uncomfortable.

Worldviews change step by step, principle by principle, choice by choice, belief by belief. Little by little, sometimes over and over again, until it holds. Forty years of consciousness research by IONS shows that humanity is shifting away from unsustainable industrial values of a linear worldview (production, evaluation, separation, competition, conflict, acquisition, certainty—a *doing* paradigm) and toward the values of a relational worldview (participation, appreciation, interconnection, interdependence, peace, sustainability, mystery—a *being* paradigm). But at the moment we're a bit stuck between the two, and, like a car's clutch grinding between gears, we're lurching our way—sometimes screeching—toward evolution. In their 2008 Shift Report, *Changing the Story of Our Future*, IONS suggests how we might rewrite our own stories, and that of our shared human family:

> Voting is good, but changing one's mind and heart is better. Our fundamental position is that reality follows the quality of our thoughts and beliefs, both conscious and unconscious, because these are what drive the choices that cumulatively result in the world we live in. By changing those beliefs, we can change the future.[11]

Perhaps you, like many people today, have already embraced an alternative worldview, one that recognizes the fundamental power of individual consciousness and the need for balance between material and soul abundance. This would put you at the leading edge of hope for the future! But that enlightenment wave won't automatically roll forward through your children unless you understand a few basic principles about what they need as they unfold their potential. We lose ground every generation because even the most conscious people have a tendency to fall back upon old programming once they become parents, because nothing can push our (old) buttons like a crying baby, a tantruming toddler or a defiant teen!

In 2000 the National Research Council and the National Academy's Institutes of Medicine published *From Neurons To Neighborhoods,* a synthesis of current scientific understandings of how children develop from birth through age five (many of which appear in this book). It called for many federal policy changes, like more funding devoted to the social and emotional needs of young children, and many "early intervention" childhood and parenting programs. That's fantastic, but the gap between such expert theory and everyday reality is usually huge. Indeed, the focus for even the youngest children in schools today is on academics rather than social and emotional wellbeing, the foundation of their healthy development and our peaceful society.

In his book *Parenting for a Peaceful World*, Robin Grille charts the fascinating—and sobering—historical connection between a society's parenting style and its propensity toward war, injustice and environmental destructiveness, pointing out that "violence is a learned response passed down from generation to generation." *What?* This sounds ridiculous in modern America; surely your parents didn't teach you violence, and neither did mine! Certainly not intentionally, but what becomes clear in Grille's meticulous research is that even our current parenting styles rely upon certain culturally sanctioned yet invisible dynamics of power and subtle violence that don't foster a child's vital, authentic, integrated self—the foundations for true adult maturity and the qualities necessary to experience and create peace. As he points out, "When we parent a child, we are parenting the world and its future."[12]

Raffi Cavoukian, beloved children's troubadour turned global restoration activist, urges that

> we need to create a culture of deep compassion, one in which the primacy of the early years guides public policy, the admired life blends

material sufficiency with more noble aims, and our children learn to
become responsible global citizens....A culture in which 'the good life'
speaks not to purchasing power but to the quality of our existence—
our relationships with one another, between cultures, and with Nature.
A culture that puts self-confidence ahead of consumer confidence and
affirms developmental health as the true wealth of nations.[13]

If you look at fundamental shifts or trends within societies, they have all
happened through the force of _individual citizens changing their minds about
what they want_. As visionary pollster Mark Penn points out in his book *Microtrends* (and backs up with many examples), "In today's mass societies, it
takes only one percent of people making a dedicated choice—contrary to the
mainstream's choice—to create a movement that can change the world."[14]
Look at the rise in popularity of alternative medical modalities such as
acupuncture. This didn't happen because expert panels announced research
on its effectiveness; this happened because average, everyday people increasingly sought it out and discovered on their own that it worked, which created
consumer demand and drove further research. Now acupuncture is far more
accepted than it was even ten years ago, much more available, and covered by
many insurance companies.

I propose the same can happen with the values around how we perceive
ourselves and how we bring children to life and to maturity. Now, the idea
that parents wield the most fundamental, lasting influence on the socioemo-
tional health of their children is not very politically correct. The notion that
there is an *ideal* toward which we might strive in any human endeavor is also
un-PC, for it runs the risk of making people feel guilty. But our politically
correct, responsibility-free mentality creates disempowerment and hopelessness
instead! This book is about hope and empowerment.

As author Dotty Coplen suggests, "The more we understand about the future consequences of what we are doing, and the intent that goes with the action, the more successful we will be in caring for our children with our own
purposes and goals of parenting in mind. Parents need to decide together what
they believe to be a healthy human being."[15]

The "Generation Peace" Profile

Our world has evolved radically, and so must our understanding of psychosocial health. Today we know through scientific research that a socially healthy

human being has a brain wired with the capacity for self-regulation, self-reflection, trust, and empathy. And, the peace I refer to is not simply the absence of violence or strife, and neither is it the stereotypical soft-focused dream scene of doves and olive branches. This peace is a state of being vibrantly at-ease, from cell to soul, steeped in the tranquil conviction *I'm a worthy participant in life... fit to meet any challenge.* Vitally engaged in both inner and outer life, imbued with comprehensive social intelligence, minimal psychological or physiological defense patterns, with an array of readily deployable capacities for manifesting the inner experience of joy in the outer world.

These key qualities include intellectual and emotional flexibility, robust imagination and the ability to devise innovative solutions to complex puzzles. Also very important, the quality of *resilience*: how does the person handle daily stresses? A child who learns to readily regain internal balance after a frustrating moment becomes an adult capable of embracing peace instead of conflict. All of these capacities rely on well-developed brain centers that govern self-regulation, sensory integration and social intelligence. Someone with a well-wired brain doesn't get overwhelmed with stress hormones, at least not for very long. They bounce back.

Peace also suggests a condition of feeling *safe*. It presumes a fundamental posture of security, wellbeing, and an orientation toward growth, exploration and connectedness, with self and with others. We know from the new field of interpersonal neurobiology that this experience of safety, of peace at the level of biochemistry, is something that can become woven into the very fabric of our neurophysiology.

This is the purpose of these seven steps and principles: they foster the optimal development of those brain centers and support the flourishing of the whole child—body and mind. As I mentioned earlier, it is less about *doing* than it is about *not doing*—not getting in the way of Nature's elegant blueprint for socially adept, relationally astute humans. This is not about us making children our projects; our children want to be received, seen, and enjoyed for who they are in the moment. But they also count on us to help them fully blossom! And since they primarily learn from who we are, our project becomes *ourselves*. But here's the amazing paradox: you can teach your child only based on what you are—*and* there's an aspect of your child that will be more than you. The fact is, Nature not only allows us but dearly asks of us to have children much better than who we are!

At this point in human history, I guess I would dare to ask, "Why be a parent if *not* to try to bring a peacemaker on earth?" It might be peace through embroidery or engineering or being a CEO. Ultimately, our consciously en-acted wish for our children becomes that they unfold as individuals with the heart to embrace and exemplify peacefulness, the psyche to experience joy and intimacy, the mind to innovate solutions to social and ecological challenges, and the will to enact such innovations. Such a human is never a genetically predetermined given, but the result of dynamic interactions between genetics and environment—with parents being the most influential environmental vari-able.

Spreading Compassion, Not Blame

I want to make something clear right up front: even though I focus here on the fundamental importance of parents for their children's development, this is not about placing blame on, or provoking guilt in, parents who did, or who are doing, their best. *Parenting for Peace* outlines a proposed *ideal*—a revolu-tionary and radical departure from how it's always been done—and is not meant to bring guilt, anguish or dejection upon parents (or adult children of parents) who did not practice these principles, nor to suggest that children not conceived, born and raised along these principles have forever missed the peacemaker boat. One of the most exciting discoveries of new brain research is *neuroplasticity*, the capacity of our social brains to change, adapt and revise when presented with more optimal conditions. This has huge implications for growth, healing and our shared evolution. But one of the primary features of the parenting for peace approach is to leverage its principles *from the very be-ginning*, so children won't have to devote their energy to intrapsychic activ-ity—first for defensive adaptation and protection, and later for remediation and healing—and instead have an abundance of available energy to live fully, to revise and revitalize our world.

This is about compassionate awareness, about understanding ourselves and our own stories: we have all been babies, toddlers and children! Those of us who had less-than-ideal experiences of being parented find that raising chil-dren offers precious opportunities for healing our own past, which is inti-mately entwined with our children's future. This is about the mysteries of our own becoming.

I explore here our personal roles in evolving our species forward, given what science knows about the influence we have over our own cells and our own destinies. This is about the twenty-first century implications of the old notion of survival of the fittest, and recognizing how "fittest" must change to meet the challenges of today, and coming decades.

This is about the unprecedented understanding of our creative power as human beings, our participation in our own evolution.

This is about the mysteries of the human adventure.

A Note on Scientific and Gender References

I put many years and countless reams of research through a fine press to extract the principles contained here. This book is meant to be a doorway to a mansion rather than the mansion itself—which ultimately emerges within each of us—and I have included resources for further exploration of the ideas presented. Also included are references for major concepts, provocative notions, and those researchers whose shoulders I'm standing on, whose noodles are in this lasagna. I alternate the use of masculine and feminine references when referring to children. And while I typically use the terms *mother* and *father*, these steps and principles are applicable in almost all cases to more fluidly gendered (e.g., gay and lesbian) family constellations. Frequently *mother* and *father* note individuals of a specific sex, but also relate to archetypal feminine and masculine principles expressed by those of both sexes. These steps and principles can also be embraced in family-building journeys featuring more biological and procedural complexity, such as reproductive technologies, adoption and surrogacy.

And now, to the doorway...

The Invisible Power Within You

Cuz I'm bigger than my body gives me credit for.
                                                    JOHN MAYER

I love speaking to young people about these ideas, because they're almost always willing to reconsider what they know. Their foundations of knowledge are still coalescing and nothing is yet etched in stone. Thus, they greet me from the position of true scientists, willing to let new information and experience modify their beliefs about the world. I can see the ah-hahs light up in their eyes, and feel the excitement brew as they begin to realize just how much power they have to shape their own futures and the future of this challenged world they will soon inherit.

My favorite teaching opportunity is as a guest lecturer each spring at a local high school's eleventh-grade cell biology class. By then the students have already learned about the functioning of our most fundamental human ingredient, the cell. I devote some time to discussing two particular kinds of cells, eggs and sperm, and about how circumstances as early as pregnancy—and even conception—can fundamentally influence the wellbeing of that new individual. We talk about the implications of this, both for children they might have in the future and for themselves in terms of their own childhood stories. They are amazed and inspired to learn how much of an influence their choices, attitudes and behaviors will have upon a child they create, and thus upon the world.

The Nature-Nurture Embrace

Technological advances of the past few decades have revealed amazing things about what really makes us humans tick, and what makes us, period. For example, after a few hundred years of the nature-nurture debate (which is the more powerful shaping force, our genes or our experiences?) it has become clear that the question itself was flawed. Nature-nurture isn't a debate but a dance, an interactive collaboration that takes place throughout the lifespan. There are windows of development when Nature leads, and others when Nurture leads, but most of the time they dance together in unison, taking cues from one another and elaborating on what each calls forth in the individual.

The Human Genome Project was expected to revolutionize our self-knowledge by counting and coding the genes that make up this amazing complexity we call a human being—and indeed it did revolutionize our understanding, but not in the way the scientists had expected. To account for all of the proteins and regulatory processes in the body, researchers expected to find at least 140,000 genes (some estimated up to two million), but instead they have found only 24,000[16]—half the genes in a grain of white rice! As it happens, *Homo sapiens* has a similar number of genes as *Caenorhabditis elegans*, a one millimeter-long roundworm. So the looming question becomes *What is it, if not DNA, that accounts for the human being's amazingly more complex repertoire than that of a grain of rice or a roundworm?*

The answer to that question, and the empowerment within its answer, is what the consciousness revolution is about: how the most microscopic centers of biological intelligence—your cells—interact with and respond to the vast intelligence of the cosmos, with your mind as the intermediary, to shape who you are and the world in which you live.[17] This mind-as-intermediary holds the keys to the palace. The nature of our thoughts, attitudes, and feelings shapes those keys. And amazingly, how we are conceived, carried, and nurtured has a huge impact on the nature of those thoughts, attitudes and feelings! It turns out that these early experiences, beginning in the womb, largely determine the potential capacities of our minds to open life's doors to us, and, which doors they will open—those to the cramped mudrooms or to the vast and limitless spaces of the great rooms.

Fascinating secrets about things that have puzzled us for centuries are being revealed by two frontier fields: *consciousness studies* and *epigenetics*. Epigenetics is the study of heritable changes in gene expression and function that occur without a change in the actual DNA code. Epigenetics recognizes that DNA is not the grand destiny maker of life after all, and identifies the mechanisms by which environmental signals (including diet, thoughts and behavior) can change the action of our genes—an unthinkable concept even just a generation ago.[18] Epigenetics findings flow together elegantly with the Human Genome Project's discovery of so few genes, and the realization that there must be some other fundamental ingredient involved in creating the breathtaking array of diverse human genetic expression. To an extent greater than ever before realized, we tell our DNA what we want it to do![19] Cell biologist and epigenetics pioneer Bruce Lipton sums up the paradigm shift succinctly: "DNA is controlled by signals from outside the cell, including the energetic messages emanating from our positive and negative thoughts."[20] (Have you seen *that* on any front pages or television news programs lately, alongside the ads for prescription drugs?)

A Consciousness Revolution

Do you remember how electrical currents and "unseen waves" were laughed at? The knowledge about man is still in its infancy.

ALBERT EINSTEIN

All great truths start out as blasphemies.

GEORGE BERNARD SHAW

This brings us to the other field making amazing discoveries about human possibilities: the untamed frontier of quantum consciousness research, which explores the nature of human thought and how it affects the physical world around us—including our own brains, bodies and experience. This is not a realm to be ventured into by those easily put off by wild possibilities and intense scientific controversy. Like all watershed discoveries through history that have struck a death blow to the prevailing worldview, the idea that our humble thoughts can wield such power stirs up quite a dust cloud of skepticism and debate. It will have to endure, like all revolutionary knowledge that has come before it—think, "round not flat world" or "sun, not earth, as center of universe"—ridicule and violent opposition before it is finally accepted. Quantum physicist Max Planck famously observed that a new truth doesn't ultimately triumph by convincing its opponents, but rather by waiting for those opponents to die, leaving a new generation that has been raised to be familiar with that truth. And here you are!

In today's world of ever accelerating change, the time it takes for innovations of all kinds to evolve has shrunk so exponentially that information revolutions that once took centuries may take only twenty years. So you may very well be the first generation to witness the entire process of ridicule, challenge and acceptance of a major paradigm shift—the consciousness revolution—within your lifetime. Indeed, there is an almost invisible transformation happening worldwide, as more and more people are coming to recognize the powerful influence their thoughts, attitudes and feelings have upon the quality and direction of their lives and those around them. Scientific research is informing spiritual matters in unprecedented ways and the results have come straight to the people.

By *spiritual* I don't mean necessarily religious, but related to the deep inner life and its experience of what exists as something more than the sum of our physical, mental and emotional being. One writer friend of mine sees the spiritual in "the catch of the breath, the sob in the throat, the shining in the eye when we feel or witness something that inspires us, moves us or heals us." Others define spiritual simply as a personal experience of the numinous, which is that mysterious, enlivening "something more." For some, this is God (by any of myriad names for a Higher Power), for others the numinous is in the transpersonal or quantum realm, such as the collective unconscious, the unified field of intelligence, or the Infinite Absolute. And for those whose faith remains focused upon the here-and-now human being—the secular humanists—it is the redeeming but unmysterious values like truth, beauty, goodness, justice, reason.

Can You Get Your Head Around This Idea About...Your Head?

The seven principles that serve as the pillars for parenting for peace are designed to inspire, and to elevate the consciousness with which we parent. Defining *consciousness* is a bit like looking into a bathroom mirror that is reflected in a second mirror, and trying to pinpoint, "Which of these infinite reflections is really me?" The most basic definition of *consciousness* is "the state of being awake and aware." (As opposed to asleep, unconscious, in a coma, etc.) But as human consciousness evolved in its varied dimensions beyond the consciousness of various other levels of animal life—with the advent of tools, and later, language, for example—new tiers of definitions emerged. My use of the term throughout this book refers to a couple of upper tier meanings. One has to do with *what that state of awareness focuses upon*: the *direction* and *contents* of consciousness. And the other, one tier above that, is *a conscious awareness of where one's consciousness is focused.* This ability to think about one's thinking is unique to the human species; it's the ability to ask, "Where's my head at?" Don't feel bad if you don't quite get it. The problem of consciousness persists as one of the big conundrums of science, philosophy, and psychology, meaning that it's one of those fundamental human phenomena—like sleep—that scientists cannot truly explain.

Mind Moves Matter

Hundreds of scientific studies exist to demonstrate that focused thought, or *intentionality*, can have a measurable effect on matter—humans, animals, plants, and even machines[21]—a fact that has particularly direct implications for healthy fertility and conception in the early steps of your parenting journey. I have included a handful of titles and links in case you wish to explore the research, and meanwhile I'll share a couple of examples here that first grabbed me about this whole idea.

Cleve Backster is a polygraph scientist and former CIA interrogator, best known for having developed the Backster Zone Comparison Test, a worldwide standard for lie detection. On a somewhat playful impulse—the kind of impulse true scientists follow, and which precedes many revolutionary discoveries, a "playing with reality"—Backster placed some galvanic skin response electrodes on the leaf of a dracaena plant that his secretary had bought to spruce up the lab. He had just given the plant a thorough watering and was curious about how long it would take the water to make the trip from the roots up the tall cane trunk and out to the ends of the long leaves. When water permeates a leaf, the natural electrical conductivity present in all living things is enhanced, and Backster figured that the electrodes would register this change. Instead, they registered something he didn't see coming.

"The contour of the pen tracing was not what I would expect from water entering a leaf, but instead what I would expect from a person taking a lie-detector test....Lie detectors work on the principle that when people perceive a threat to their wellbeing, they physiologically respond in predictable ways....So I began to think about how I could threaten the well-being of the plant."[22]

The idea came to him to burn one of the leaves with a match. "I didn't verbalize, I didn't touch the plant, I didn't touch the equipment. The only new thing that could have been a stimulus for the plant was the mental image. Yet the plant went wild. The pen jumped right off the top of the chart."

Cleve Backster says his own consciousness changed irrevocably that day, and he devoted himself to studying this phenomenon that he came to call *primary perception*. He went on to study interspecies biocommunication with other forms of life such as bacteria, eggs, and most notably for our purposes here, human cells. White blood cells taken by scraping the inside of someone's cheek and put into a sterilized test tube with sterilized gold electrodes, responded in step with their donor's activities and emotions regardless of how far removed from them the person was. (The furthest distance tested was three hundred miles.)[23] Although Backster and his discoveries got some fleeting popular attention in the '70s, featured in the book and documentary *The Secret Life of Plants,* he suffered the kind of professional ridicule and exile typically delivered upon scientists who venture too audaciously into frontier territory. But the evolution in his own consciousness was worth it to him: the recognition that even one single human is more influential, and more interconnected with the rest of the world, than ever suspected.

What dawned upon one of my eleventh-grade students was the realization that her thoughts and feelings aren't just hers: how she feels, thinks and acts carries an impact that extends beyond her own self and into her wider world. Our consciousness can even have an impact on things we don't normally consider as being alive, such as water, and even machines! Bernard Grad at McGill

University had patients suffering varying severities of depression hold vials of water for thirty minutes. That water was then used to water carefully monitored houseplants, and there was a measurable difference in plant growth that correlated with the various mental and mood states of the vial holders.[24] Human intention can also influence machines: For the past thirty years, scientists at the Princeton Engineering Anomalies Research labs have conducted rigorous studies showing that we can affect both mechanical and digital machines through our thoughts. For example, a random number generator (RNG) left unattended will produce a roughly equal distribution of 0s and 1s, consistent with the statistical expectation. However, when a person is asked to intend for the RNG to produce either more 0s or more 1s, this results in a small but tangible effect on the stream of digital information.[25]

Psychologist William Braud has done extensive studies of this kind within the human realm, in which subjects influence various physiological systems of distant individuals (for example, their heart rate or blood pressure) through mental intention.[26] Although this entire area of mind-matter research is continually dismissed by skeptics as pseudo-science, the sheer volume of serious studies seems to challenge not only the skeptics, but also our culturally accepted framework of how our world works, and how we fit into that world. Writes UCLA psychiatry professor Jeffrey Schwartz, "A century after the birth of quantum mechanics, it may at last be time to take seriously its most unsettling idea: that the observer and the way he directs his intention are intrinsic and unavoidable parts of reality.[27]

We Are the MVPs in Our Own Evolution!

As revolutionary as it is, the idea that each of us has a powerful say *today* in how we and our children evolve *tomorrow* isn't a brand new idea. It has been researched and expressed in many previous centuries by progressive thinkers whose ideas have simply been waiting for us to recognize their brilliant relevance. Notable among them is Pierre Teilhard de Chardin, a paleontologist whose life spanned the nineteenth and twentieth centuries, and who was present at the discovery of the famous bones of Peking Man. He was also a Jesuit priest and a philosopher—a man whose life and work embodied the science-meets-spirit movement so popular today. Teilhard's writings expressed a view of evolution not as the series of random mutations that characterizes what we know of Darwin's model, but as both a scientific and a holy process steeped in what he called *orthogenesis*—the divine, collaborative, upward drive of all things, living and not, toward increased complexity and consciousness.[28]

Teilhard's explanation of human evolution is compelling in its correlation with actual events, many of which have happened in the decades after his death. He saw two stages of what he called the "planetization" of humans. The first is the *expanding* stage, when humans spread and populated far-flung regions across the earth, when they multiplied and diversified into races and cultures that were very different and isolated from one another. The second (which began in the twentieth century) is the *contracting* stage: once most of the earth has been occupied, the races and cultures begin to converge, with all of the challenges and opportunities that brings. Information, commodities, wars and dreams, are no longer confined to single races or regions, but are shared among diverse peoples of Earth. Teilhard also saw this as a unifying stage, and envisioned something wild and amazing as the primary evolutionary leap of this stage.

Keeping in mind that Teilhard wrote about this at a time when the concept of personal computers was still science fiction, let alone the internet, he pictured the earth encircled by an interdependent system of collective thought that he called the *noosphere*, which is up the evolutionary ladder from the earlier established interrelating system of physical life known as the *biosphere*. He saw "the Earth not only covered by myriads of grains of thought, but enclosed in a single thinking envelope so as to form a single vast grain of thought" with many "individual reflections grouping themselves together and reinforcing one another in the act of a single unanimous reflection."[29] Can you imagine a more prophetic (or lyrical) description of the World Wide Web? Or a more inspiring image than his description of the noosphere as the "very soul of the earth," a "living membrane which is stretched like a film over the lustrous surface of the star which holds us"? Think about *that* the next time you log on!

From this perspective, we are in a transition—always a time of crisis—between the expanding stage and the contracting, or unifying, stage. This is when all the rules seem to change, particularly the famed "survival of the fittest" slogan of popular Darwin theory. Like many of today's futurists, Teilhard saw that humanity will survive—and indeed thrive—only by embracing and cultivating the abilities needed for interdependence and unification, suggesting instead, as Bruce Lipton puts it, "survival of the most loving." Indeed, Teilhard wrote, "Someday, after we have mastered the winds, the waves, the tides and gravity, we shall harness for God the energies of Love. Then for the second time in the history of the world, man will have discovered fire."

This brings us back to the power of this moment for evolution within each of us right now, and as we bring our children into the world and raise them. Post-Darwinian biologists recognize the significant role in evolution played by a living being's own efforts. One such biologist sees the "psychic life" of the organism as a "most powerful creative element in evolution."[30]

Many fields of research tend to affirm that we humans are indeed at a crucial moment in our evolution, and our survival is going to depend upon our realizing, deeply, that our true security is rooted in connectedness, in our relationships, in healthy interdependence with our fellow humans and with our natural environment.

It is a moment that requires thoughtfulness, fortitude and faith.

It is a moment for us to embrace, together.

It is a moment that is here now.

Let us gather our courage, our Cliff Notes, our hero's grit… and embark on the transformative adventure of parenting for peace.

Resources

Inclusive Psychology: inclusivepsychology.com.

Kurzweil, R. *The Singularity Is Near*. New York: Penguin, 2005.

"The Plants Respond: An Interview with Cleve Backster," www.thesunmagazine.org/archives/1882.

Mayer, Elizabeth Lloyd. *Extraordinary Knowing: Science, Skepticism, and the Inexplicable Powers of the Human Mind*. New York: Bantam, 2007.

Step One

Pro-Growth Choices— Cultivating a Fertile Mind and Body

Are You Creating, or Recreating?

We are what we repeatedly do. Excellence, then, is not an act but a habit.

ARISTOTLE

One of the biggest challenges we face in creating the lives we want—for ourselves, our partners, our children, and for our larger community and world—is that our basic attitudes and perceptions of the world were shaped in the earliest days, months and years of our lives, long before we had a chance to form our own opinions about things. Our basic understandings of who we are and what the world is all about are a series of neural perception templates that were pretty much molded *for* us, by our earliest experiences with the people and environment around us.

For example, you're a tiny baby, and you're hungry. (For an infant, hunger is not the diffuse, easy-to-ignore situation it is for an adult; it is a rapidly escalating sensation of actual pain.) You cry, and before too long someone picks you up, soothes you, and feeds you. As this happens again and again, some of your perception templates become shaped around such basic tenets as *I have an effect on my world...People are there for me...I can trust...Being close to someone feels safe.*

This is what we call the *implicit memory* system at work: during our pre-verbal early months, over the course of repeated experiences, the brain subconsciously distills the constant themes that underlie those experiences.[1] This results in a kind of surreptitious learning that psychiatrist Daniel Siegel calls "memory masquerading as fact."[2] Wrestling with these implicitly learned, habitual patterns of thinking or reacting is a little like having someone give you a great computer, but discovering it's got some basic operating programs you don't like, but you can't seem to uninstall them! Nature designed us this way so that children could survive when we were prey for animals out on the savannah: Neanderthal toddlers quickly and automatically came to associate an approaching low growl with tensing up and running from the tiger, exactly like Mom, Dad and Uncle Ork did. And after we evolved beyond being possible main courses, this kind of invisible, wordless learning has been part of how children adapt to the emotional and behavioral idiosyncrasies of their particular clans, which can also be fundamental to psychologically surviving modern family life.

Because this learning is indeed survival-based, it features a kind of bad-news bias. Rarely have sweet, pleasurable experiences been fatal*, so our primitive brain systems pay much more attention to unpleasant experiences, detecting, imprinting and cataloging them—because until very recently in human history, our survival depended on remembering every detail of how we survived bad things. However, in the twenty-first century and beyond, our survival may instead depend upon prioritizing the *positives* of human experience—joy, appreciation, and connection. Not because we're living in a Hallmark card, but because this is how we will upgrade our own evolution and effectively address the multiple crises facing humanity. We can, we *must*, for

---

* My point is somewhat undermined by the fact of STDs, of which there has been a deadly one present for most of human history.

the first time in human history, unfold the *full* potential of our brains, including what one scientist calls the angel lobes—the prefrontal cortex, the seat of introspection, intention, conscience and civilization.

You Are Always Self-Creating

When we focus our consciousness toward gratitude, beauty, and communion, what emerges is joy. Thus we can weave peace into our very cells. This isn't just flowery sentiment, this comes from leading-edge research in the fields of positive psychology and mind-body science. Peace emanates upward, outward, omniward, as we grow peaceful children and cultivate a peaceful world. Human development visionary and author Joseph Chilton Pearce teaches us that our biology is fully equipped to enact our self-perfected evolution. We have the hardware—the uniquely human prefrontal cortex of our brain, driving our uniquely human capacity for self-reflection—to uplift our own species into new realms of previously unimagined glory.[3]

But we've been running desperately outdated software! It's time to upgrade our SelfPerception, HeadFocus and HowWeParent programs and embrace our own magnificence. When we understand our powerful role in our own evolution and use that knowledge to take conscious control of our destiny, we turbo-charge the evolution of all humanity.

Near the end of my hour with the eleventh-graders, after our discussion of the fundamental shaping power they will wield when they decide to bring children into the world, comes a moment I savor: I inform them that they needn't wait one more minute to put these principles to work in their lives, because each of them, right this moment, is pregnant! Cue the shocked looks and nervous laughter. That's when I discuss the process of cell regeneration, and ask if they realize that the cells of their taste buds live for only a few hours, white blood cells for a maximum of ten days, muscle cells for about ninety days, and red blood cells for four months. The students are fascinated to hear that about 1 percent of all of their cells die and are replaced every day, meaning that at the cellular level they have *new bodies about every three months!*[4]

The same environmental and experiential influences that shape a newly developing individual person also exert great shaping effect on the health and quality of each one of our newly regenerated cells. Thus, we are all pregnant with our future selves, always participating in our own self-creation!

Where's Your Head At?

Whatever we surround ourselves with becomes a shaping force on our very being. Peacefulness, order and beauty in our environment support our inner wellbeing and health, from cells to organs to the whole bodymind system. Clang, clutter and chaos, on the other hand, can also become embodied physically and mentally. As without, so within.

What we put our attention on increases. When we focus on the positive—beauty, possibility, enjoyment—just as when we zero in on the negative—criticism, losses, everything that's wrong—it's like putting water and fertilizer on it, making either the positive or the negative flourish and multiply. This isn't just fuzzy "power of attraction" stuff; this is also Brain Function 101: when we tune our attention in a certain way—either positively or negatively—we initiate a flow of biochemicals that carve brain pathways for more neurons to travel down that same pathway in the next minute, hour, day, year. Our attitude and focus also create a subconscious template of perception that filters the millions of incoming bits of life's information and captures those bits that match our initial proposition.

Can you see how quickly this becomes a feedback loop, spiraling either up or down? Let's say I've just missed out on getting a job even though I was sure I had nailed the interview, my cat is throwing up all over the apartment, my rent payment is overdue and the landlady is getting harder to avoid. Each of these situations individually could unleash streams of brain chemicals (what neuroscientist Candace Pert calls "molecules of emotion") to edge me toward upset, and when they happen all together, it wouldn't be unreasonable for me to have a bit of a meltdown. That's understandable, normal and human. The trick here is to find an exit ramp before I go completely off the rails: a short trip on the FreakOut expressway is okay as long as we take control of the wheel and get ourselves back onto the tree-lined avenues of Life.

While it can feel so weirdly satisfying to wallow in our misery—replaying the upsetting events over and over in our minds, complete with all the perfect comments we wish we'd made; talking to friend after friend about the awfulness of it all; holing up at home and cranking up the heavy metal—this emotion recycling makes it harder to make our way back to a positive outlook, simply by virtue of how our brain chemicals work. I'm not suggesting that you ignore your feelings, or cover them up with some fakely nice façade—

yikes, that's a fast track to real mental problems!—but that you engage your healthy will and power of choice in deciding when the pity party is over.

Revising Old Programming

There are many simple and effective ways to do a pattern interrupt on spiraling negativity, whether it's sadness, stress, anger or whatever—and each time we make a choice to exit that negative brain pathway, we rewrite those old operating programs we don't want, installing healthier ones. Here are a few that are tried and true:

Breathe. Put your attention on your breath and mindfully take in some slow, deep breaths, holding each one for a few extra counts. (This encourages extra oxygenation of the blood going to your brain to help it cope with the neurons firing away like crazy in this intense moment.)

Notice and name. The simple act of observing and identifying your emotions can help the brain structures driving those negative feelings to self-correct, and help you find your way back to a lighter, freer emotional tone. It also helps lasso your mind back from rehashing the past or rehearsing the future, to situate you in the present moment, the only place where true serenity can be found.

Focus on appreciation. Think of something that pulls up the "appreciation" feeling from your mental file cabinet, and immerse yourself in that feeling now: it can be the memory of an event that made you feel wonderful, or the thought of a person whom you deeply love, or something exceptionally kind someone did for you. This is especially helpful when you're in the grip of angry feelings, because as sophisticated an instrument as your brain is, when you're in a stressed or highly emotional state, it becomes fairly primitive and can deal with only one thing at a time—either anger *or* appreciation. Research demonstrates that appreciation brings us into inner alignment at the levels of the brain, heart and mind.[5]

Smile. When we smile—even if it at first feels forced, because we're really in a funk—we do get happier. This puts the brain's own impressive pharmacy to work!

Nourish yourself. Omega-3 EFAs (essential fatty acids) are the equivalent of motor oil for the healthy functioning of the brain. As our national fish consumption has dropped over the decades, our depression rates have indeed risen, and scientists think there is a connection. Getting your omega-3s is simply an enlightened, basic health practice—just like brushing and flossing.

Connect with others. Spend some time in the real (not virtual) presence of someone with whom you feel comfortable, supported and safe, someone who ideally is grounded and centered. Thanks in part to *mirror neurons* (recently discovered by scientists in the field of interpersonal neurobiology), another person's calm can be contagious, and by simply being in their presence we can feel better. (It's important to keep in mind that emotional moods and social modes are contagious, so hang out with those people whom you want to be more like!) Humans are biologically designed to be in physical proximity to one another as a way of mutually regulating our inner physical and emotional states.[6]

But modern technologies seem intent upon prying us apart with the allure of awesome gadgets that are, ironically, designed and perceived as "connecting" tools. In today's iTwitterFaceLinkedInPod world, blogging, texting, IMing and tweeting are today's accepted modes of reaching out and touching one another, yet studies have found that people become more depressed and lonely the more time they spend "interacting with others" online![7] While electronic communication is amazingly convenient for sharing information, there is something fundamentally missing in those disembodied cyberspace encounters for the aspect of us that needs the full human connection. *Social Intelligence* author Daniel Goleman cautions, "This inexorable technocreep is so insidious that no one has yet calculated its social and emotional costs."[8]

One of the primary qualities that will characterize Generation Peace is *resilience*—the capacity to weather tough times and challenges with physiological, psychological and behavioral equanimity. Meaning, we don't collapse, freak out, or smash things when the pressure's on. It bears noting that people who score high on resilience feel comfortable reaching out, and that the interdependence of asking for help (and giving it back when help is asked of you) is one of the healthiest capacities a person can develop.

Do something. I love a saying from Constructive Living: "Accept your emotions as they are and do what needs to be done." If the dishes need to be washed, wash them. If the floor is nasty, sweep or vacuum. It may require an act of will, but tackle that messy corner of the room you've been avoiding. You can borrow a secret that poets and magicians use, the law of analogy: "As I am doing this, may this be done unto me." So, as I am ironing out the wrinkles in my shirt, may my inner turmoil be smoothed away. An activity as mundane as scrubbing the bathtub can be surprisingly restorative when we immerse ourselves utterly and completely in each moment's movement: the warmth and hum of the water, the pitted texture of the sponge, the tangy smell of the cleanser, the stretch of the arm muscles when reaching to the far side—and the satisfaction of the gleaming, ring-free final result.

Which brings us back to appreciation!

The Power of Appreciation

The suggestions listed above aren't just for crisis moments, but are fundamentals for cultivating mastery of our inner lives, which is fundamental to wellbeing and peacefulness. Two themes prominent in all those activities are *connection* and *appreciation,* both of which have emerged as superstars in human health research. The field of positive psychology finds that the single most potent means of amping up our joy—and also our physical energy and wellbeing—is to cultivate gratitude. Scientists talk about keeping a gratitude journal, writing gratitude letters, and an exercise one doctor calls "three blessings," in which you take time each day to write about three things that went well, and why.[9]

Even more simply, though, appreciation can take the form of noticing more fully some of the numerous things we normally take for granted in daily life. For example, the small act of eating a piece of fruit can take on a whole new dimension when we turn our attention to what is embodied in that apple— seasons of nurturance by rains, sun, and those who cared for its tree—and to the amazing fact that the flesh of that fruit will be transmuted into *us* in the coming hours and days. When we consider the research on the effects of human consciousness upon plants and water, it doesn't seem like such a bad idea—indeed, most likely a wonderful idea—to appreciate an apple (or anything else) as we prepare to make it part of us!

The very phenomenon of a shower is an amazing, deeply pleasurable thing. People in many parts of the world would find a shower utterly miraculous. It can be a wonderfully centering (and surprisingly challenging) practice to shower with full engagement: rather than rehearsing for the day ahead, or replaying yesterday, or detouring to any of the gazillion places our minds tend to pull us when we shift into auto-pilot, try to keep all of you, mind and body, in the present as you soap up, shampoo, rinse and repeat. Engage fully in each of the delicious sensations a shower offers. It becomes almost impossible to not feel gratitude for such a sensuous treat. This level of noticing and appreciating lies at the heart of P for P Principle #1, Presence, and will serve you richly through-out your parenting journey. When we bring our presence to the current mo-ment, we adjust our brain to be most able to engage in the other principles as well.

What Head Are You In?

Having a basic idea of our brain landscape is critical to understanding the ori-gins and development of peacefulness, social intelligence and innovation in human beings. The late renowned neuroscientist Paul MacLean gave us the "triune brain" theory, which recognizes three distinct brain systems within our single modern brain.[10] MacLean, working at the National Institute of Mental Health, traced how these three brain levels mature in seven-year stages (birth to seven, seven to fourteen, and fourteen to twenty-one).

One hundred years before McLean, Austrian philosopher and scientist Rudolf Steiner taught about the "three-fold nature" of the human being, and how we evolve in a series of stages related to age and physical, emotional, and intellectual growth that align remarkably with McLean's portrait of the brain and its interrelated, sequential development. Steiner drew upon esoteric as well as medical and philosophical science to paint a picture of human devel-opment as a gradual process of incarnation, a sequential maturing and un-folding of each of three "bodies"—*etheric, astral, and "I"** —in addition to the physical body present at birth. Steiner's discoveries formed the basis for his Waldorf education system, and a bumper sticker for Waldorf provides us with the most concise possible crash-course in the triune brain: "Education for the head, heart, and hands." As you'll see in my primer below—and as will be ex-

---

* These three bodies can be seen to correspond to *chi, soul, and Spirit.* Steiner used the terms *"I"/Spirit* and *ego* interchangeably; his *ego* differs fundamentally from Freud's in that Steiner sees this highest self as being imbued with Spirit, the individual's connection to the Divine. Also, contrasted with Freud's view of the ego emerging in a child's first year, in Steiner's model the ego doesn't unfold and fully incarnate until age twenty-one.

plained in more depth as we go along—each brain system relates to a fundamental aspect of the human being that needs to be supported in its full flowering in order that he or she is equipped with the robust capacities of a peacemaker.

This Is Your Brain, in Three Acts

Our three brains reflect evolution itself, as nature never stops remodeling her creation. Each new addition has been devised to update and improve upon limitations of the previous brain, and—ideally—to both propel and accommodate leaps in evolution. But as with most remodeling jobs, sometimes the joining of old and new isn't quite seamless. It is still very possible for any of the systems to become dis-integrated from the others, pushing them aside and predominating with its own agenda, usually in response to threat, either real or perceived.

We have all experienced this kind of mental hijacking: You've just gotten distressing news and you careen into a sort of automaton mode where suddenly neither people nor consequences seem to much matter (you become reckless on the road, reach for the junk food, go on a yelling rant). This is the mode in which violence happens—on large scales and micro scales—because the primitive, reactive, survival-based areas have taken over and shoved aside the prefrontal cortex, the seat of empathy, higher-order thinking and the assessment of future consequences. The extent to which our three brain dimensions are able to remain integrated and operating smoothly together—rather than any of them hijacking the others—lies at the very heart of this endeavor of raising Generation Peace, for reasons I will point out as we go along.

Meet your three brains, in order of their development in human history and in your own life:

The Sensing-Doing Brain – The brain stem and cerebellum together comprise the sensory-motor brain, which governs our senses—to bring in outside information from the environment—and our muscles—to move in response to that information. This most ancient, primitive region is dedicated solely to physical survival and is entirely unequipped for anything like emotions or future consequences. It also controls basic bodily functions and regulation such as heart rate, digestion, respiration, temperature, etc., and reflexive, habitual (i.e., unconscious) responses to the environment. MacLean calls this the reptilian brain, and indeed, anything you might think of as cold-blooded is governed by this primitive brain center. For example, deception is an ancient instinctive survival behavior developed eons ago to elude predators; this aspect of our brain enables us to be two-faced, to lie, fake or cheat—particularly when we feel threatened in some way (like a chameleon changing its colors).

The Feeling-Knowing Brain – While the primitive brain is concerned with monitoring and responding to the outside world, this emotional brain (or *limbic* system as it is often called) maps and monitors our own inner responses to and perceptions of that world, in other words, emotions—likes and dislikes, appetites, feelings. It mediates fear, which is one of the thorniest issues when we speak of cultivating peace; housed here is an almond-sized structure—the amygdala—dedicated to archiving the details of everything we're afraid of. The feeling brain governs *relationships* of all kinds. Anything that is rooted in past experience is a limbic function; memory itself is governed by the limbic structures. (You can like, fear or desire something only based on a remembered or imprinted experience of it.) We share this newer brain with mammals, so a handy reminder list of the capacities of your feeling-knowing brain is things your terrier can do: sulk, play, whine when you leave, mother her pups, whimper in fear, attack an enemy but not a friend, "sing," enjoy sex, and...*learn*. Yes, many people mistakenly assume it's primarily a function of the highest brain center, but perhaps the most critical of all human endeavors is mediated by the emotional brain: learning. Why? Because all learning relies upon memory, and always happens in the context of relationship!

The Thinking-Talking Brain – The neocortex ("new brain") gives us access to language and the ability to elaborate on what we've learned and imbue it with multiple dimensions of substantive meaning, to decode abstractions, to understand cause and effect, to plan ahead. Indeed, while the sensing-doing brain relates to only the present tense, and the feeling-knowing brain relates to both present and past, the neocortex gives us the ability to project into the future and *envision anew*—a new answer, a new invention, a new recipe. A new garden landscape, a new furniture arrangement, a new exercise routine. A new leaf, a new attitude. But also, a new worry, a new anxiety, a new worst-case scenario. This ability to project ourselves into a theoretical future can bring with it the *what if?* backlash—lots of mental hamster-wheel spinning that can generate "I'm in danger" feelings that can prompt the doing and feeling brains to take over. That is, unless we have a very well-developed portion of the neo-cortex that is so special it gets its own entire section.

The Prefrontals (Human.04, the Upgrade)

Nature's most recent addition to the brain—appearing roughly 40,000 years ago, an evolutionary nanosecond—and the one that has been steadily grow-ing larger over all those years relative to the other brain regions, are the *pre-frontal lobes*, which sit just behind the brow area, at the most *front*al portion of the neocortex. They are the seat of those virtues we think of as the pinnacle of humanity—creative intellect, compassion, empathy, understanding, con-science. The qualities that make us civilized. But unlike the earlier three brain regions, the prefrontals do not govern within their own isolated sphere (sens-ing-doing, feeling-knowing, thinking-talking) but rather work *in concert* with each of the earlier, foundational structures. As such, they develop in phases throughout childhood that parallel the sequential development of the doing, feeling and thinking brain areas. They act like an upgrade feature to enhance, augment and lift the three earlier brain structures up to new levels of seam-lessly integrated, high-function potential—*if their development is fostered early in life!*

A recent news story told of a man who, driving over 100 mph in a 55 mph zone, hit and killed a seventeen-year-old bicyclist, and then sued the boy's family for damage to his Audi. This is an individual who, I can confidently diagnose from afar, has poorly developed prefrontal lobes. He is an example of the sophistication of the neocortex (thinking brain) being hijacked into the service of the lower functioning levels of the doing and feeling brain, rather than being primed by the prefrontals for elevated acts of empathic thought-fulness. The result is a drastic lack of humanity. While this may seem to be an extreme and isolated case, it really isn't. How often do we witness (or ourselves participate in) situations in which the importance of *things* or *projects* or even *ideals* (especially involving money or power) eclipses what neuroscience now knows is our most valuable treasure—our ties with other people?

Paul MacLean called the prefontals our "angel lobes," and they are, truly, our ticket off this ride of repetitive cycles of human-on-human aggression, war and misery.

The Only Question, Always: Growth or Protection?

If you remember only one point from this book, this is the one, since it per-vades and informs each moment of your existence: At every level and every stage of life, an organism is either in growth mode *or* in protection mode. Ex-panding or contracting. Reaching out or withdrawing in. Unfolding or rein-forcing. The entity may be a single cell, a community of cells that is a person, or a community of people that is a family, an organization, a community, a country. When we perceive a threat—either real or imagined, either conscious or below the level of our conscious awareness—our nervous system's collection of sensory processing neurons, receptors, and signaling proteins and hor-mones—together more simply called the *stress axis*—shifts us into gear for protection, as our feeling and doing brains call for a dose of fight-flight-or-freeze hormones. This kicks off an intricate cascade of survival responses throughout the body and the mind: pupils narrow to focus on the threat, blood vessels constrict to minimize blood loss from the anticipated injury, the heart and lungs speed up to oxygenate the system for optimal performance, and, typically, the more instantly reactive lower brain centers take over, push-ing aside the wiser but slower-acting neocortex. (Don't expect a very fright-ened, anxious or angry person to remember a phone number or calculate a 15 percent tip.) The threat doesn't have to be a tiger about to pounce, or an in-truder coming through the door; it can be a project deadline nipping at your heels, or an insulting relative on the phone.

Another handy way to think of the growth vs. protection posture is to think in terms of being connected or disconnected. Next time you're stressed out (if you can remember), check in and ask yourself, "Am I feeling connected, or disconnected?" Funny enough, very often the simple act of tuning into your-self and asking that question helps you feel connected again! You don't need to wonder, "Connected to what?" When we're really connected, it's at all levels from cellular communication channels to organ functioning to the direct neu-ral communication continually taking place between the coordinated nervous systems residing in our brain, heart and gut,* to our relational human impulse

---

* Though still not widely popularly recognized, scientists in the fields of neurocardiology and neurogastroenterology have known for a decade or more that our intestines and our heart each function as "small brains" in connection (and sometimes *dis*connection) with our "big brain"; thus, having a gut feeling or the experience of your heart just knowing is grounded in hard sci-ence. The website www.heartmathinstitute.org is a good source of information on this.

of reaching out to others. When we're connected, we're in growth mode; when we're disconnected, we're in protection mode.

Our stress system is designed for occasional activation by a stressor followed by a resolution of the stress. This resolution initiates a cascade of pleasure hormones which gives us that *Ahhhh* feeling we've all had when we were preparing for something terrible ("I forgot to feed the meter, and it's afternoon tow-away time!") and then discovered that the something terrible didn't happen ("My car's still there!"). When stress is not intermittent but constant and unremitting, healthy growth is inhibited; indeed, cell biologist Bruce Lipton points out the mutually exclusive postures of protection (the survival posture adopted under stress) and healthy growth (only possible in the absence of threat or stress).[11] As you'll soon see, this "growth or protection" concept will become one of your most helpful parenting tools!

The organ most vulnerable to growth impairment due to stress is the brain, *particularly the healthy development of the prefrontal lobes!* The ways in which this is so—and more importantly, what we can do about it—will become clear in the coming pages. For lo these 40,000 years with this wondrous, potentially uplifting addition to our neural architecture, we as a human race have thwarted its development—and thus our own glorious evolution—through our threatening actions, both subtle and extreme. And many of those actions have taken place in the context of parenting.

Installing the Upgrade

As you continually give birth to your future self with hourly, daily, monthly cell regeneration, you have a powerful influence on the quality of that growth. Recognizing that your thoughts, attitudes and emotions have a direct impact on the functioning of every cell, tissue and organ—and particularly the brain—you have the power to harmonize them all into coherent, integrated, and purposeful function. Here's a little experiment I like to do with the eleventh-graders, so I invite you to connect with your inner high-schooler and try it with me: Imagine there is a bowl of Sour Skittles on a table next to you. Imagine reaching out and grabbing a handful. Feel the slight roughness of their sugary coating between your palm and fingers, and glance down to appraise the mix of colors. Now toss them all into your mouth and bite down.

If you felt saliva bubble forth, you have just experienced the power of thoughts in your mind to make things happen in your body. This is a most auspicious time to understand and harness that power. As Joe Dispenza puts it, every time you have a thought, you make a chemical.[12] You are at the helm of your ship, the master of your destiny to a far greater degree than scientists ever before realized (but many philosophers knew).

It is a choice, and not always an easy choice. Our culture doesn't warmly welcome the cheerful person (calling them Pollyanna or branding them on sitcoms as the silly or naïve one), and instead fosters pessimism, cynicism, criticism and other forms of collective negativity. Our very way of life ultimately organizes around consumerism, and it is far easier to sell things to people who are feeling down. Indeed, from birth onward, we are enculturated to the idea that pleasure and security have to do with things rather than connections with people. This engenders a materialist drive: getting more and more. But the late George Leonard was acute in his observation about the hollow core of materialism: "You can never get enough of what you really don't want."[13]

Cellular Genius

Here's a quick and dirty cell biology primer, because understanding a few things about this most basic level of your physical being will help you make choices that invite health at every other level. Individual cells possess intelligence. To grasp the truth in that statement, it helps to have a solid, working definition of that word *intelligence*: "the ability to bring in information and respond to that information for one's own wellbeing and continuity." This can be applied to a cell, an individual, a community, a nation, a race, even to humanity itself. It is a primary fulcrum on which this entire platform of raising a peaceful generation balances. At every step and through every principle we are seeking to foster the greatest possible intelligence according to this powerful definition.

So, back to cells. They are intelligent, meaning they have the ability to bring in information about the environment and respond to that information for their own wellbeing and continuity. There are three basic kinds of "information substances" in the body—peptides, transmitters and hormones.* Collec-

---

* These relate to the conventionally accepted chemical-molecular model of cellular communication; there is an emerging paradigm that includes a physical and atomic aspect to cell communication, which includes what is referred to as *energetic,* and opens the delightful can of worms of electromagnetic fields and their role in this. Bruce Lipton is a great source of understanding the role of energy in cellular communication and intelligence.

tively these chemical messengers are called *ligands*. Ligands tell our cells (and thus our tissues and organs) what they need to do, based on information coming from our selves inside as well as the world outside.

There are thousands (and for some cells hundreds of thousands) of switches on the surface of the cell (the membrane) that engage with ligands to constantly adjust the nature and functioning of the cell to suit the demands of the environment. You can imagine these switches as parking spaces encircling the perimeter of the cell, and the ligands carrying information into the cell as infinitesimally tiny vehicles. But not just any vehicle can park in any space—specific types of cars fit into only their specifically shaped spaces. A pleasure hormone can't park in a stress hormone space, for example. But if it finds an available pleasure hormone space, it pulls in, and when its front wheels tap the curb, this signals the cell to adjust itself to more relaxed, pleasurable circumstances. This continual parking-signaling process is the basis of how we exist, function and grow—a neverending parade of ligand "cars" parking in receptor "spaces" on the membranes of each of our fifty trillion cells. The complex intricacy with which these fifty trillion cellular geniuses orchestrate our existence and expression is mind-boggling.

Now, it's only partly true that hormones and other ligands have specific shapes that fit into specially shaped receptor spaces on the cell membrane. Just as several sizes of round pegs can fit into a particular round hole, and even some square pegs—if they're small enough—can fit into that same round hole, some receptors can serve as "parking spaces" for a variety of ligands. (Here's an example that you can put into practice immediately: Neurobiologist Candace Pert points out that the rhinovirus, the cause of the common cold, enters cells via the same receptors as the neurotransmitter norepinephrine, which is widely believed to flow in more abundance when we are in a joyful state of mind. More receptor spaces occupied by norepinephrine means fewer vacant receptors available through which the cold virus can enter the cell!)[14]

A Glitch or a Glimmer in the Works

In some cases the communication between the environment and the cell is straightforward: When we're exposed to the sun, certain ligands park in certain receptors, signaling for melanin to be produced to adapt our skin to sunny conditions. When we see, hear, feel, or smell an immediate threat (a hissing snake, an earthquake, a fire) torrents of ligands flow, dock in receptors, and trigger an arsenal of fight-flight-freeze hormones so that we can effectively respond to the threat.

But in most cases, especially in our modern world, the communication between the environment and the cell passes through an intermediary: your mind. It is through your mind that you *perceive* your environment, that is, you tell yourself a story about it. In this way you amplify, diminish or even fundamentally redirect the ligand responses to many of your experiences. Our human ability to think inventively is a double-edged sword—the more painful edge is our ability to invent *negative perceptions* to environmental circumstances, which we have a natural, survival-based tendency to do. The driver didn't simply pull in front of you without signaling; he deliberately dissed you and put your life in danger. The electricity didn't simply disappear due to an outage; it confirmed that "everything's conspiring against me today!" The telemarketer didn't simply call during dinner; she demonstrated that there is no civility or privacy anymore and that civilization is crumbling. You get the idea.

This is where Nature's brilliant design runs into some snags in the twenty-first century. The way our bodies and brains operate has remained virtually unchanged since we stood upright on the savannah, and yet our world and our worldviews have changed dramatically. For most of us, the grave physical threats faced by our distant ancestors have been replaced by more mental and psychological insults (usually made far more insulting by virtue of the story we wrap them in), and this results in a derailment of what used to be an adaptive survival response. In more primitive times, the routine act of running or fighting or even screaming used up all those hormones (adrenaline, corticosteroids, epinephrine) designed to give you quick energy, make you think fast, run, fight or scream with the most power and effectiveness possible, or successfully feign death. But today we typically don't express the actions we're biologically primed for during stressful circumstances; in fact, we actually suppress them to remain civilized. This is one way that stress puts wear and tear on our bodily systems—it's like driving a car with one foot on the brake and one on the gas.

Making it ever worse, we were originally designed to respond effectively to major but occasional threats. Today's turbo-paced, traffic-jammed, technopowered, instant-access, cell-phone-fax-web, information-overloaded e-world is peppered with one mini-threat after another, with little time in between for all those activating hormones to abate. Chronic stress can shrink brain cells, harden arteries, raise cholesterol, and impair immune function, among many other negative effects, so it isn't surprising that stress has emerged as a strong contributing factor to most chronic or degenerative diseases, as well as common acute illnesses like colds and flu.

Because of this, stress has gotten a really bad rap—however, if we banished it altogether, we'd quite literally collapse, physical and mentally. A balance of tension (stress) and relaxation (calm, pleasure) allows us to stand up, to move, to create, and to be curious; even that most lofty of human endeavors—learning—requires a certain (ideally very small) dose of stress![15] In terms of those more relentless, unpleasing stresses that tend to beat us up, research consistently turns up glimmers of empowerment: rather than wringing our hands over the unavoidable pressures of modern life, we have the ability to *choose which story we tell ourselves* about whatever is going on—to perceive with consciousness, and thereby shape our own being.

Growth-Protection Regeneration Gap

Remember, whatever we put our attention on grows. This truth drills down to the cellular level. The distribution of receptor spaces on a cell's membrane isn't a fixed design, but one that is constantly being revised on an as-needed basis. The cell's intelligence, propelling it to respond to environmental information for its own wellbeing and continuity, interprets an abundance of circulating stress chemicals (remember those tiny cars?) as evidence that the environment is dangerous. This in turn behooves it to generate more receptors (parking spaces on the cell's membrane), and to make the signaling curbs of those parking spaces even more sensitive to the tap of the wheels—to speed the process of receiving and responding to this critical information. This, very simply, increases the individual's chances of surviving in dangerous circumstances. As a complement to this brilliant survival strategy, the cell will also reduce the number and sensitivity of receptors for chemicals that trigger feelings of pleasure and contentment, since stopping to smell the roses in a threatening world would put an organism at serious risk.

Do you think this cell is in growth mode or protection mode?

Recalling the rapid cycle of cell death and renewal, consider that each time this cell duplicates itself, the new cell will reflect the revised, protection-mode arrangement of receptors. Over time, with the uninterrupted, routine stress and joylessness that so many people experience these days, this person's reactivity and sensitivity to stress heightens ("irritable"..."can't sleep") while his biochemical capacity to feel calm, content and happy erodes ("in a funk"..."depressed"). A nasty domino effect is created that undermines health and wellbeing: the need for more and more receptor spaces to respond to all of his stress hormones means fewer spaces are available for the chemical messengers responsible for signaling basic cell maintenance processes, let alone growth. And forget feeling pleasure. He feels worse and worse. And with each cycle of renewal, more growth-diminished cells are regenerated. Thus, a decline in this man's wellbeing begins as a weakening of his individual cells, since critical growth-oriented cellular functions are pushed aside in favor of the mandate to respond to stress. The past decade's discoveries in this area have gone a long way to explain the long-observed but little-understood connection between stress and a long list of human ailments, including acute illness, chronic and degenerative disease, depression, infertility and premature aging.

Cells Are Excellent Students

Research in psychoneuroimmunology (the study of the mind-body* connection) has given us astonishing illustrations of the power of our minds to effect "cellular instruction," such as:[16]

- Subjects given a harmless substance but told it is something to which they are highly allergic, develop asthma attacks.
- Hypnotized subjects touched on the forearm with a piece of chalk and told it's the lit end of a cigarette, develop "burns" on their skin.
- Patients with multiple personality disorder have differing physiological profiles depending upon which personality is active—including optical prescriptions, allergies and even diabetes in one personality but not others.
- Patients with high cholesterol levels reduce them by 35 percent solely through daily, fifteen-minute mind-clearing sessions.
- The *placebo effect*, while complex and subject to a variety of factors, has a long and impressive history of demonstrating the powerful role of a

---

* Candace Pert, who made the landmark discovery of the brain's opiate receptor and is one of the pioneers in the study of how mind and emotions are expressed in the body, points out that it's not accurate to think of mind *over* body, or even as mind *affecting* body, but as mind's outward physical manifestation *being* body. As such, mind-body is more accurately expressed without the separation-suggesting hyphen; Pert prefers, and I henceforth use, the term *bodymind*, which reflects its inseparable unity demonstrated by her research.

patient's mind when she has expectations that a treatment will work. One study found that up to 75 percent of the effectiveness of antidepressants was due to the placebo effect rather than the treatment itself.[17]

We are walking pharmacies, able to produce our own powerful drugs to treat everything from pain to sadness to fear. (Endorphins, those mood-lifting pleasure chemicals that flow when we indulge in exercise, lovemaking, or chocolate, take their name from *endogenous*, meaning "from within," and *morphines*!) In fact, the way that drugs work (all drugs, prescribed or self-prescribed, including alcohol) is to park in cell receptor spaces designed for our own internal chemicals of communication. While not exactly accurate, you can think of it this way: tequila molecules hog spaces that would normally be used by messengers involved with sense perception, self-control, motor coordination, etc., meaning that these signals don't get delivered and their associated functions decline as a result.

Our brain and nervous system do not know the difference between something we imagine or something we experience "in reality." Elite athletes have long known this and use focused visualization to augment their physical conditioning and practice. Whatever you spend time thinking about and envisioning—regardless of whether it's something you hope *for*, or something you're complaining about or hope *against*—is what you're igniting with mental energy and thus ordering up from the grand menu of Life: *This is what I'll have, thank you.*

As Bruce Lipton details so remarkably in his book *The Biology of Belief*, this is the power of imagination: your neuro-endocrine system lines itself up in service to your thoughts, perceptions and intentions about yourself and about the world! With this awesome power in your service, you engage 24/7 in a nonstop dialogue with your fifty trillion brilliant cells, telling them about the world they need to adapt to. As those cells continually regenerate to make the neverending story that is you, the question becomes, *What are you instructing your fifty trillion cellular geniuses to be?*

Cultivating Fertility

Once we've oriented ourselves toward optimally healthy growth within our own organism, we can begin to consider the amazing notion of growing a completely new organism. Recall the fundamental question always being asked, at the level of every cell, tissue, organ and beyond: *Do circumstances warrant devoting my energies toward optimal growth, or do I need to protect and defend myself?* Life itself also asks this of those who might be entrusted with bringing new life into physical form.

As it becomes more and more clear that human health is shaped to a great extent during intrauterine life and that prenatal pollution is a significant threat to the health of future generations, we humans will undoubtedly, someday, come around to such considered physical preparation before conceiving children. But you can begin today! A woman's body is like the soil in which a prize seed is planted. Rich, fertile soil doesn't happen overnight, but over months of enriching, tilling and patience. And prize seeds are the result of knowledgeable tending of the source plant. The first acts of enlightened parenting can take place many months—even years—before a sperm is embraced by the ovum, as you both strive to nourish yourselves with wholesome foods and eliminate such toxins as cigarettes, drugs, alcohol, and chemical contaminants from both your internal and external environments.

More on pre-conception nutrition next step, but women want to see to it that they're getting enough omega-3 fatty acids; 400-800 mcg. of folic acid, which is found in leafy green vegetables, beans, peas and lentils, liver, beets, Brussels sprouts, nutritional yeast, wheat germ, mushrooms, oranges, asparagus, broccoli, spinach, bananas, strawberries, and cantaloupe; and enough calcium.

Detoxifying your immediate external environment is highly recommended and not that difficult. Both women and men who are contemplating conceiving are well advised to avoid chemicals, regardless of "proven" evidence of their safety or toxicity, and eliminate them from your home. They are often found in garden products, paint, new carpeting, many kinds of flooring, and furniture laminates. (Just one example: over-the-counter insecticides have been associated with lower testosterone in men, as well as DNA damage and impaired sperm motility.)

For those interested in advanced levels of preparation, it means detoxification of your inner environment, including body-borne stores of heavy metals, chemicals and other toxins. One approach to this—which is simple, but requires a significant commitment of time and money—is replacing dental fillings with mercury-free versions. Another approach to further preparing a purer reproductive environment, developed by physician Michel Odent, a pioneer in primal health research and the ecology of the womb—is the Accordion Method of pre-conception preparation. It is based on the premise that the majority of the synthetic chemical toxins that pose hazards to conception, embryonic and fetal development accumulate over decades and are stored in adipose (fat) tissues, leading to the potential for a time-bomb effect. The program is designed to facilitate "lipid mobilization" through a series of short, repeated semi-fasting sessions.[18]

The growing rate of fertility challenges is a complex phenomenon with myriad interacting causes, but one significant contributing factor is certainly the proliferation of environmental toxins to which we are continuously, invisibly exposed. Flame retardants, pesticides, fertilizers, plastics, and cosmetic and personal care ingredients like phthalates and parabens—they are everywhere and it takes dedication to avoid them and to significantly reduce them in your daily living or working environment. In the most serious cases some of these toxins—such as those mimicking estrogen—can cause structural and functional impairments of the reproductive system. But even in cases of milder exposures, again it is important to keep in mind a basic principle at work in fertility preparation: Nature is looking for her best possible shot at a healthy new member of the species, and her intelligence (working 24/7 within each of your cells and organs) assuredly registers toxins, sub-par nutrition and severe stress as cues that the environment will be unfriendly for a new organism. The ongoing "growth or protection" assessment may come down on the side of "don't grow"—thus, don't procreate.

For example, when a woman's percentage of body fat drops below about 22 percent, she stops ovulating and menstruating. Her bodymind's intelligence perceives that a baby conceived in such circumstances could easily suffer malnutrition. Along these lines, it's interesting to note that in Harvard's massive longitudinal Nurses' Health Study, it was found that healthy fats are important in preventing infertility due to ovulation problems. According to the authors of *The Fertility Diet*, "The more low-fat dairy products in a woman's diet, the more likely she was to have had trouble getting pregnant. The more full-fat dairy products in a woman's diet, the less likely she was to have problems getting pregnant."[19] Fast-burning carbs (white bread, potatoes, sodas) also impaired fertility, but the largest fertility decline was seen in women who ate trans fats (such as those found in margarine, doughnuts, French fries)—an ingredient that is created through the man-made reengineering of natural fat to enhance its shelf life. As the old commercial (ironically for Chiffon margarine) used to exhort, "It isn't nice to fool Mother Nature." Indeed.

Fertile Mind, Fertile Body

Through the nonstop cellular instruction dialogue just described, our inner life (mental, emotional, spiritual) becomes reflected in our biology, including the delicate hormonal balance of fertility. Understandably, based on Nature's assessment of the environment as mediated by our perceptions and thoughts, chronic stress is associated with diminished fertility. When you experience stress, hormones inform your bodymind that there is a threat "out there." In a process similar to menstruation cessation, the experience of chronic stress (so often mediated by perception) reports to the bodymind of an external environment that is neither conducive to optimal, healthy life nor to generating new life.

Our endocrine, immune, and nervous systems are intimately connected and are influenced by our every thought, attitude and emotion, especially the ones that we're not aware of having. Keeping in mind the implicit perception templates with which we become programmed during our early months and years, some of our most potent attitudes and responses to life are automatic and reflexive. Now is the time to really look at your inner responses, dialogues, and perceptions with the question, *Do they invite growth and life, or not?*

Some of our most critical early programming has to do with our reproductive capabilities, many of which are formed decades before we decide to begin a family! Along with parental attitudes about the body and its creative functions, as young children we perceive and internalize basic attitudes about such things as

- how babies come into our family (with ease, difficulty, crisis, etc.)
- whether children are loved and valued in our family
- whether it's safe and desirable in our family to have a child
- whether it's safe and desirable in our family to be a child.

Our endocrinology (hormonal profile), so critical to healthy fertility, adjusts itself to enact whatever our mental-emotional perceptions dictate. The late bodymind fertility pioneer Niravi Payne suggested that when a doctor (or even just conventional wisdom) tells a woman that she's too old to conceive, she will have an immediate bodymind response whereby her hormonal profile falls into line with that belief.[20] Research finds that our healthy bodymind balance can be especially keenly affected by "feelings we don't feel," repressed emotions often related to unrecognized trauma or loss in childhood. Here are a few examples:

Ellyn* had been trying for a long time to get pregnant, and though there was nothing medically wrong, it just wasn't happening. An adoptee, Ellyn had wordlessly learned a fundamental bodymind lesson throughout her growing-up years: *women in our family don't get pregnant.* After working with a counselor to consciously reconnect with and claim the fertile part of her past—the birth mother whom she had met some years earlier—Ellyn was finally able to conceive.

Maya suffered repeated miscarriages, and her doctor could find no physical cause. In charting her family history it became painfully clear that she and her sister had been "throwaway" children, left behind in their native India when their parents emigrated seeking a better life in America. Maya gradually came to understand how she was reenacting—in classic bodymind fashion—what her mother had done: Maya allowed herself to get pregnant but then "left the children behind." In making the connections, detective-like, with the truths of her early life, and experiencing and releasing the repressed sorrow, fear, anger, etc., Maya changed her biochemistry and ultimately had a healthy, full-term baby boy.

Sometimes inner shifts happen more spontaneously and mysteriously. We have all heard stories about "infertile" couples who spend many years and untold dollars on reproductive technologies with no success, then adopt a baby and end up conceiving naturally, by surprise. People who offer infertile couples the infuriating advice "Just *relax!*" point to these stories as evidence for their theory. Yes, hopping off of the conception-go-round can improve one's stress biochemistry, but it also has a lot to do with their biology adjusting to reflect their new feelings, behaviors and devotions: *they were mothering and fathering.*

One of my favorite stories is of a woman who, after a year of grueling rounds of IVF (in vitro fertilization) and two miscarriages, was faced at forty-three with the dismal expert diagnosis that she was too old and all of her eggs were bad. She decided to get some cats. Indeed, she got several cats and smothered them with unconditional love. Six months later she was pregnant with her son, who is now a healthy eight-year-old.

With each decade that passes, it seems that we humans have a harder time having babies. The number of people facing fertility challenges appears to be

---

* Names in this section were changed.

reaching epidemic proportions of anywhere from 15 to 30 percent, depending on where in the complicated grab bag of statistics you look. Fertility has become a major industry; most of the information available on the internet comes not from scientific researchers but from doctors, clinics and institutes for whom fertility treatment is their (big) business.

The medical model tackles infertility as a primary problem to be wrestled into compliance through a barrage of drugs and technological procedures, much as it addresses high cholesterol, heart disease, and all manner of chronic aches and pains. Rather than regarding these as *symptoms of imbalance* in the organism's system, and seeking to address the (much more invisible) underlying causes, our cultural norm is to simply eradicate the evidence of imbalance—in essence, to shoot the messenger—while leaving the deeper causes untended. What would happen if we reframe the very idea of fertility with this in mind? What if we consider fertility as an essential *vital sign*, like heart rate, blood pressure, temperature, and inflammation? When we're willing to follow the vital sign of infertility to where it might lead us—when we are willing to trade in a "Fix me, Doc" mentality for the responsibility of being a creatively active participant in cultivating our own reproductive health—we empower ourselves.

It may be important for us to do some inner investigation into the invisible answers we may be carrying to basic questions about how fertility, pregnancy, birth, and children were perceived in our family of origin, so that we can journey ahead into these realms in full growth mode, right down to our cells. (And, engaging in the creative process of mastering your own inner life is the best preparation not just for conceiving a baby, but also for parenting in general.)

Once you realize how you carry on a continual dialogue with your fifty trillion cells—consciously and unconsciously—you can aspire to cultivate an inner ecology that is truly fit for life. And when you consciously practice presence, cultivate gratitude and focus on appreciation, you are teaching yourself to be peace.

You are being the peace you seek.

You are changing the world.

PRINCIPLES TO PRACTICE

Presence – To practice this principle, try to gather all of yourself—body, mind and spirit—to whatever activity you are engaged with at the moment. It is sometimes referred to as *mindfulness*. The easiest activities to practice presence with are the ones that tend to completely absorb you without your effort, activities you are passionate about: surfing, painting, playing a musical instrument, tuning an engine, dancing, writing, computer programming, electrical engineering—any of those pursuits during which time tends to fall away. Mihaly Csikszentmihalyi described this phenomenon in his landmark book *Flow: The Psychology of Optimal Experience*. The most challenging—and thus the most transformative when we can bring presence to them—are the mundane activities: chopping celery, cleaning the toilet, shopping for groceries. Rather than letting your mind wander while the rest of you does the chore, devote your full, undivided attention to it. If we perceive them as an empty series of motions, it's hard to keep our attention on such basic tasks, but once we begin to unfold layered dimensions of the experience, it becomes more engaging. Think of it as weaving a relationship with that activity, object or substance: one of the first things we do when initiating a relationship is to express interest in the details of the other. Like showering and eating a piece of fruit, it's good to choose one or two things you do all the time, to which to bring your full presence as richly as you can.

- Meditation is the granddaddy of all the presence practices, and has emerged in the research as one of the best things you can do for all aspects of your health and wellbeing. One of its central purposes is to afford us the chance to practice in concentrated form, for those fifteen, twenty, or thirty minutes*, the level of presence we then seek to carry with us into our daily activities. It also opens a space within which your own powers of intuition can take root and grow; meditation over time becomes like a cosmic hotline to a level of knowing that is simply unavailable anywhere else. And just as physical exercise changes the way your body metabolizes for the entire rest of the day, so too does meditation uplift and unfold your consciousness long after you get off the mat (or sofa or chair or bed), expanding your inner resources for whatever the day brings.
- Drinking your daily morning glass of water is a great activity with which to start bringing more presence to routine activities. As you pour the water, notice

---

*Renowned meditation and mindfulness teacher Jon Kabat-Zinn wrote that it's better to meditate for three minutes every day, than for thirty minutes hardly ever. This has provided me reassurance over the years!

how it never falls in a straight line, but rather flows in curving arcs—oh, what water can teach us about the fastest way between two points! You might also reflect for a moment on the miraculous properties of water[21] that make all life possible; focus on gratitude for this most extraordinary elixir. And as you drink it down, you can imagine—even participate in—the delight of your body.

- Another simple but powerful practice of this principle is to bring mindfulness to your own body in space as you perform routine tasks, such as opening and closing doors quietly, or seeing how much care and mastery you can bring to the very use of your eating utensils at mealtime, making as little noise with them as you can. When we cultivate our capacity—and ultimately our tendency—for this level of presence, we are preparing an incomparable gift for our children, whether they are already here or yet to join us. Our presence is ultimately the most basic nourishment for their most robust, resilient development. We also give ourselves a very tangible gift of neurological and psychological wellbeing: an Oxford study[22] found that when a volunteer subject performed a habitual task on "auto-pilot" it resulted in the disengagement of his higher brain centers. This kind of disengagement can lead surprisingly rapidly to diminished brain tissue volume in those areas, which in turn can contribute to depression—the distinct opposite of what is cultivated with mindfulness! The awesome opportunity highlighted by that Oxford study was this: after watching the subject's higher brain activity go largely dark as he worked on auto-pilot, the researchers asked him to once again bring his full attention to the task he was doing (it was a numerical keypad sequence), to act as if he were once again figuring it out for the first time. He did, and his higher brain centers quickly reengaged and all the lights came back on! Buddhist monk, teacher and peace activist Thich Nhat Hanh didn't need fMRI scans to recognize the power of presence to reshape us, and his book *The Miracle of Mindfulness* is a wonderful primer on cultivating this principle in daily life.

- While bringing presence to everyday tasks and striving to reduce the habit of multitasking (which necessarily requires auto-piloting), give some thought to what for you are those flow pursuits—activities that stir your soul's passions and utterly absorb you. Fostering your connection to these pursuits is a gift to your future children.

Awareness – Bringing into awareness those things that we typically overlook or take for granted is an excellent practice for every aspect of your inner life.

Developing the depth and acuity of your awareness will serve you throughout your parenting journey.

- Cultivating conscious awareness of what are normally unconscious bodily functions is exactly what the yogic adepts do, who can sit naked in the snow while maintaining their body temperature and other aspects of metabolism normally outside our conscious control. This is a perfect time to begin developing awareness of such normally out-of-consciousness processes as the wonders of your breathing and the beating of your heart—and, if you're a woman, the ripening and release of each month's egg from one of your ovaries.

- Together with your partner, share memories, stories, photographs related to your families, particularly around the topics of your childhood experiences and how you feel they might influence your parenting choices. Exploring your childhood experiences and developing a coherent story about them is one of the most potent ways to positively impact your child's healthy development—it cultivates important circuitry in your social brain, which in turn provides the model for your child's social brain development! Interpersonal neurobiology pioneer Daniel Siegel points out that it isn't whether your story is wonderful or difficult that has an impact upon your child—what's important is how you come to make sense of your story. Becoming more fluent with your own story, and how your early relationships and experiences impact you today, is how you can liberate yourself from the generational repetition of parenting patterns that happens by default if we don't dedicate ourselves to this important exploration.[23] It isn't enough to consciously decide, "I'm not going to parent like my parents did," because when the heat is on and your toddler is having a tantrum—or your teen is revolting—your unconscious programming *will* kick in and your best intentions will be eclipsed by limbic imprints (or as Siegel calls it, "the low road"). I would invite you to begin this exploration before you're actively parenting, beginning with the "Questions for Parental Self-Reflection" on page 133-134 of Siegel's book *Parenting from the Inside Out*.

- Another area of awareness to tend to is the roots of your own feelings, beliefs and attitudes about sex, intimacy, and reproduction. Explore within yourself and together with your partner what's been passed down your family line regarding how children come into your family—with struggle or tranquility, health or crisis, etc. Make a family tree chart going back two or three generations (to your grandparents and even great-grandparents) in which you notate everyone's reproductive details, such as ease or difficulty in pregnancy, type of delivery, miscarriages, abortions, childlessness.24 Consider questions like, *Are children loved and valued in my family? Was it safe, secure and desirable to be a child in our family, or was it otherwise?* If you think these answers are unavailable, try meditating on them and see what arises. This information lives within your cellular intelligence and somatic memory, informing your fertility; cultivating fluency and making peace with your history helps cultivate a biochemistry more attuned to new life.

- Engage in expressive art forms that can reveal material you "knew but didn't know you knew." Quiet your mind, let the rest of the day fall away, sit before your medium of choice and fill yourself with the inner question, *What wants to be expressed?* And then just embark...
- Record your dreams and explore them for insights.
- Along with the above ideas for cultivating inward awareness related to yourself and your partner, it refreshes and expands you to develop a "reaching out" awareness toward others; tune in and notice if the clerk at the market...or the woman passing you on the sidewalk...or the neighbor's dog...seems to be having a bad day; silently let them know you notice and care.

Rhythm – Rhythm is a fundamental life principle, and one of the best things we can do for our children and ourselves is to develop appreciation and compassion for the ebbing and flowing processes of our bodies and psyches, especially as we travel such a momentous path as new (or contemplated future) parenthood. This tends to be a radical choice in our fastfasterfastest technoautomated world. Early people knew they had to understand nature's cycles and work with them, particularly the cycles of the sun and moon: during the waxing moon is when all things needing to grow must be tended to, and the new moon heralds the harvesting of crops and reaping of results.

- Notice the rhythms surrounding you in nature (waxing or waning moon, flowers budding, leaves dropping, birds nesting), and also going on within you. There is rhythmicity to your breath, your heartbeat, your digestion and elimination; there are even regular tidal movements of the fluids within your tissues, spinal cord and brain—one of which cranio-sacral therapists call the "long tide."
- Women, try journaling, charting, or other ways of tracking your energies, thoughts, and moods related to your menstrual cycle, noting any rhythms that emerge, and also their relationship to the moon phase.

- At any moment we choose, we can begin to reclaim our native connection to the earth, the moon and our own sacred, cyclical, powerful natures. Begin to experiment with seeing how differently (more successfully) big projects and important events tend to flourish when contracted on or scheduled for a waxing (filling up) moon, and how much more intimately we can "go deep" with friends, lovers, children—and most of all, ourselves—during a waning (emptying out) moon.

Example – In countless disciplines and traditions there is the concept of a master, teacher or guide, one who has dedicated him or herself to the mastery of its principles. A would-be initiate—whether it be an artist, a tradesperson, or a spiritual seeker—apprentices with this advanced individual for a period of time typically far longer than it would take for the master to teach the student all of the finer points of the discipline. The more subtle but powerful learning process is a result of *time*—time spent in the presence of the master, whereby the natural process of emulation works its magic. Thanks partly to the recently discovered mirror neurons in our brains, the experience of another to whom we are close becomes as if ours. We become more like them!

- Whom do you admire? Make a list of these people, and note the specific reasons for your admiration.
- Read a biography of someone whose qualities you would hope to emulate.
- If there's someone who is accessible to you whom you admire, sit down with him or her and have a conversation in which you ask questions such as *What do you think made you able to…?* and *What was it about you, do you think, that interested you in…?*
- Who are those who have inspired you so far? Pause and give them thanks.

Nurturance – Think of this principle, at this step, as an audition for the energies of Life, who might be wondering how you will love and nurture a child it might bring to you. The relationship between a child's parents is the foundation, the nest, and this is an excellent time to feather that nest! Self-care is also key: It is so common to be caring for others, but to put ourselves last on the "To Take Care Of" list. Only a parent who is well nourished—physically, emotionally, spiritually—is truly fit to raise children steeped in the atmosphere of strength and flexibility required for a generation of peacemakers. There are infinite ways to demonstrate your unique love and caring of yourself and your partner, so to list only a few is like singling out just a few stars in the vast night sky. But just to prime the pump of your own ideas…

- The single most extraordinary, effective form of nurturance is *empathy*— putting oneself in the place of the other, perceiving and caring about the other's experience. It is a mode of deeply seeing the other, so that the other "feels felt."[25] Practice empathy with your partner, yourself, the telemarketer who calls at dinner, even your plants and cooking pots!
- Find out the things you do that feel most nurturing to your partner, and share with him or her what makes you feel loved; Gary Chapman's book *The Five Languages of Love* is a wonderful guide in this exploration.
- Eating a nutritious, well-rounded diet that includes your favorite treats in moderation is a fundamental form of nurture.
- Whatever cleansing, detoxifying and health renewal you engage in now is a way of nurturing your future child, as your vitality becomes reflected and expressed in optimal sperm and ova.
- When buying clothes, pay special attention to how different fabrics make you feel throughout the day; you might discover natural fibers—cotton, silk, wool—nurture your skin best.
- The colors, sounds, and images you surround yourself with are a basic opportunity for loving care; with this in mind, consider your home décor, music choices, etc., with the question, *Does this nurture me? Nurture us?*

Trust – Recalling that trust is "calm reliance upon processes outside of your immediate perception and control," this is probably the most subversive principle of all for those of us weaned on the information revolution. Our instant access to infinite amounts of data on any topic has had a steroidal effect on our deeply ingrained conviction that by virtue of our vast intelligence we can figure out and be in charge of everything in our lives. But Life can quickly be drained of vitality beneath the weight of a ponderous intellectual force that quashes any sense of the mysterious or unquantifiable. Begin now to cultivate a fond taste for mystery and the unfathomable, to ensure that by the time your child gets behind the wheel of a car—and you need trust like never before—it will be well-established and enduring, like a beautiful rosebush whose roots can reach deep beneath drought-ridden topsoil to find life-sustaining water. Trust brings you to an unparalleled source of strength, paradoxically called "surrender," which might just be the most important resource in your parenting toolbox!

- If you are a list-maker, experiment with foregoing your "To Do" list for one week, with the conscious intention of inviting unseen energies within and outside yourself to organize what takes place. Yes, you'll forget some items, but what a delight to be guided into unplanned activities. (A frequent side effect is when you realize that the things you forgot were more fruitfully done a following day in light of new circumstances.)
- Make friends with your uncertainties and worries: *Hi, there, I know you well. Thank you for reminding me that* <fill in blank with situation heavily on your mind>. *I'm trusting it will all resolve in the way that's right.*
- When we want to develop an attitude more fully (such as trust), it helps to strive toward being worthy of that same virtue. One of the simplest yet most potent ways to develop trust is to build within yourself your own trustworthiness. Try to make your words and actions coincide with what is. If you say "I'll meet you at three," then be there at three. Don't exaggerate ("It took *forever* in line at the bank" is really "I waited much longer than I was expecting to") and don't "ultimize" ("I'll *never* do that again"…"It was the *worst* thing *ever*"). This powerful precept from esoteric spiritual science comes with a promise: practicing this kind of self-mastery will imbue you with a natural inner authority. And you'll be many steps ahead when your children become preteens and teens, and fervently want their parents' words to align with what truly is.

Simplicity – Famed Supreme Court Justice Oliver Wendell Holmes said, "I would not give a fig for simplicity this side of complexity, but I would give my life for simplicity the other side of complexity." Shallowness, superficiality and paucity of meaning are what we are left with if we settle for the simplistic, which is simplicity "this side of complexity." Discerning what is this side or the other side of simplicity is indeed the heartbeat of this principle; therein lies the practice! In many disciplines—mathematics, physics, philosophy— the solution considered best is the one that is most elegant, i.e., the simplest. Designer John Maeda offers one guideline that I particularly like for how it relates to this role of discernment: "Simplicity is about subtracting the obvious and adding the meaningful." It is possible to have a very simple, uncluttered room that is at the same time devoid of meaningful elements, which is not the point, eh? "Rich simplicity" is a portal to joy, and joy lies at the very foundation of health, wellbeing and peace.

- Consider the objects you have in your living space, assessing their meaning-to-space-taken-up ratio, and streamline to those essentials with a high meaning/low clutter ratio.
- Think about your plan of things to do in a given day, and see if you can trim it by a third.
- Most of us have become inured to a barrage of sounds in daily life; tune in to the idea of simplifying your aural sensory experience by mindfully tending to the sounds with which you fill your space.

Resources

Social Intelligence, by Daniel Goleman. This book, by the author who educated us all about EQ (emotional intelligence), is essential reading about the science of human relationships.

The State of Ease (Free booklet from the HeartMath Institute). Accessing your personal space of "inner-ease" can be done with minimum practice and in just a little time. When operating in an ease-mode, it's easier to choose less stressful perceptions and attitudes and cultivate growth mode throughout daily life: www.heartmath.org/state-of-ease.

Resiliency expert Karen Reivich's great website offering practical tools for helping children (and adults) cultivate the important GenPeace capacity of resilience. The best example I've seen of leveraging big business money for good (as this is a Pepperidge Farm site): www.fishfulthinking.com/Fishful-Thinking/WhatIs.

Two informative, easily digestible articles on stress:
- newsinhealth.nih.gov/2007/January/docs/01features_01.htm
- www.msnbc.msn.com/id/15772952

www.TheFertileSoul.com

Step Two

ATTUNED CONCEPTION—
A QUANTUM
COLLABORATION

*In every phenomenon the beginning remains always the most
notable moment.*

THOMAS CARLYLE

It seems crazy but it's true: we typically breed our prize animals with more
conscientious care than we breed ourselves. Think about it—in everything
from purebred dogs and cats, to horses and farm livestock, to exotic pets like
birds and fish, attention is paid to nourishing the physical health of the breeding stock before mating, since this results in more robustly healthy offspring.
There is also, at least with mammalian species, care given to keeping the pregnant mother in a calm, secure environment, and having an uncomplicated
birth.

In this step I invite you to approach this momentous event by attuning on
the physical, psychological and spiritual levels. Taking (at least) nine months

before you choose to conceive will help align you with Nature's highest vision, which wants your body vitally healthy to provide the best possible "mother earth" growing ground for the prize seed and egg that will grow to be your baby. Also, we now know that optimal health and fertility flourishes best when you have consciously explored, within yourself and with your partner, your reasons, dreams, fears, fantasies and ideals behind having a child.

Maybe it will reassure you to know that almost nobody feels quite ready to be a parent; in order to feel completely ready, we would have to feel relatively finished as a person, all done with our own development. According to this formula, we'd all seek to postpone having children until our nineties! Happily, it is not a parent's completeness or perfection that is of central importance to their children's optimal wellbeing or to finding joy and success in parenting— it is their *striving*.

A promising approach to take, once you feel at peace and resolved in your (relative) readiness, is to reconsider the standard postures of "We want a child" and "We're ready to have a baby." Taking a cue from Buddhist monk and mindfulness teacher Thich Nhat Hanh, who points out that "the vitality is in the question," you might consider living *these* questions over those months: "Does a child want *us*?" and "Is there a baby ready to join our family?" The curiosity and reverence inherent in such a rapport with Life may even cultivate within you an attunement that will allow you to perceive the actual moment of conception. (But please do not feel like you failed if you do not notice or feel it; it is quite rare to do so!)

Womb Ecology, World Ecology

A good place to embark on your journey into reproductive fruitfulness is by exploring your own life history related to your body's creative functions. How did your early experiences with puberty go? What was your mother's attitude toward her period? For men this may have left you with certain attitudes, most likely outside your awareness, about the elemental aspects of female reproductive function. For women, it can set the tone for how we embrace, or subtly (and not-so-subtly) reject, our generative powers as females. This then informs our bodymind's orientation toward creating life. Are our bodies a locus of integrity, honor, and power, or are they reservoirs of "unfresh" odors that need to be tamed with FDS? Are we empowered by the life-giving forces of our miraculous, mysterious bodies, or are we diminished by the onslaught of cultural messages that casually characterize those forces as "the curse," and by commercials that counsel us about the best product to medicate away the entire experience, cheerfully pronouncing "Your period is more than a pain—it's bloating as well!"? And, saddest of all, are we too familiar with apologetic monologues in which uncomfortable mothers hastily explain to their embarrassed daughters about "that time of the month" in terms that engender disgust and shame (or at the very least, apprehension) rather than a sense of the sacred privilege and power of fertility unfolding within them?

True, privilege and power aren't typically associated with our visit from Aunt Flo! But the late environmental and birth activist Jeannine Parvati Baker urged us to reconsider the true meaning of our monthly moon time: "Menstruation is the red flag that salutes the hard work of the preparation for another conception. Modern women suffer premenstrually because they do not fully comprehend the magnitude of the psychic and nutritional preparation that is required to build a healthy lining for an embryo. Your body has not slackened off from its commitment to reproduction and pulls from every cell to fulfill this mandate."[1]

In other words, a woman's body and psyche work hard to create conditions for new life and our obliviousness to that fact can bring suffering, which we've labeled PMS. In traditional cultures that abide by natural cycles of many kinds, menstruating women withdraw from many of their regular duties and activities to have time and space for contemplation and self-nurturing. It makes sense that the modern cycling woman might become irritable or snappish as something primitive in her urges her toward solitude, while her culture presses her to be machine-like: an unpausing, linear automaton rather than a cyclical, sacredly fertile woman.

In her writing and worldwide teaching Parvati Baker decried our modern alienation from our own bodies, from our knowledge of them and our trust in them. She devoted her life to raising (or more accurately, *restoring*) women's—and men's—awareness of their connection to the earth and its cycles, and of the innate wisdom and power that resides in each of us. She invites us to "an increased sense of trust and appreciation of [our] reproductive cycles—an invitation to reflect upon these cycles as a means of soul-making and spiritual development that will vibrantly color all aspects of our lives."

Some conscientious self-inquiry can pave the way for healing the intergenerational passage of less-than-empowering attitudes about our role in Life's big picture.

Attuned Conception—A Quantum Collaboration with Chaos

> *You think because you understand one you must also under-*
> *stand two, because one and one make two. But you must also*
> *understand "and."*

> —RUMI

Because we can observe it, we think we understand conception. But is fertil-ization (the merging of sperm and ovum) all there is to conception? We tap into a powerful dimension of human development when we broaden our per-ception of what really takes place surrounding this minute, secreted process—and, indeed, when we heed Rumi and ask ourselves if fertilization equals conception. Yes, the "one" of the sperm and the "one" of the egg come together to initiate a new being, but is there something about the "and" we have yet to understand, a less observable "something else" going on at conception? Re-search is suggesting yes.

Recalling the impact of our consciousness upon all the cells of our body, it isn't such a leap to realize that it would also influence cells in a mother's body during the process of reproduction. Indeed, neonatologist Jean-Pierre Relier highlights embryological research showing that as early as the two-cell stage of development of a newly fertilized zygote—after just one division following fertilization—the distribution of IGF^2 (insulin-like growth factor) receptors on its cell walls can vary, in part based on the mother's "psychoaffective qual-ity."[2] This means that her mental and emotional state can enhance or diminish the action of IGF^2, which governs the vascular organization of the placenta—the wellspring of embryonic and fetal development. A healthy placenta pre-vents early miscarriage, toxemia, maternal hypertension, intrauterine growth retardation and prematurity—the latter of which can saddle the offspring with lifelong challenges. Relier writes that these data "point out the fundamental importance of a real psychoaffective equilibrium of the parents, conscious and unconscious, in the quality of early growth of the embryo and placenta."

Recent research strongly supports Relier's concern: while it has long been known that stress in pregnancy increases the risk of giving birth prematurely, a 2009 study of 1.34 million births over twenty-three years in Denmark sug-gests that stress *prior* to conception can also seriously increase that risk. Severe life events in close relatives in the six months before conception increased the risk of preterm birth by 16 percent; and severe life events in the mothers' older children in the six months before conception increased the risk of preterm birth by 23 percent *and the risk of very preterm birth by 59 percent.*[3]

These are just two pieces of research among hundreds demonstrating that an individual's optimal lifelong health can be powerfully influenced this early. Although the catalog of such research, most recently compiled for the public's eyes in Annie Murphy Paul's book *Origins: How the Nine Months Before Birth Shape the Rest of Our Lives*, rarely includes much about conception, we're currently seeing more investigation into this issue by virtue of the soaring rates of IVF (*in vitro* fertilization) and some related developmental concerns now coming to light.

Researchers have long wondered whether there might be subtle changes in an embryo that is grown for several days in a petri dish, as IVF embryos are, and if so, whether there would be any consequences. Tentative answers are starting to emerge: some studies indicate that there may be some abnormal patterns of gene expression associated with IVF and a possible increase in rare but serious genetic disorders linked to those unusual gene expression patterns.

My intention is not to put down or create undue fear about IVF,* but rather to point out the technoscientific hubris that permeates our era: because we had the sophisticated means to join sperm and egg outside the body's natural processes we went ahead and did it, without a full understanding of the intricate developmental processes we were supplanting with pipettes and petri dishes. Richard Rawlins, director of the IVF and assisted reproduction laboratories at the Rush Centers for Advanced Reproductive Care, says he never gets questions about the possible consequences of growing embryos in the laboratory. "I have never had a patient ask me anything" about it, he said, adding, "For that matter, not many doctors have ever asked, either." He has "gradually become slightly less optimistic about the things that are known about the health of the children" born after IVF and related procedures.[4]

Relier cites research emphasizing the importance of the fallopian tube in conception and implantation, describing its developmental role on five different postovulatory days, including the secretion of specific long-chain proteins, the preservation of sperm motility, and activation of genomic expression. "This action is essential for the first steps of growth but almost absent during

---

* I believe that all of the principles in this step, regarding the impact of attunement and consciousness on cellular processes during conception, can fruitfully be applied when undergoing IVF.

in vitro fertilization, reducing the efficiency of this technique with possible long-term consequences after birth."[5] Along with those five days in the fallopian tube that are eclipsed with the use of assisted reproductive technologies, might there be other unrecognized forces at work at conception, something that might beckon to those of us seeking to bring new beings to life who are organized for peace and vibrant growth from the very beginning?

A Most Notable Moment

Many ancient spiritual traditions teach us that conception matters. It was written thousands of years ago in the Vedas that conception is a process of tremendous importance for the incoming being, that it captures and reflects the nature of the consciousness of the parents, and lays that portrait down as a gossamer watermark upon the new being—intangible, yet lifelong, a fundamental organizing principle underlying all else: conception as the one developmental window marked by near-infinite potential and possibility.

Data from embryology, cell biology, neonatology, epigenetics and even quantum physics suggest that circumstances at conception do indeed carry lifelong implications. It also suggests that conception involves more than just physical fertilization—the joining of the matter of sperm with the matter of ovum—something less quantifiable, having to do with forces that organize and inform the unfolding of the new being. I think of it as the "and" of Rumi's verse above—the elusive, often unfathomable "something else," variously referred to by such terms as the vital spark, entelechy, even soul. Within a vitalistic framework, such as chiropractic and other holistic healing models, this force is the inherent intelligence within the bodymind, which, if unimpeded, continually animates and motivates the organism toward healing and growth.

It is likely that this force lies in the realm of waves (energy) rather than the realm of particles (matter), and our conventional scientific understanding of the role of energy fields in human development and functioning is in its infancy. Perhaps some of the most compelling insights into how energy is involved in the informational signaling of cellular processes come from research into the subtle and not-so-subtle derangement of those signals and processes by EMFs (electromagnetic fields), discussed later in this step. Outside of the alarming and largely quashed research on reproductive effects (such as sterility and birth defects) of radar, microwave and radiowave exposure to both military and civilian workers in the mid-twentieth century, we are in largely uncharted territory when discussing the role this energy may play in human conception.

The Power of Gracious Thought

Einstein and his colleagues founded modern physics on the principle that the simple act of observation changes the nature of a physical system, leading them, as parapsychology researcher Dean Radin puts it, to think deeply about "the strangely privileged role of human consciousness."[6] I discussed in Step One how our emotions, beliefs, attitudes and perceptions can affect our own biology, but there is significant research on how they can also affect systems outside us—what scientists call nonlocal mind-matter interactions, the effects of *directed intention* (such as prayer or meditation) on *distant biological systems* such as plants, bacteria, human cells, and humans in other locations.

Recall from the introduction Bernard Grad's research on the effect of mental-emotional states on plant growth: He had people suffering varying types of depression hold vials of water for thirty minutes, after which the water was put on plants, which were carefully monitored. There was an appreciable difference in plant growth that correlated with the severity of the mental and mood states of the vial holders. You may be familiar with Masaru Emoto's compelling research on the power of words, thoughts, and music to affect the molecular organization of water and its symmetry when frozen into crystals. He is the first to disclose that his studies are not done following rigorous scientific protocols, but his findings are nevertheless instructive.

Different kinds of messages—spoken, written or merely held in mind—influenced the molecular shape of water crystals as revealed when frozen. Messages such as "You fool" or "I hate you" resulted in disorganized, messy crystalline structures, while messages such as "Truth" and "Love" resulted in symmetrical, organized water crystals. For example, Emoto had people pray for polluted water from Tokyo's Fujiwara dam—by which its crystals changed from incoherent and random to symmetrical and beautiful. He took distilled water and applied messages to their vials ("You fool"…"Beauty"…"You make me sick, I will kill you"…"Appreciation") then recorded their effects on the shape of the water when frozen.[7] His finding that "Thank You" had the most consistently positive influence on water's crystalline structure directly lines up with research from the field of positive psychology about the life-enhancing power of gratitude.

Emoto's inventive work sits on the sharp, glistening edge where old and new worldviews face off. He, along with such visionary scientists as William Braud, Marilyn Schlitz, Larry Dossey and many others, has ventured outside the "cult of the Randomized Controlled Trial"* to chart less quantifiable, reproducible phenomena. In so doing, they are contributing to an emerging understanding of how much vaster and more miraculous we humans are than we've been led to believe—than we've been enculturated to believe, through a reductionist "flat-human theory" that permeates our institutions and our culture. Let's explore a few ideas about how we might more richly unfold as a human family if we conceive our babies, our future generations, from this vaster awareness.

Simply, Let Us Pay Attention

In light of the growing body of research demonstrating a multitude of ways that focused thought or directed intention can influence biological systems, and the psychoneuroimmunology findings about the influence of our mental and emotional life on our own bodies, the desirability of mindful attunement to the process of conception might seem downright self-evident. And yet even the most holistically oriented, natural-living, spiritually evolved folks among us seem in the grip of a collective cultural blind spot when it comes to bringing consciousness to conception.

I recently attended a talk by a spiritual teacher whose name is an international household word, and who has written brilliantly about bringing prayerfulness to all aspects of daily life. Since the talk was specifically about peace, and this was an uncharacteristically small gathering in light of the speaker's fame, I raised my hand during the Q&A portion of the evening. Delighted to

---

* Thanks to Chris Kent, DC, JD, for that fitting phrase. Within a paradigm that acknowledges the effects of consciousness on biological and mechanical systems, such conventional scientific parameters as *random*, *control* and *double blind* become at best challenging, at worst blinding; nevertheless, Emoto's findings were reproduced in a 2006 double blind study. Whether it was performed in response to skeptic James Randi's offer of $1 million to do so—and whether Randi ever paid up—is an open question. See www.explorejournal.com/article/S1550-8307%2806%2900327-2/fulltext.

be called upon, I spoke of the need to seed peace in our incoming children from the very beginning, which ideally includes bringing attunement and intention to the process of conceiving. I'll never forget the look of disdain and the glib words of mocking dismissal I got in return, from this visionary who urges us to pray over everything from bathing to money to sex. It was in that moment that I realized how insidious, how glaring and how gripping this collective blind spot is, regarding taking responsibility for how we invite in, welcome and incarnate our next generation.

Laura Huxley and Piero Ferrucci write in *Child of Your Dreams* about the routinely overlooked miracle of conception, the triumphant process that violates all statistical logic:

> when the sperm…finally arrives at the longed-for destination. In some kind of unknowable alchemy a miraculous quantum leap occurs. From a predictable biological happening springs the beginning of a human life, an individual who is capable of loving and hating, of thinking and dreaming, of making wars and composing symphonies. This is the moment of the beginning. And all beginnings carry in themselves something hopeful and happy. Beginnings should always be accompanied by enthusiasm, and good wishes, and a loving care, and faith, and thoughts that all is well and shall be well.
>
> Yet consider what most often happens instead. The most basic and sacred moment of an individual's life is surrounded by the most hurtful of all human attitudes: indifference.[8]

Gabor Maté points out that the origins of the word *attend* is the Latin *tendere,* "to stretch," and suggests that to *attend* means to extend, to stretch toward—"attention as an active form of loving."[9] What if we were to love our children in this active way beginning at the very beginning? Recalling Cleve Backster's findings of the responsiveness of cells of all kinds (human, plant, bacteria) to human thoughts, emotions and intentions, and keeping in mind that we're about 70 percent water, and a newly fertilized zygote is probably closer to 95 percent water, might we take a cue from Emoto and Grad? Their findings illuminate a process whereby the subtle bioinformational aspect of water—conveyed to Grad's plants and captured in Emoto's crystalline portraits—was calibrated by the human consciousness to which it was exposed.

These avenues of frontier research suggest how the parents' inner atmosphere surrounding the act of conception may be communicated to the created individual, and should urge us to wonder about how parents' thoughts and feelings might affect egg and sperm cells, and the mysterious processes that unfold as they unite. Remember that cells are always expressing intelligence—responding to information for their own wellbeing and continuity—and continually engage in the process of reading the environment and adapting to its signals. Recall the unceasing question of all life, beginning with cells: do current environmental circumstances warrant devoting my energy toward optimal growth, or do I need to protect and defend?

If a single cell possesses this fundamental intelligence, so too does the barely visible zygote, newly conceived and floating down the fallopian tube. It "begins to pick up on subtle cues in its environment. It then canvasses its own genome, switching genes in different cells on or off according to the signals it receives. At this moment, 'nature' becomes malleable, and genetically identical cells set off on different journeys."[10] Environmental cues can be biochemical via a mother's moods, nutrition, and environment, or energetic through the parents' thoughts and electromagnetic fields. They let the new being know whether it's a safe, secure environment or a threatening one.

Might this then be one causal pathway involved in such connections research has found between unwanted conception and a higher risk of neonatal death, or of schizophrenia?[11] Or on the positive side, perhaps this illuminates processes involved in the association between planned conception and higher infant functioning?[12] When at the age of only a few cells, the zygote may perceive the environmental message, "The world is safe—*grow* robustly"…or, "Things out here aren't so great—marshal your energy and *don't grow* so vigorously"? These are not rhetorical questions. We are a long way from having definitive, proven explanations or answers.

I would invite us all in the meanwhile to seriously consider *consciousness as an organizing principle*. Reorienting ourselves toward bringing in new life based on this principle carries no risk or downside, and a most extraordinary array of potential upsides. For one thing, the research out of the psychoneuroimmunology (bodymind) and positive psychology fields is virtually unequivocal: mindfulness, gratitude, attuned interdependence are the master keys to individual happiness. And indications from many disciplines suggest that such an orientation also carries brave new implications for human development at its very beginning: an opportunity at conception to offer the new physical being thoughts and intention that invite harmonized, healthy organization and growth from the earliest moments of its formation!

In the Realm of the Spiritual

There is a fascinating collection of researchers' findings around the phenomenon of parents having experiences of visitations—through dreams, visions, inner voices, "subtle knowings"—by their children *prior to conception*, sometimes years prior.[13] Elizabeth Hallett's *Soul Trek* and Sarah Hinze's *Coming from the Light* explore these fascinating phenomena. Such accounts lead toward the undeniable possibility of a continuum of spiritual existence punctuated by embodied lifetimes, which would harmonize with the teachings of esoteric spiritual traditions.

One interpreter and teacher of such esoteric traditions was Bulgarian philosopher Omraam Mikhaël Aïvanhov, who emphasized the great impact that pre-conception preparation and conception consciousness can have on the incoming being: "The very best way is to make sure that your thoughts and feelings, indeed your whole attitude and way of life, are such as to attract exceptional beings into your family.... [Parents] have this tremendous power, the power of choosing their own children—and most of them are totally unaware of it."[14]

Omraam anguished over the fact that rather than preparing themselves for months or possibly even years, and then consciously choosing the occasion under conditions of peace and lucidity for conceiving their child, parents often "pick a moment when they are besotted by alcohol and not fully conscious of what they are doing. This is the 'sublime' condition of many parents at the moment of conceiving a child!" Omraam suggests that the supreme act of conception is "something for which they should call on Heaven, asking the angels to come and help them to attract a powerful, luminous being into their family."

The Persistence of Primal Memory

Of only a handful of authors who have explored the psychospiritual dimensions of conception, body psychotherapist Albert Pesso writes, "To have a place in the world of the mind, we must first exist as an image in the mind of another. That is, we must first be given a place in the mind of another..."[15] According to psychiatrist John Sonne,

> babies are conceived psychogenetically at the same time that they are conceived physically. The manner of their conception becomes an *unthought known* as part of their being—something known but out of awareness—that will prenatally and postnatally influence all the baby's postconception experiences, including the baby's relationship with himself or herself, with others, and with God.[16]

Working in the world of adoption education, and being an adopted person myself, I have often witnessed in adult adoptees the deep resonance and recognition and sense of relief when we talk about the lived experience of a conception that wasn't intended: somehow feeling, at your deepest core, *wrong*, in the most basic, existential, yet intangible way—never quite legitimate, never quite enough. Feeling like we have to keep earning and demonstrating our right to be here. For some it includes going through life apologizing for intruding: "Sorry to disturb you," "Sorry to interrupt," "Are you sure you really want me to come to your party?"

While it is almost impossible within a brain-centric framework to consider the possibility of retaining memories of the atmosphere around conception, our current understandings of how memory actually works lead us to fathom it. Candace Pert points out that to understand the capacity of the body to retain life memories, we must keep in mind science's fairly recent discovery of peptides, transmitters, and hormones (again, collectively termed *ligands*—information substances) and their receptors throughout the body. She suggests "their distribution in the body's nerves has all kinds of significance, which Sigmund Freud, were he alive today, would gleefully point out as the molecular confirmation of his theories. The body is the unconscious mind!"

Indeed, "Biochemical change wrought at the receptor level is the molecular basis of memory," according to findings by famed neuroscientist Eric Kandell and his associates at Columbia—and provides us the basis for understanding what is sometimes referred to as *cellular memory*, a process that pervades our entire body, right out to our skin's surface. "When a receptor is flooded with a ligand," Pert explains in her book *The Molecules of Emotion*, "it changes the cell membrane in such a way that the probability of an electrical impulse traveling across the membrane where the receptor resides is facilitated or inhibited, thereafter affecting the choice of neuronal circuitry that will be used."[17] So, our very *cells* prefer and opt for what is familiar! (Our bodymind's inclination to follow this path-of-most-familiar keeps us stuck in ruts with our old buttons getting pushed.)

Prenatal psychologist Simon House writes, "However it happens, [early fetal memory] is a wonder that echoes chaos theory. Even in one single-cell zygote, 'a butterfly's wings,' as it were, can be so disturbed as to cause 'a storm' in a trillion-cell human being decades later!"[18]

Within the conventional Cartesian worldview, the size of something is directly related to its importance and significance, and there is the tendency to think, regarding conception, *How could anything have a lasting impact so very early, when there is just one or two or twelve cells?* But when we recognize that human beings are dynamic systems whose workings can be illustrated by chaos theory…when we consider chaos theory's central tenet of "sensitive dependence on initial conditions"…and with a small but quantum shift in how we look at it…wouldn't it make sense that the influence of a very positive, or very negative, environmental message would bear the most pervasive influence *upon a tiny, emerging system, at the very beginning*, considering that each cell division will replicate that cell's knowledge again and again?

How We Begin

There are two paths along which we can seek to understand fertilization—the quantitative biological facts about what physically takes place, and the qualitative exploration that mines the deeper meaning of those facts. I will now attempt a crash course that synthesizes both. (This is a complicated maneuver—don't try this at home.)[19] The first two weeks of human physical existence, marked by fluid movement and rhythm, pressure and release, inward and outward impulses, can be seen as a template for all basic developmental gestures the organism will express lifelong. It is our first hero's journey, the "most delicate of human operas," writes ecologist Sandra Steingraber, and thus "the language of embryology has a heroic, epic resonance."[20]

The sperm and the ovum embody the paradoxical polarities inherent in all that we encounter in life. We perceive sperm as sheer perpetual motion, almost frantic in their propulsive action, and the ovum as utterly still, passive, waiting. But the less visible reality is that a sperm cell's interior is virtually inert, and

within the "quiescent" egg is found a bustle of purposeful activity. Men develop new batches of sperm continuously—beginning in adolescence, about
one thousand per second!—while a woman's ovaries, which have carried millions of immature eggs since she was in her own mother's womb*, release one
egg to mature every moon cycle (although new research suggests that the old
story of a woman having a finite supply of eggs may not be the whole story,
and that mammals may have the ability to generate new eggs).[21]

In a single act of intercourse, up to five hundred million sperm are tasked
with reaching a singular, newly ripened ovum.† Contrary to our perception
of the sperm penetrating the egg in aggressive, conquering fashion, there is a
profound mutuality to the process whereby the ovum, by virtue of the all-important receptors on the surface of the zona pellucida (the protective casing
surrounding the ovum‡), chooses a sperm to invite in. When the sperm and
ovum unite, the union of their reciprocal polarities ignites the embodied yin-
yang dynamic underlying all life. One of the most astonishing things I learned
in studying the phenomenon of fertilization is that the cell membranes of both
sperm and egg *remain intact*; rather than a piercing of the egg by the sperm,
there is, again, a *reciprocal incorporation* of each by the other. The outer layer
of the sperm head dissolves and then the genetic material fuses with the egg
membrane and is incorporated into the egg's cytoplasm.

The fusion of the two nuclei marks the creation of our first cell—the zygote—and the end of fertilization, roughly twenty-four hours after the sperm
and egg united. (Prior to this it can take anywhere from a few hours to several
days following intercourse for the sperm to make its journey to the egg.) In
Tibetan medicine the initialization of the heart chakra—and bliss—happens

---

* Says embryologist Michael Shea, "Depending on which book you read it could be as many
as 14,000,000 eggs at the beginning in the embryonic embryo and by the time a female baby
has been born it is trimmed down to about 100,000 to 1,000,000. Then only 400 get released
from the ovaries in a woman's lifetime. To me this speaks to the imprint carried in the female
womb of death as a natural process."

† Here's scientific irony I find amusing: although it is the largest cell in the (female) body, and
the only human cell visible to the naked eye, the ovum was the last human cell "discovered"
and identified, in the 1800s.

‡ Before the sperm and ovum's membranes merge, the sperm must release enzymes to dissolve
the hard casing surrounding the ovum—just like with a chicken's egg, whose shell you crack
and inside which there's that thin, stretchy membrane—that's a good way to visualize the relationship of the zona and the egg's membrane.

now. I consider this fusion of egg and sperm—the coalescing of fluids, molecules, information, and energies—as the vitalistic big bang that echoes through us forever.

The zygote now cleaves into two cells called blastomeres, then those two cleave into four, and so on (our first multiplication lesson!), with each division occurring approximately every twenty hours. Despite all this growth and cell division going on, the size of the embryo remains the same—still encased within the same protective shell of the *zona pellucida* within which the ovum began. The ovum is the only human cell visible—just barely—to the human eye: it is about the diameter of the width of a piece of printer paper. After three or four days, when the embryo has divided into sixteen cells, it is called a morula (Latin for "mulberry" which this little ball of cells resembles). It is still the same size as the original ovum was, with each of its dividing cells having gotten smaller and smaller with each cleavage. The compression is intense.

Then, at four or five days of physical existence, when we have multiplied several more times, we engage a fundamental principle of development that will follow us lifelong (and that will profoundly inform our parenting): *there is no growth without resistance.* The very pressure of compaction within the unyielding boundary of the zona pellucida stimulates our first developmental milestone at the end of the first week: the differentiation of our cells (that are still all roughly the same) into two different shapes that will go on to fulfill different developmental missions. In very general terms, this first differentiation gives rise to the first stem cells that will become our further developed embryo and fetus and those that will over the next couple of months become our placenta. These different types of cells continue dividing—each into more of their own lineage of either being the inside of the embryo or being the outside of the embryo. They grow to their respective places within the zona pellucida, leaving a hollow space in the middle filled with fluid, the future yolk sac; the embryo is now called a blastocyst.

This adventure has all taken place while we've been rolling down the fallopian tube, gently fanned on our way by rhythmically pulsing hair-like cilia. It was on about day five that we spilled from the tube in a sort of controlled freefall into the uterine cavity. Tiny cracks begin to form in the zona pellucida.

Near the end of the first week, the blastocyst is still in the same small quarters of the zona pellucida with its multitude of highly compacted cells. It excretes an enzyme that carves open an escape hatch through the cracks in the zona pellucida, and the ball of cells squeezes out ("hatches") and begins wafting its way, jellyfish-like, through the dark fluid sea and up to the uterine wall. Microscopic images of this scene reveal something very much like the landing of a lunar module on the moon. But prior to that landing, the glistening, quivering little space explorer spends up to two days suspended in the vast open space of the uterine cavity. Joseph Chilton Pearce has said that eight to ten days is a common point of spontaneous miscarriage, and biodynamic embryologist Michael Shea explains why: this is an important point of choice for the pre-embryo, because it requires a tremendous amount of energy to accomplish its next big task, implantation.

Upon landing and nestling into the nutrient-rich uterine lining lavishly prepared each and every month in case just such a potential human should happen along (and is shed as the woman's menses should fertilization not take place), we must tackle two jobs of life-or-death importance: excrete chemicals outward to placate our mother's immune system so we're not gobbled up by white cells who might (accurately) identify us as a foreigner, and excrete chemicals downward to excavate into our mother's uterine tissue, resulting in tiny tide pools of maternal blood—the first tendrils of our future placenta.

What happens next is largely inscrutable yet important to at least fleetingly grasp, as it is yet another lifelong developmental principle that is essential for parents to understand if they want to make their jobs easier and more joyous. Near the end of the second week, when we're still basically just two layers of differentiated cell types, the inner layer of the future body grows out to the periphery as it begins to differentiate into yet more different kinds of cells with different functions. For example, some are angiogenic cells—cells that will later build a heart, but for now express the beginnings of embryonic blood. The function of blood precedes the formation of our heart structure. Other cells arise to perform enzymatic and hormonal functions, many days before the formation of the structures of a liver, kidney or adrenal glands.

It is practically a mantra for Michael Shea, and it will inform every stage of development from now until we pass out of this life: *Function is projected into the periphery until the structure is built inside.* We will see this dynamic of "projection of function outside before internalizing the capacity" recur vividly in infant, toddler, early child and even adolescent development; it never ceases to operate, no matter how old we are. It will help us immensely to be more compassionate with our children, with ourselves, with everyone, if we really take this in and understand it: we need help with basic tasks until we develop the ability to take over and do it ourselves.

Nourishing Conception

Though every pregnancy book says it, the importance of folic acid is worth repeating here, due to its key role in healthy development of your baby's spinal column and brain. Because the critical window of this development often occurs before a woman realizes she's pregnant, enough folic acid should be in your diet as part of your healthy fertility and pre-conception regime.

The importance of sufficient EFAs (essential fatty acids) cannot be overstated; this family of nutrients (omegas 3, 6 and 9) is key to the development of your baby's brain and nervous system—which begins in the earliest weeks of pregnancy—and also to the functioning of your own cardiovascular, reproductive, immune, and nervous systems. The body needs EFAs to manufacture and repair cell membranes, enabling the cells to obtain optimum nutrition and expel harmful waste products, and to produce prostaglandins, which regulate body functions such as heart rate, blood pressure, blood clotting, fertility, conception, and play a role in immune function by regulating inflammation and encouraging the body to fight infection.

Many Americans are deficient in omega-3s, so a pregnant (and soon-to-be-pregnant) woman might need to pay extra attention to them.*[22] Fish is a primary source, and while there are concerns about the levels of mercury found in some fish, research finds that the advantages of sea fish consumption in pregnancy by far outweigh the theoretical risks associated with mercury contamination.[23] A host of studies has found that sea fish consumption helps protect against preterm labor and certain psychiatric disorders, and is associated with robust nervous system development, cognitive functioning and a cascade of other positive health criteria. The key to low-mercury seafood consumption (in pregnancy and in general) is to eat fish lower on the ocean food chain— smaller fish such as sardines, anchovies, flounder, and small ("light") tuna.[24] Wild salmon is also on the safer side. Vegetable sources include nuts, leafy greens, and flaxseed.

The question of whether to supplement or not is complex, with ambiguous findings emerging about whether or not vitamin and mineral supplements are

---

* One concern about many fish-oil-based omega-3 supplements is the potential for the oil to turn rancid in the punishing environment of the stomach, not only defeating its healthy purpose but also turning it potentially carcinogenic, so do keep this in mind as you're researching omega-3 supplements.

a sound way to go. That unintentionally ironic margarine commercial I mentioned earlier was so correct when it chastised, "It's not nice to fool Mother Nature"; there's research to indeed suggest that trying to isolate and encapsulate specific nutrients in supplement form is shortsighted and possibly unhealthy in the long term: in their whole, food-borne state, vitamins and minerals occur together with other important micronutrients that interact, synergize and optimize their intended actions in the body. That said, adequate folic acid is a critical enough issue that if you're not confident you can get 400-800 mg. in your daily diet, supplementing might be wise.

Laying the Foundation for Success

As prenatal specialist Laura Uplinger points out, "Your pregnancy will run on the habits you developed for your body before pregnancy. These habits set your body on a specific course. Ideally, naturally occurring vitamins, mineral salts, and omega-3s are a part of your diet before you conceive." Michel Odent routinely cites research that indeed found, for example, that fish consumption during pregnancy had the fullest cascade of positive effects when the woman had already been eating fish before conceiving. It is very much like exercise in this way; while no midwife or obstetrician would discourage some form of healthy exercise during pregnancy—even a gentle walking, swimming or stretching regimen that is brand new for the woman—most agree that the level and intensity of exercise that is beneficial during pregnancy is optimally established in a woman's lifestyle prior to conception.

Political scientist Amanda Rose learned through rugged experience that the toll of a woman's subpar diet can finally come due when she's faced with the physiological rigors of pregnancy. A whole new body is being formed out of the raw materials your body provides, and it's imperative to realize that the baby comes first in nature's hierarchy: prenatal development will draw nutrients to the baby even if it means leaving you deficient in key vitamins, minerals or essential fatty acids. This is likely a drastically under-recognized contributor to maternal depressive symptoms, both postpartum and during pregnancy. Dr. Rose had never suffered from depression, but it hit her during her first pregnancy and afterward.

> I spent the formative years of my life on low fat diets of bagels and imitation cheeses. Nary an omega-3 was to be found. I proceeded

through life managing nonetheless until my body was charged with making an entire new person. As my first son's brain developed in my womb, he sucked the limited omega-3 stores out of me and I went bananas from the lack. I produced the food that grew him out of his infancy as well, a food that also required omega-3 fatty acids and many other nutrients. It took about six years to recover from my task of producing him. I was seriously deficient in omega-3 fatty acids, B vitamins, and magnesium, all nutrients that can at least aggravate depression if we do not have enough in our diets. Zinc is another culprit as is iron in the case of postpartum depression.[25]

After she suffered debilitating depression, the painstaking research Dr. Rose did during her arduous journey back to health is a boon to all of us, as collected for her website and book *Rebuild from Depression*. Some of the depression-buster foods she has identified (those supplying key nutrients pregnancy can deplete) are salmon, walnuts, eggs, lamb, beef, sesame seeds, clams and liver.

Sensitive Dependence on Initial Conditions, Part 1

Nutrition comprises a fundamental message to a woman's bodymind about the circumstances in her world, and whether they would support the growth of a baby—thus informing fertility and the healthiest beginnings for a child to be conceived. So too are a woman's emotions, attitudes and perceptions informing the intelligence of her bodymind about the nature of the environment and whether it will provide new life with an optimal—or even passable—growing ground. There is a relatively newly discovered biological phenomenon called *genomic imprinting*, through which a mother's experience of her environment—as downloaded via stress or pleasure hormones, for example—begins shaping the development of her child *as early as ovulation*.

In genomic imprinting—so far studied in the mammalian realm only as high up as mice—the same genes carry different imprints depending upon whether the genes are maternally or paternally expressed. In English, this means that there is a whole variety of genes—for such traits as musculature and neural development—that are carried by both a mother and father whose egg and sperm are going to unite to cooperatively form a new member of their species; the process of genomic imprinting determines whether it's the mother's version or the father's version of these various genes that are expressed in the offspring. The mechanism and the meaning are still poorly understood, and most conventional biologists have cast it as a competition between the mother's and father's genes as to whose will prevail in shaping their fetus' development most profoundly.

They do understand the basics of *how* genomic imprinting works: when the genes are paternally expressed, mice grow considerably larger; but paternal expression can be thwarted and trumped (again, using the language of competition) by the maternally expressed genes, which direct thriftier growth.[26] The "conflict theorists" chalk it up to evolutionarily programmed, gendered agendas: Dad wants big, strong babies, and Mom wants to protect her resources for building more babies.[27] Cell biologist Bruce Lipton sees it differently from his more conventional biology fellows.

"Everything that they perceive is taken in the vein of competition. I don't see this at all; nature is cooperative. There is a reason for the smaller and larger size as I see it right now."[28] Lipton postulates, in line with his encompassing theory of *adaptive mutation* that maternal and paternal interests, embedded as they are in the species' drive toward evolutionary survival, lie in cooperatively creating offspring as perfectly suited for successful life in the current environment as possible. What many of the "larger, paternally designed versus smaller, maternally designed" findings on genomic imprinting don't usually point out is that, for example in mice studies, the mice with smaller bodies have bigger brains—especially forebrains. The mice with larger bodies had smaller brains, with the hindbrains relatively larger than the forebrains.[29] The paternally directed mouse can be seen as a mouse suited to (*designed* for?) a more dangerous environment, with bigger, stronger bodies and brains more geared toward survival-oriented reflexive behavior than toward complex, rational thought. The maternally directed mouse is better-suited for a more peaceful, supportive environment, in which reasoning, reflecting and relating are more useful than brute strength and impulsiveness. "It's a differential expression," says Lipton, "and it's not just 'larger'; if you look at just one parameter then you're missing the meaning of the whole thing."[30]

Lipton suggests that the same hormonal and other maternal signals that drive fetal adaptations in the womb also drive the intra-ovum potentiation of either paternally or maternally expressed genes, signals elicited not simply by the environment itself, but by the mother's subjective *perception* of the environment: as safe, supportive and loving, or chronically stressful, disconnected and threatening. In light of this compelling characterization, the maternal-paternal conflict theorists end up sounding a bit on the simplistic side. Explains Lipton, "They're not considering the more important understanding, which is that the organisms are intimately adapting to the environment."[31]

This theory bears huge implications for pre-conception care and consciousness! Nature and nurture engage in a complex, iterative co-creation of states and traits. Together with my colleagues in the field of prenatal and perinatal development, I have met with considerable resistance to the notion that this dance begins well before birth—that people are affected, not just physiologically but psychologically, by circumstances during fetal development. Imagine the stir were we to discover that the perceptions a woman has about the relative safety or danger of her circumstances could direct fundamental aspects of her future child's physiological and neurological development *before she even ovulates?!* But it makes perfect sense within a framework that remembers that *Homo sapiens,* just like all other animals, is evolutionarily driven to adapt to its environment. What more elegant way than to wait until just before ovulation to induce the first of the environmental adaptations that will make the individual as well-suited as possible to its present environment?

A Twenty-First Century Concern: EMFs

Whenever we hold a cellphone to our ear, use a Bluetooth headset, or simply hang out in a space equipped with wireless, we're participating in an ongoing experiment about the effects of EMFs (electromagnetic fields) on human health and functioning. We as a technoculture have enthusiastically embraced all this gadgetry without really knowing what it might be doing to us. One of the challenges of the EMF issue is its extreme complexity. Not only are there myriad frequency levels and strengths of different kinds, but the variety of interactional possibilities is virtually infinite. Testing the effects of a single unchanging frequency, for example, is largely irrelevant outside the lab, where synergistic effects inevitably occur in the latticework of today's everpresent electromagnetic web. The EMF danger is a tough sell—to public policymakers, to many scientists, to the public. It's hard to wrap slogans around, tricky to grasp.

Nevertheless, the facts are available to those who dig a little and find the work of intrepid researchers who've have had the mettle to amass evidence for the human immune, reproductive, and bioregulatory effects of our growing worldwide carpet and canopy of multistrength, multifrequency electromagnetic fields. The late UCLA brain researcher Ross Adey—who in the '60s developed for NASA the telemetry technology that allowed for EEG monitoring of the effects of weightlessness on brain function in astronauts—was among the first, and most vocal, to recognize the double-edged aspect of bioelectromagnetics. Carefully deployed, they hold exciting promise for many healing and communications applications, but the proliferation of uncontrolled, multiple daily doses of them in the form of ubiquitous electrical and wireless devices presents very real health concerns.

In Step One I discussed the most basic definition of intelligence—the ability to bring in information and respond to it for one's own wellbeing and continuity. Adey's many streams of research were all tied together by the theme of communication in the body—and what happens when that communication is interfered with. Stress is one well-documented such interference. Current research focuses on the effects of stress on neurotransmitters—hormones and other information substances—and views these at a *molecular* level. (Recall the tiny cortisol cars parking into their specific receptor sites on the cell membranes of the stress axis.) Adey's work demonstrated, however, that all communication in the body takes place at a molecular *and atomic* level (some refer to this as "energetic"), where infinitesimally weak electrical signals alter cell membrane permeability to allow the transfer of millions of ions back and forth in milliseconds. Adey's new paradigm of cell communication allows us to comprehend numerous well-documented observations that cannot be explained by Newtonian physics, or earlier accepted laws of thermodynamics that govern ionic flux.[32]

ELF (extremely low frequency) fields and pulses seem to be of greatest concern, since they can be so similar to the tiny bioinformational frequencies going on within our own bodies, and can therefore more insidiously perturb them. Having studied brain neurons' response to ELFs, Adey found that some pulse levels can change calcium flow in the nervous system; such a disruption in calcium *efflux* interferes with concentration on complex tasks, disrupts sleep cycles, and changes brain function in countless other ways. He pointed out that this relates to disruption of delicate molecular processes at the site of the cell membrane, the cell's "window on the world around it." He saw evidence of EMFs disrupting the "private language of intrinsic communication by which cells may 'whisper together' in activities such as metabolic cooperation and growth regulation." Such a perturbation of information flow is a corruption of the most basic intelligence in the human body, an assault on the infinitesimal foundations of peace.

Even in the absence of consensus on EMF effects, it makes sense to choose "the path of least regret," especially during the unfolding of a brand new human being. Try to use (old-fashioned, I know!) corded and wired devices rather than cordless and wireless. To be without a cell phone is akin to living in cultural exile, but take precautions. Consider choosing a phone with a lower level of absorbed radiation, and getting a "Blue Tube" (as opposed to Bluetooth) wired headset, or use the speaker so you keep the phone away from your head. Move your bed so that your head is three to six feet away from any electrical outlets or devices. Before going to sleep, turn off everything electrical or wireless (ideally in your entire house, but at least in your sleeping areas), including WiFi, cell and cordless phones.

The Radiance of Our Inner Life

Besides managing external electromagnetic fields, we need to tend to our internal ones. One of the premises from which energetic healthcare pioneer Milton Morter works is that a person's health—from the prefertilized egg until death—is dictated by two primary factors: 1) the presence or absence of defense physiology, and 2) positive or negative forces of internal and external electromagnetic fields. He believes that both of these factors influence the development of the embryo and fetus from the very beginning.

> If the mother of an unborn child is in defense physiology brought about by emotional or nutritional stress [or stress due to EMR effects just mentioned], the development of the child is affected. Likewise, if the internal and external electromagnetic fields of the mother are disrupted by negative thoughts, attitudes, and emotions, the development of the unborn child is affected...thoughts are the strongest single influence on health. Thoughts "make or break" the stability of an individual's personal electromagnetic field. When a pregnant woman's field is disrupted, the field controlling the development of cells, tissue, organs, and systems of her unborn child is also disrupted. When the energy projected by the mother (or any other individual) into her field resonates in harmony with that field and the universal field, health is mandated."[33]

Conceiving Peace

Though we optimize our animals through conscientious physical preparation before breeding, it may be that we will realize the highest potential available to us as humans only when we include in our pre-conception preparation that most unique, human intelligence, *the power of imagination*. In the realm of imagination, we hold the reins, we can decide, we are free. And at no other moment of human development is that freedom more potent or palpable than at conception. To willingly welcome Life's plans for another being on earth is a momentous choice.

The opportunity at conception can be compared to throwing a pebble into a lake: the freedom to determine its path and destination is virtually unlimited up until the moment it leaves your hand—when it settles to leave its infinite crown of ripples on the lake. Conception sets a point of departure and a trajectory for the pathway of becoming. What would happen if we conceived our babies with the same vital, generative intentionality we bring to so many other projects that we deeply believe in? Might we unfold a whole new unimagined realm of evolutionary promise for our global human family?

The idea of bringing consciousness, awareness, even reverence, to the act of sexual union may seem antithetical to passion, but it need not be so. No cumbersome rituals are needed—and are of use only if they that have true meaning for both partners. No sprinkling of rose petals, smudging with sage, or burning of incense required! Just the simple, and simply powerful, awareness that you are participating in the most important, auspicious and mysterious collaboration of all, the inviting of new life to grow—within your shared life and within the body of the mother.

Your pre-conception awareness and conception consciousness ideally takes whatever form that is meaningful to you, and can be as uncomplicated as this, from Laura Uplinger as published in *The Marriage of Sex and Spirit*:

> During the months leading to the conception of my child, I was aware that my body was to become a vessel for the making of a new human body. My husband and I sent out a call to the universe—as if posting an ad on a galactic website—stating who we were and what we could offer to a soul who wished to join us. We carried on our daily activities in a mood of solemn expectation and profound surrender: was a soul going to be drawn to us?

On a clear May morning when the air was full of the scent of spring blossoms, we welcomed the soul of our child as we conceived. "Dear One," I recall saying inwardly, "if we are conceiving your physical body this morning, may you have a vast and luminous life."[34]

———— **PRINCIPLES TO PRACTICE** ————

Presence – As you practice this principle in your daily life, you will reveal new dimensions of your own being. Through practicing presence you become imbued with the impressive *quality* of presence—described with such terms as charisma, poise, self-assurance, self-confidence, and a certain force of personality. As in, "what a presence she has." Remember Aristotle's promise— "we are what we repeatedly do." So presence becomes not just *how* you are, but *who* you are. This reinforces its status as Peace Parenting Principle #1, since the latest interpersonal neurobiology research attests to the fact that who we are is of even more far-reaching significance to our children's wellbeing and success than the specific words we say or parenting techniques we employ.

- One of the qualities of presence is the ability to be here now—the willingness to say an inner "Yes" to whatever Life has brought us, wherever Life has taken us. This could be for an instant, an hour, a month or a lifetime. In a moment in which you're feeling annoyed, impatient, dissatisfied, take a deep breath and see if you can find that space of grace in which there is a shift toward acceptance of the moment just as it is—a surrender to what is—and the tranquility that can come with that.
- Treat yourself to periods of silence. Our lives are so filled with wall-to-wall sound that we can become noisy inside, less able to hear the subtle callings of our inner knowing—our intuition. As a couple, spend some time in silent presence together. It is especially in communion with your beloved that you can experience the relief of conscious silence (which might at first not feel like relief, but awkwardly unfamiliar). Let the silent space between and around you fill up with the potency of your feelings for one another in that moment, be they tender, passionate, loving—or maybe a mixture of those along with "negative" feelings such as disappointment, annoyance. Silence is like water—so soft and yet such a potent force for eroding off life's and love's rough edges.

- Let each of you, together or separately, devote time to consciously be present to vivid thoughts of those qualities you admire and love in your partner, particularly in the light of your coming parenting adventure together. Begin making an imaginary home video of you parenting together, seeing him or her in action with your child engaging those aspects you so adore. Focus on and steep yourself in the feelings that arise in you as you envision your future life.

- Allow yourself to be present to the history of the womb you're inviting life into, including past reproductive health issues, painful periods, and especially any abortions, miscarriages or stillbirths. Just as you might clear the energy and bless a new home before moving in, consider tending in this way to your womb, and your heart, if there is grief or loss there. The detailed ceremony suggested in Niravi Payne's book *The Whole Person Fertility Program* can guide you, or give you ideas for creating your own process for clearing and blessing the womb.

- Continue the process of getting present with your past—for instance, engaging in the "Inside Out Exercises" in Siegel and Hartzell's *Parenting from the Inside Out.*

Awareness – You are inviting Life to multiply you. Engaging in an ongoing exploration of who indeed you are is your most important preparation—a fact corroborated in the subtitle of Siegel and Hartzell's book: *How A Deeper Self-Understanding Can Help You Raise Children Who Thrive.*

- With your partner, contemplate such questions as *What do we have to offer a child who will come to us? Which of our talents, aptitudes, and qualities will the child be attracted to? What should we enhance within ourselves in order to welcome our child?* This will pay dividends once your child is here, wanting more than anything to know who you are.

- Continue to investigate the sometimes shy, tangled roots of your feelings, beliefs and attitudes about love, family, and the big questions of what makes a fulfilling life. If you find that some preprogramming from your early life doesn't harmonize well with your conscious values and vision, consider the healing approach of Emotional Freedom Technique (EFT), whose guidelines are free to all, and which has trained practitioners all over the world. It is powerful, transformational and very effective in a short period of time.

- Notice the multiplicity and profusion of life around you. Colors, lights, plants, people, clouds, breezes, animals, soils and stones, all weave their energetic tapestry in which you live, love, and evolve. Ponder on this, let it inspire you. Bring a bit of it into your home as a reminder that, as theologian John Cobb puts it, "The power of life is not limited to clearly living things, and we may think of life as exerting its gentle pressure everywhere, encouraging each thing to become more than it is."[35]

- As part of cultivating fluency with our inner lives, it is helpful to enrich the vocabulary with which we understand and express our feelings and our needs. The Center for Nonviolent Communication's website offers an inventory list of feelings and needs to help us expand our awareness of these important aspects of our inner life. You are your children's first teachers of the language of relationship; the quality and tone of your communications together becomes their lifelong template.

Rhythm – Some of the most fundamental rhythms in our bodies are found in the cyclic processes devoted to reproduction. Men have the multiple ongoing cycles of continuous sperm production together with the four to six weeks it takes for the new sperm to mature. Women, whose cycles get far more (bad) press, have the noticeably rhythmic experience when, every month, one ovum matures in the ovaries and is released to its voyage down a fallopian tube and onward into the uterus, whose nutrient-rich lining is shed as her period if conception doesn't take place. This intricate series of events is controlled by various hormones whose fluctuating levels have taken the blame for mood swings.

- Take a few moments to give some thought to the automatic processes taking place rhythmically within you, such as respiration, heartbeat and digestion. (In Chinese medicine, for example, each organ has its own two-hour period of peak energy; many have discovered this for themselves when their liver activity—which peaks at three a.m.—awakens them after an evening of overindulgence!) For men, consider your impressively abundant sperm production and the ongoing rhythm of their maturing cycles. For women, find a way that works for you—journal, notes on a calendar or on your chosen electronic data device—to tune into, observe and chart signs of ebbing and flowing fertile periods during your cycle.
- Enlist the greatest energy there is in your conception preparation: when you can, greet the first rays of the sun—the conception of the day. (In Portuguese *sunrise* translates as "birth of the sun.") Depending on where you live (please avoid frostbite!), to go out barefoot in the morning, to feel the morning dew, to bask in the early morning sun, can be fabulously enlivening. It is said that this is the time when the cosmos offers us the most *prana*. A sunny dawn

symbolizes a beginning, a start, and you can ask nature to awaken in you the rhythms of receiving light and life.

- Tune into the various rhythms that envelope you—day to night, sunrise and sunset, tides, the rotation of the seasons—and take note of which aspects you're drawn to more strongly. Taking a cue from Waldorf education's nature table can be helpful; choose a small spot in your home where you gather a few beautiful objects that evoke and express the current season. Through your own affinities, you may be getting a sense of when your child wants to come. Consider, for example, will you conceive at dawn, at noon or at midnight? One mother I know came to realize she had to conceive in spring. One thing to keep in mind is that as with all beginnings—as with planting seeds, launching key projects, signing important contracts and throwing successful events—it is advisable to conceive during a waxing moon (which affects the biological distribution of water in our bodies, making for optimal conditions for growth).

Example – Learning by consciously seeking out worthy examples prepares us for the role we are stepping into *as* worthy examples. There is a dynamism in both following examples and being an example, through which the growth cultivated by each feeds into the other—an enriching feedback loop.

- Find an example in nature of vitality and fertility—a plant, a pond, a bird or other animal—and apprentice with it!
- Choose images to put on your wall that embody life, fertility, and beauty.
- As you engage in attuned conception you set a profound lifelong example of consciousness for your child, with the imprint of an organizing principle that continues to reimprint over and over, like launching a fractal* wave that continues to flow throughout development. This opens an avenue of cohesion from the very beginning, woven into the very fiber of the child, drawing him or her toward a path of consciousness and attunement later on in life.

Nurturance – Parenting is all about nurturing and ways of showing love. There are many ways to let nurturance preside over the very initiation of your child's physical life.

---

* Fractals are self-similar patterns that repeat themselves throughout every level of growth and organization in the natural world; patterns expressed in lower tiers of development help organize, and are reexpressed in, subsequent tiers.

- Cultivating discernment in choosing products will be an important form of nurturance as you parent. You might begin by looking at the ingredient labels in the soaps, lotions and moisturizers you are using to nurture your skin, ensuring there are no toxins such as parabens, propylene glycol, parahydroxybenzoic acid, DEA, ethylene oxide, which typically appear in many conventional cosmetic products. Also pay attention to packaging; new research shows that prenatal exposure to bisphenol A (BPA)—found in polycarbonate plastic and in the coating of most food and beverage cans—was associated with more anxious, depressed behavior and poorer motor control and inhibition in children at age three.[36]

- Let your gestures, even when nobody's watching, generate connection to whatever it is you are engaged with—a pet, a pear, a skillet, a room, a car. Let your voice, your gaze, your touch be nurturance for whatever is in your company. Eventually, when this becomes second nature for you, your child will absorb, emulate, and carry out into the world this second-nature nurturance!

- Jeannine Parvati Baker believed that the "lack of attention to the care and maintaining of this planet is sharply reflected in the way we have ignored the messages from our own bodies." Womb ecology, world ecology. One way to nurture Mother Earth while tuning in to your body is to return your monthly flow to the earth, which—as weird as it sounds to us modern gals—isn't that hard and is surprisingly satisfying. I used to drop my organic cotton tampon into a cup or so of warm water in a pitcher dedicated to this purpose… let it soak awhile… then squeeze it out completely into the water. This elixir was an awesome fertilizer for my roses! But more importantly, points out Jeannine, it's a good way to get in touch with your period. As she wrote, "Handling your … blood helps to discharge lots of our self-disgust, so inculcated by media, myths and poor health. …Blood will cease to 'freak you out.'" This is earthy nurturance that brings blessings in perpetuity.

- As noted above, there are no dictates or prescriptions for attuned conception, but to be present and compose with the forces that surround you in the moment. The only real requirement is to have love in the embrace; I would also invite you to see the divine in each other—the God in him, the Goddess in her. An initiatic principle relevant to conceiving Generation Peace asks you to consecrate your act of love to something vaster than your own physical pleasure—to an ideal (raising a peaceful generation!), or to the uplifting of those who don't know this joy. This gives intercourse a completely different tone of meaning; as one friend says, "It then becomes food for the angels."

- While there are few prescriptions, there are a few proscriptions: avoid conceiving during times of electromagnetic disturbance, such as during very windy weather, or when there are many clouds; and during the waning moon. (For example, wood that is chopped during a waning moon is more prone to rot than that cut in a waxing moon; there are many ways of respecting and working with Nature, which is what I'm proposing throughout this book.)
- It is also best, when you're seeking attuned conception, to not make love intoxicated.
- If statistics were available on this, we'd see that it is very common for conception to take place during breakup sex, make-up sex, angry sex, or even violent sex, for reasons having to do with our biochemical programming. For evolutionary, species-survival reasons, the hormonal turmoil that attends these high-arousal emotional states—especially anger and fear—can help facilitate fertilization.[37] (This is also why apprehensive first sexual experiences disproportionately often result in pregnancy.) With Generation Peace intentions at heart, it is best to wait until such a stormy moment has passed and you have regained emotional equilibrium as a couple before conceiving your child, so as not to include such a hormonal upheaval as part of his or her beginnings.

Trust – Trust is a miraculous antianxiety potion, a powerful antidote to the stream of messages from our consumerist culture that seductively whisper to us that we're not quite enough—but that something we can purchase will make up for our lack.

- Befriend the unknown, the process, the miracle, and, as the *Desiderata* mentions, remember that you both are children of the universe. Lean into the great mystery and let it embrace and strengthen you.
- To inspire you as you cultivate this principle of trust, take in the words of poet Kahlil Gibran from his classic book *The Prophet:* "Your children are not your children. They are the sons and daughters of Life's longing for itself." Recognizing that you are a collaborator with Life, detaching a bit from the intensely personalized notion of *our* children, can help refresh the atmosphere surrounding conception with a more expansive perspective and the comfort of knowing you are not on your own!
- Each step of trust is a call to practice surrender. Befriend the forces at work in you and with you as you attune to the mysteries of conception.
- When couples are trying anxiously to conceive I share what I've learned from working with couples anxiously awaiting an adoption placement: the trans-

formation, the tranquility, and confidence that emerges when prospective parents are able to shift from a self-focused orientation (*How soon can we get a baby?*) to a baby-focused orientation (*I wonder when a baby will need us as parents?*).

Simplicity – This principle works hand in hand with trust, each reinforcing the other: it is easier to embrace simplicity once you have tapped into a well of trust, and the joy found in simplicity nourishes trust. It's one of the most enlivening feedback loops you can get going, like a blessed boomerang of serenity! By contrast, without trust it is almost impossible to release ourselves from the 4G grip of our culture's incessant "new, improved, faster, mightier, flashier" siren call. Then the locus of engagement shifts from inner to outer, from process to product, from people to things (i.e., we find ourselves slipping back into the grip of an industrialist worldview). But we can always begin again, find our center—a new center, in which, paradoxically, we are always enough even while we continually strive upward. To even think of having a baby is humbling, and there is immense freedom and relief in embracing that we are simply who we are, ready to join forces with Life as our partner in composing our children.

- The question of finances has perennially been on the minds of people as they contemplate beginning a family—frequently as a source of worry. Certainly the economic climate in which I'm writing this book is one of the most challenging of our modern history. The riches needed by a child for her healthiest development don't rely upon great or even moderate wealth; there are many budgets that will accommodate an excellent experience of parenting. Honest conversations about your priorities and your intentions toward simplicity, combined with research about financial realities and alternatives, are an important aspect of this stage of preparenting.
  - The upside of simplifying in this economic climate is that it's in style! And, there are currently lots of information sources for ways to stretch your money so that your principles and not your stuff are the centerpiece of life. Author Jeff Yeager found that so-called cheapskates regret only about 10 percent of their purchases—compared with 80 percent for a typical American. The idea that less stuff can provide more contentment is one of simplicity's delicious gifts. Yeager's books, as well as *10,001 Ways to Live Large on a Small Budget*, are just two of the resources on this subject.

- A colleague attending a conference of the International Society for Prenatal and Perinatal Medicine in 1991 in Krakow heard a presentation by a Scottish doctor renowned for his IVF clinic. He laid out his research, discussed his practice, described the details of the various IVF protocols. He then reported the rates of success, which featured an astonishing finding: *the pregnancy rates of the IVF patients were identical to the pregnancy rates of those couples who were waiting to enroll in his IVF program!* The simple, reassuring knowledge that they were soon to be helped by this remarkable doctor may well have adjusted their biochemistry toward the growth mode that tends to accompany the perception that "All is well." So do remember to often remind yourself—sometimes in seeming contrast to all outward appearances—that "All is, and will be, well."

- Zen tradition sees that suffering comes from the state of *grasping,* and paradoxically also from the aversion to grasping (i.e., a grasping at the cessation of grasping—still with me?)—and so we might see the Zen concept *detachment* as the principle of simplicity as applied to the inner life. Detachment is not the same as indifference; with detachment we do what we do with care and engagement, but without worrying about the results, which in our humility we recognize are out of our hands. Strive for this inner simplicity of detachment as you attune to conception, surrendering to *what is,* at each moment of the adventure. Josephine and her husband pursued conception for many months, months that turned into years. All the while Josephine strived to practice detachment. As she put it, "Wanting a child is all about wanting to express love. There is nothing I imagined more frequently and more vividly than holding a baby to my heart with his head resting on my shoulder. Once I fully settled into the awareness that love is always there ready to be expressed in any relationship regardless of the age, gender or blood ties of the person in front of you, how could I continue focusing on who was not there, on what was lacking? I allowed myself to cherish that image, all the while surrendering to whether or not it would materialize, and trusting that all was well and in perfect order."

Resources

Verny, Thomas, and John Kelly. *The Secret Life of the Unborn Child.* New York: Delta, 1982.

Chamberlain, David. "When Does Parenting Begin? An Introduction." Association for Prenatal & Perinatal Psychology and Health, birthpsychology.com/free-article/when-does-parenting-begin-introduction.

McCarty, Wendy. *Welcoming Consciousness: Supporting Babies' Wholeness from the Beginning of Life.* Santa Barbara, CA: Wondrous Beginnings Press, 2009.

Aïvanhov, O. M. (1990). *Education Begins Before Birth.* Frejus, France: Prosveta.

Association for Prenatal & Perinatal Psychology and Health: www.birthpsychology.com.

Primal health essays by Michel Odent: www.wombecology.com/index.html.

Healthy Child Healthy World – Empowering parents to protect children from harmful chemicals, from before conception onward: www.healthychild.org.

Masaru Emoto's work with water crystals: www.masaru-emoto.net/english/ephoto.html.

Masaru Emoto's current applications toward peace: www.geocities.jp/emotoproject/english/home.html.

Life's Greatest Miracle (Nova video): www.pbs.org/wgbh/nova/miracle/program.html.

Information on vegetarian sources of omega fats: goodfats.pamrotella.com.

Rebuild from Depression: www.rebuild-from-depression.com/blog/depression_food_and_nutrients.

Cell phone radiation research and resources from Dr. Mercola: products.mercola.com/blue-tube-headset.

Emotional Freedom Technique: www.eftuniverse.com.

Center for Non-Violent Communication's Feelings Inventory List: www.cnvc.org/Training/feelings-inventory

and Needs Inventory List: www.cnvc.org/Training/needs-inventory

Waldorf nature table description: www.naturalfamilycrafts.com/2007/06/what-is-nature-table.html.

Step Three

RADIANT PREGNANCY—
HARNESSING THE POWER
OF THE WOMB

We can't build the future for our youth, but we can build the youth for our future.

FRANKLIN D. ROOSEVELT

We can no longer afford to consider pregnancy a nine-month grace period before parenting begins. On the contrary, pregnancy is like Nature's Secret Head Start Program for your baby! When a woman is pregnant, her baby's organs and tissues develop in direct response to grow-or-protect lessons they receive about the world—lessons that come from Mom's diet, her behavior and her state of mind. Mounting evidence tells us that circumstances in the womb program us in critical, life-altering ways. The prenatal environment is equally as important as genes, perhaps even more important, in determining lifelong physical and mental health.[1] U.C. Berkeley professor of integrative biology Marian Diamond cautions, "If we're putting millions of dollars into Head Start, which begins at three, four, or five years of age, and haven't developed the appropriate brain to receive that education, it will be a waste of money. It is important to be sure that the brain has developed well *in utero*. So when you start with formal education, you have the nerve cells and the dendrites that can respond."[2] And brand new research suggests that attention to health factors during prenatal development may prevent childhood aggression, teenage delinquency, and violence in adulthood.[3]

Prenatal parenting empowers you with the ability to make conscious choices to equip your child with the fundamental capacities required for experiencing abundant peace within and promoting innovative peace without, throughout the many years of his or her life.

The Wonder of Embryonic Development

As in the first two weeks of embryonic development described in Step Two, over the next six weeks the embryo takes shape during a series of processes whose innate intelligence and unfathomable intricacy cannot help but inspire awe.* The differentiated strands of cells that will form both the placenta and the embryo continue to pursue their individual paths of growth. (While it is the embryo we usually focus upon, the importance of the placenta's healthy, robust development is paramount. The quality of the mother's diet, metabolism, circulation, and psychological wellbeing help determine the integrity of the baby's development.)

An astonishing intelligence within the organism directs the cells to specialize themselves to become future bones or liver or heart or brain, all while the embryo still looks, at the beginning of week three, like a featureless little trilayer disc—a bit like one of those tiny round batteries, with a diameter about the size of the thickness of a quarter. During weeks three through eight following conception all of the baby's different organs develop, materializing from stem cells that began as identical.

Recall the effects of positive versus negative mental states, thoughts and words upon the health of Bernard Grad's plants or the structure of Masaru

---

* In this book I use an embryology calendar, which begins at conception and makes gestation a roughly thirty-eight week process, as contrasted with the obstetrical calendar, which pronounces a woman pregnant as of the first day of her last menstrual period and considers pregnancy a forty-week affair. Since this is what your caregiver will likely use, simply subtract fourteen days (two weeks) to align with the embryological timeline.

Emoto's crystalline water droplets, and the research mentioned last chapter regarding the higher risk of neonatal death in unplanned pregnancies. Now is when the inner atmosphere cultivated prior to conception—marked by joy, gratitude and a calm surrender to the tide of Life—serves to foster progrowth development in the embryo at one of the most critical stages he or she will ever pass through.

Instructions for Growing

This period of organogenesis (making of the organs) is the time when the developing baby is most vulnerable to teratogens—the wide range of substances that can cause malformations. (One theory is that pregnancy sickness, which peaks over these weeks of organ formation, is an evolutionarily adaptive mechanism that protects the embryo from everpresent toxins in plants as well as the pathogens and parasites in spoiled animal products.[4] It tends to restrict the mother's caloric intake in the first trimester, which also serves to encourage more breadth in the growth of the placenta—an auspicious factor pertaining to the term delivery of a strong and healthy baby.

Think of a teratogen as noise on the channel that finds its way into the information pipeline to corrupt the flow of instructions directing the embryo's growth. Teratogens do their damage by disrupting any of the countless minutely intricate events taking place to unfold the new human during these weeks of organ formation. One such sophisticated maneuver is *programmed cell death* (also called *aptosis*) whereby certain cells know to self-destruct to help shape the human form, as when the webbing between the fingers and toes gets trimmed away. Another barely fathomable dance is performed by primitive brain cells: they stack themselves to form *cortical ladders* up which freshly minted neural cells climb to reach their level, exit the ladder, and migrate to their assigned space in the forming brain. It is thought that when something disrupts this process—a teratogen—cells may get stuck on the ladder, blocking the way for new climbers, resulting in developmental abnormalities. It is strongly suspected that disruptions in this laddering process are involved in schizophrenia, dyslexia and certain kinds of personality disorders.[5]

It's important to realize that our scientific knowledge about teratogens is in its infancy, and the mechanisms at work in teratogenic effects on the embryo and fetus are not well understood. What is even less understood—yet strongly suggested by significant bodymind research—is how much protection might be conferred by a mother's unrelenting intention to cultivate a state of appreciation and joyful expectation during this time when she is a vessel of creation for her baby.

The list of known teratogens is long and accessible on many websites, but in general they include: many prescription and nonprescription drugs; viruses such as influenza, measles, and herpes; recreational drugs like cocaine, meth and heroin; environmental toxins such as pesticides, solvents, radiation and lead, mercury and other heavy metals; caffeine; cigarettes; alcohol. The two most everpresent and studied of threats to fetal development are cigarette smoking[6] and alcohol,[7] which compete in the experts' opinion for the distinction of being the most serious threat to an embryo or fetus.

Possibly the most damaging of all teratogenic influences is the combination of prenatal alcohol exposure in conjunction with maternal stress, particularly when it occurs early in the pregnancy.[8] It is clear that stress, a potent teratogen by itself, can also be a powerful amplifier of other harmful influences. The effects of smoking, alcohol, and stress that are of greatest concern to parenting for peace are those that play the greatest role in predisposing the individual for later violent behavior and diminished creative, flexible thinking, thereby sabotaging the spectrum of brain-based capacities needed in a generation who might see us skillfully and joyfully into a flourishing future.

Risk in the Mirror: Teratogens in the New Age

It wasn't long ago that the list of teratogens was pretty straightforward: the spectrum of outside agents listed above. But nowadays teratogenic properties are turning up in the midst of our most everyday, mundane, popularly unsuspected experiences. In the "old age" of our understanding of teratogens, the distinctions between what was safe and what wasn't safe (to the extent that we knew at the time) were clear: *If I stay away from smoking, drinking, drugs, cat feces, caffeine, German measles, peeling leaded paint, and chemicals of all kinds, it'll be okay.* In our current era, we're finally understanding that some of the most potent dangers to (and opportunities for) our fetuses aren't Out There, they're In Here, they are in us, they are *what we do, feel and think* or *do not do, feel and think.* To quote the beloved, satirical comic figure Pogo, "We have seen the enemy, and it is us."

Perhaps the most pervasive, insidious of all teratogens is stress. Stress has become almost like white noise: it's so everpresent as a concept and experience in our lives that we don't give it much thought. The very word itself is so small and unimpressive. It doesn't even sound scary, like *carcinogen* or *polychlorinated biphenyl* (PCB). But cortisol, the primary hormone produced when we are stressed out, is a highly potent neurotoxin—meaning, it kills brain cells. And in consistently high amounts during pregnancy, it wreaks havoc with a staggering array of developing structures and systems in the embryo and fetus.[9]

Hans Selye's landmark 1976 work, *The Stress of Life,* put stress on the map—named it for the first time, and offered a most elegant definition, "the non-specific response of the body to any demand." In the final pages of the book, he challenges future researchers to extend what he had begun with his revolutionary findings. His words could not have been more eerily predictive of what later researchers would learn about the effects of maternal stress on fetal development: "Such defensive measures as the production of adaptive hormones by glands are built into the very texture of the body; we inherited them from our parents and transmit them to our children, who, in turn, must hand them on to their offspring, as long as the human race shall exist."[10]

Belief in this principle goes back to ancient times: Empedocles (480 BC) said that an embryo's development could be guided and interfered with by the mental state of the mother; and Caraka, an Indian embryologist, wrote before 1000 BC that psychological factors in the mother may cause mental disturbance in the fetus. The Chinese have long recognized the mother's influence on the fetus, and in their history have had prenatal clinics established to keep the mother tranquil and to maintain the psychological health of the fetus.[11] Let's look at the basic mechanism at work behind the extraordinary and unprecedented opportunities we have to raise a generation of peacemakers.

My Mother's Psyche, My Self's Psyche

Science now recognizes that physiological and psychological health are intimately entwined, each one supporting and reinforcing the optimal expression of the other. Indeed, there is far more to an individual than his or her physical body, and along with lifelong physical health, the personality begins to be organized during fetal development.

This concurs with findings from the field of prenatal and perinatal psychology, which have long suggested that circumstances surrounding conception, pregnancy, labor, birth and the postpartum period have profound influences on lifelong mental and emotional wellbeing.[12] There are countless fascinating case histories in the literature to support the connection between experiences *in utero* and certain affinities, compulsions, behavioral patterns, fears and fascinations in later life. Most such stories on record are ones demonstrating the negative possibilities of prenatal influence, since they come to light when the person is in crisis, and therapists become involved.

The field of prenatal and perinatal psychology indeed grew its roots in psychoanalytic and psychotherapeutic clinical research, when over a hundred years of patient reports of memory traces from birth and before finally could not be ignored; further, when the memories were addressed and processed, patients' symptoms resolved.[13] The primal,* bodymind memory processes described in the last step govern the impact various prenatal milestones can have on the developing being. If you are a child who is planned, the *discovery* phase, when your mother learns she is pregnant, is a time of great welcome, a celebration of your existence, an affirmation that you belong and that your presence brings joy. Many in prenatal psychology see a mother's reaction upon discovering her pregnancy as the first and possibly most significant marker for the child's future self-esteem. This is when you learn that you are welcomed, you are received, you are affirmed, or not. If you were not planned, and aren't a "happy mistake," discovery is when your existence becomes a Big Problem. This is when you may first feel unseen, overlooked, unacknowledged. Now is the time when a mother's feelings of anger, blame, fear and, sometimes, even thoughts of abortion, can lay a foundation of existential rejection and terror in the developing child.[14]

For example, there was an interesting, small study of suicidal young men that found that their suicide attempts were taking place at the same time of the year as when their mothers had tried to abort them. None of the adolescents had been told or consciously knew of their mothers' attempted abortions, which were verified by the mothers when later interviewed.[15]

But then there are the delightful accounts of enduring prenatal influence, like that of Canadian symphony conductor Boris Brott, who in a radio interview years ago related a story from early in his career. He was puzzled over the fact that he simply "knew" certain new pieces of music, every note and tempo—that the cello line in particular would just "jump out at him," and

---

* Different writers define *primal* in different ways; I consider it to apply to that period of a person's life that precedes their fluency with language—prenatal to about age three.

he could tell where the piece was going before turning the page of the score. He mentioned it to his mother, figuring as a professional cellist she would be intrigued. She was. But when he told her with which music he'd had this odd sense of precognition, the mystery was solved: they were all pieces she had played during the season when she was pregnant with him.[16]

One reason we have precious few success stories of prenatal influence, and so many bleak ones, is, again, that our evolutionarily mandated memory processing apparatus is designed first and foremost for survival: beginning in the womb and continuing during our early years in the world, it is primarily *negative* experiences, ones that are highly emotionally charged, that indelibly mark us in ways so lasting that those memories will keep us alive when the danger returns. For the toddler this may be a hissing snake or a growling dog: his imprint of fear will help him remember to avoid those things. For the fetus, such an imprint occurs when the "interchange of satisfactory maternal-fetal emotion, so reliably good as to be scarcely noticed, is interrupted by the influx of maternal distress," wrote British physician and prenatal researcher Frank Lake.[17] Psychiatrist Thomas Verny in his landmark book *The Secret Life of the Unborn Child* vividly describes what the prenatal baby learns, and how she is changed, when "successive hormonal jolts" perturb the dynamic harmony that is the optimal state of the womb.

We have little research thus far about the effects of extremely *good* prenatal experiences as mediated by the mother (such as spiritual ecstasy, living in conscious bliss, regular meditation, etc.), other than anecdotal reports from those who are disinclined to do scientific research about a process they simply live—such as the handful of deeply spiritual parents Joseph Chilton Pearce talks about in his lectures, while showing photographs of their peaceful, precocious children whose prefrontal brain structures are so robustly developed it is obvious to even an untrained observer gazing at their impressively expanded foreheads.[18]

Indeed, we don't have any randomized double-blind studies of the effects of a pregnant mother's joy on growth and wellbeing of her fetus, why? The wisp of cynic in me says for the same reason we have so few studies on how to lower your blood pressure or cholesterol through natural means: joy cannot be trademarked, patented or sold. But the reason is probably not quite so bleakly mercenary. Science as a discipline is only just beginning, tentatively, to mature toward the depths plumbed by literature, music or art. Writes physician and primal health researcher Michel Odent about his fellow scientists:

We have to overcome a major obstacle: although many emotional states have been studied in a scientific way by physiologists, psychologists, epidemiologists and other scientists, the concept of joy has not. Explore scientific and medical databases: the keywords "anxiety," "stress," "depression," "psychological distress" or "fear" bring up thousands of references. "Joy," on the other hand, remains as a sterile keyword.

Today scientists do not hesitate to penetrate the realm of poets and other artists. All sorts of emotional states, including love and the connections to the sacred, have already been "scientified." One day the concept of joy will be studied with scientific methods. One day the function of joy in pregnancy will appear as a serious topic. Meanwhile, we can indirectly study joy in pregnancy by looking at the opposite pole of the emotional spectrum.

High levels of cortisol have been found in states of chronic anxiety, depression, bereavement, chronic stress, and "maternal psychological distress in pregnancy." In daily, simplified language, we can claim that whatever facet of unhappiness one considers, the level of cortisol is high. It is well understood today that cortisol is an inhibitor of fetal growth, particularly of brain development.[19]

The S Word

The brain development needed to equip an individual with the kinds of capacities fundamental to peace and prosperity—self-regulation, creative innovation, mental flexibility, robust will—does indeed begin during pregnancy, and it isn't just diet and lifestyle choices that influence it. A pregnant woman's thoughts and moods have a significant impact upon the brain development of her baby in the womb. While I'm confident that scientists will soon "prove" what so many wisdom traditions and cultures have long known about the role of *joy* in optimally prenatal development, what we do now know for sure is that a pregnant mother's chronic *stress* has enduring negative effects upon the developing fetal brain.

Fetal (and infant) exposure to maternal cortisol—when it is chronic and unremitting as opposed to the occasional doses that are part of normal life and development—can reroute the trajectory of an individual's development in devastating, though often subtle and not immediately recognizable, ways.

I've become such a proponent of lighting candles rather than cursing the darkness, it pains me to catalog the truly staggering series of developmental derangements that can be caused by significant maternal stress during pregnancy. So here is the bleak litany to throw you back in your chair—and then I'll discuss some of these in more detail: altered gene regulation and expression; altered cell migration leading to malformation of neural circuitry; destruction of synapses, particularly in the hippocampal and amygdala areas, affecting memory; impaired development of corpus callosum; impairment of sexualizing hormones, feminizing males and masculinizing females; inhibition of dendritic branching, reducing learning potential; reduced brain weight; diminishment and suppression of immune system; up- or down-regulated stress circuitry; diminishment of oxytocin circuitry and increase of vasopressin circuitry; reduced brain size.

A pregnant mother's chronic stress is associated with prolonged fetal heart rate disturbances and is a strong predictor of low birth weight, prematurity, and "irritable" infant temperament[20]—which itself is an entire constellation of neurophysiological and psychological hypersensitivities; these in turn predispose the growing child to more anger, frustration and interpersonal conflicts, which bodymind research tells us means more risk of a number of chronic degenerative health conditions over the lifespan. Low birth weight and prolonged fetal heart rate reactions are associated with later heart disease,[21] and major stress midway through pregnancy has been associated with a higher autism risk.[22]

Let's all take a nice, cleansing breath at this point, and turn the dial out to a bigger picture of all this, a metaview that more constructively relates to our intentions for raising joyful, peace-oriented individuals. Hang in there with me, because understanding what's really at work here is a) pretty simple, and b) quite empowering.

When a baby in the womb is continually exposed to maternal cortisol (the major stress hormone), he expresses his distress with an accelerated fetal heartbeat and hyperactivity, while his developing brain's set points for the ability to effectively manage stress are permanently being down-regulated: the hormonal feedback system designed to keep his experience of stress within normal levels is damped, leading to lifelong hypersensitivity to what would normally be benign stimuli.[23] Along with this hypersensitivity to minor environmental stimuli that is hardwired into the baby's brain by prenatal stress, there is also impairment of the baby's (calming) opioid system;[24] in other words, the brain-based ability to experience pleasure and contentment, or what Peter Kramer calls "hedonic capacity," is corrupted.

So not only is he going to be more prone to experiencing the environment as stressful, but he will get little relief from the action of the brain's pleasure axis, which would normally help mediate the effects of stress by engendering feelings of satisfaction, reward, and contentment. This person loses wellbeing from both ends, so to speak—feeling hammered by distressing stimuli while never quite able to feel much at ease or gratified. No wonder it is suspected that the down-regulation of these fundamental neurochemical receptors is present in depression and other mood disorders. Also of central importance to raising Generation Peace is that this reduction of opiate receptors during fetal development is associated with lifetime changes that include increased aggression, lower cognitive performance and decreased exploratory behavior—all of which equals a protection-rather-than-growth profile that is not consistent with the innovation, ingenuity and empathic interpersonal capacities needed by a peacemaker.

(Interestingly, chronic stress during pregnancy also has a negative impact on the mother's own opiate system; it disables the mother's natural internal pain-relieving capacities that are needed during labor, greatly increasing the likelihood of anesthesia use.[25])

You see, Nature in her wisdom has decreed that while we're in the womb, our brain develops in direct response to our mother's experience of the world. If a pregnant mother's thoughts and emotions are *persistently* negative, if she is under *unrelenting* stress, the internal message—delivered to the developing baby—is, "It's a dangerous world out there," regardless of whether or not this is objectively true. The baby's neural cells and nervous system development will actually mutate (adapt) to prepare for the unsafe environment it perceives it is going to be born into.

Chronic stress in pregnancy tends to sculpt a brain suited to survive in dangerous environments: short of attention, quick to react, with reduced impulse control, with a dampened capacity to feel calm and content. This makes for a temperamental baby, difficult to soothe, a baby who is challenging to parent—and thus the seeds can be sown this early for parents and child to get stuck in a sad but common vicious cycle: dealing with the baby is frustrating for Mom and Dad. This generates a spectrum of strong feelings within them, which further activates the baby's heightened antennae for threat, makes him even more agitated, and may distance exhausted, exasperated parents from their baby. With no positive interruption of this negative feedback loop, the child has limited opportunity to internalize the self-regulating capacities developed through the intimate, engaged, face-to-face and skin-to-skin contact that fosters healthy development of the social brain. Once the toddler is considered "a handful," there are likely to be consequences to make the child mind, punishments whose shame basis further thwarts peace-oriented brain development, hardwiring it instead to thrive in a threatening world. Later, the child's impulsivity gets labeled, and his sense of alienation—from himself, from others, from Life—grows. And it is in the womb that this insidiously downward-spiraling cycle so often begins.

One primary piece of fetal learning involves the maternal heartbeat: development of key brain centers organizes around the drumbeat of the mother's heart.[26] If she is generally centered and peaceful—feeling connected, loved, happy to be pregnant—her heart will drum a rhythmic, regular beat. (Renowned child psychiatrist Bruce Perry tells us that this is why people across all cultures instinctively tend to rock a baby at roughly eighty beats per minute—the resting heart rate of a pregnant woman! The baby responds internally with a sense of, "Ah, I know that, that's familiar," and she settles down.) But if a pregnant mother is under constant stress, or besieged by persistent anxiety, her heartbeat will be dysrhythmic and irregular, and her baby's primitive brain structures imprint this heart-rate variability as their baseline state. Thus, there is no familiar, at-home rhythm with which to rock the baby, and he is far more likely to be born with what Perry calls a state-regulation problem: he's irritable, difficult to soothe, hard to engage. In turn, the parent can get frustrated and overwhelmed, and as Perry puts it, "Instead of having this smooth, synchronous interaction, you have kind of this bad fit. It leads to problems with normal social emotional development."[27] Frequently experienced stimuli become familiar, and familiar—even if it's negative—becomes comforting, so we gravitate to it. We all know people who feel at home with turmoil, and this is how early that affinity can begin!

It has been conclusively shown that chronic stress is a potent teratogen that corrupts prenatal development in myriad ways, via mechanisms that the researchers themselves admit they don't yet fully comprehend. But what about chronic joy? True, there have been no clinical trials, but research from such disciplines as psychoneuroimmunology, cell biology, positive psychology and epigenetics reveals that joy allows for optimal functioning of our organs and psyche; by simple logical extension, we can confidently hypothesize that joy during pregnancy allows for optimal development of each fetal organ. When the brain in particular develops optimally during gestation, this predisposes the baby—and her parents—to better self-regulation, attentiveness, responsiveness, and serenity. Such peace-oriented traits constitute the foundations of lifelong personality.

Nature's Elegant Survival Scheme

I have just described Nature's perfect adaptive system for keeping offspring alive in the animal kingdom: if a giraffe is pregnant during a particularly heavy lion season, for example, her calf will need two primary brain-based traits to remain alive: 1) the hyper-reactivity of an acutely sensitive stress response, to detect and respond to all of the predators stalking him, and 2) a hard-wired disinclination toward experiencing pleasure and relaxing to enjoy the finer things in life, such as calmly sunning in the warm grass, or sipping contentedly at the watering hole, lest he be caught unawares and end up as dinner on the savannah. The biochemicals produced by his mother's chronic stress during pregnancy, constantly fleeing all those lions, shapes his brain for those survival traits.

Makes sense, right? But we have a difficult time grasping the reasonability of this process at the human level. All of us (at least in the Western world, and definitely in the U.S.) are expected to be well-adjusted, productive—and certainly happy—citizens. But meanwhile, we conceive and carry our babies under conditions of frazzling twenty-first century stress and wonder why we have an epidemic of ADHD, depression and a host of other psychosocial ills plaguing our young people. While it is tempting to lay the blame on the advances of our technological wizardry and the resulting cacophony of information and interventions, we humans throughout history have always insisted on throwing monkey wrenches into Nature's exquisite plan— through our social structures, our laws, our religions, our mores and taboos, and yes, now our technologies as well.

The evolutionary process that helps organisms develop adaptations over time to their environment hasn't kept up with *homo sapiens'* warp speed thrust into the techno-info-cyber age: the human being's brain, nervous system and hormonal machinery have not yet evolved the automatic ability to distinguish the difference between a threat in the form of an upsetting Tweet (2012 AD) and a threat in the form of a charging mammoth (18,000 BC).

The stress system of the account executive—who happens to be seven months pregnant—who gets an electronic message alerting her that she is expected to make her presentation this afternoon despite the fact that her PowerPoint file just crashed, will experience activation of her fight, flight or freeze response just like that of the Stone Age woman fleeing a deadly animal. But the modern woman doesn't fight or flee, at least not physically; maybe she curses at the company's computer guy, or tries vainly, full of exasperation, to reschedule the meeting. (Some clinicians who work with trauma theorize that the act of fighting or running—or otherwise having the opportunity to act in a physical way to meet the threat—diffuses the destructive effects of a mobilization response that otherwise becomes essentially "frozen" in the nervous system.)[28] And meanwhile, she is unwittingly flooding her baby with the chemical message, "It's a dangerous world out here." And his brain is shaping itself to prepare him to survive in it. (Because I can feel the panic rising in my readers—*How do we avoid stress?!*—let me again mention that if this is a once-in-a-while occurrence, it is not something to worry unduly about—because for one thing, we don't need more worry! Chronic and consistent experience sculpts the baby's brain, not occasional events.)

Here, it seems, we see science and spirit intersecting: research from the field of neuroscience is now giving empirical credence to what many wisdom traditions have been saying through the ages—that during the time when we are being knit together in the womb, we are wired with lifelong lessons about the world and how we'll best fit into it: in peace mode, or in protection mode.

Sensitive Dependence on Initial Conditions, Part 2

While poring over old birth and death records in his native England, a mystery captured David Barker, an epidemiologist. (Epidemiology is the study of health and disease in populations.) He found that men who had lived their lives in the poorest cities were most likely to die of heart disease—which was puzzling, since it's considered a disease of affluence, usually associated with too much good living (food, drink, etc.) and too little exercise. Back then, men in poor cities worked hard physically and didn't eat rich food. The plot thickened when Barker realized something else: these poorer areas of England not only had higher rates of cardiovascular disease, they also had higher rates of infant mortality.

Barker's team developed a radical hypothesis to explain the paradox of poor men dying from a "rich man's disease": since infant mortality is an indication of negative circumstances affecting the fetus and infant, they suggested that babies who suffered nutritionally during fetal development were more prone to suffer from heart disease in later life. Their guess turned into a theory with huge Generation Peace implications—called "fetal origins."[29]

Basically, the mechanism goes like this: if a pregnant mother is poorly nourished, the availability of oxygen and essential nutrients to the fetus will be less than optimal. To protect the most important organ of the developing fetus, blood is diverted to the brain, leading to constrained growth in the blood vessel systems, liver, pancreas, and other tissues. One of Barker's telltale clues turned out to be the ratio of a newborn's abdominal measurement (girth) to its head circumference: many babies who made fetal adaptations to poor nutrition in the womb had a high head-to-abdominal-girth measurement ratio at birth, and this reduced abdominal girth turned out to have lifelong implications, including higher blood cholesterol decades later. (Reduced abdominal girth indicates a smaller liver, which plays a central role in regulating cholesterol.) A second marker for Barker was birth weight: the likelihood a man will die of heart disease, Barker found, is increased by over 50 percent if his birth weight was less than 5.5 pounds, compared with a man who weighed 9.5 pounds at birth. The third clue was the presence of a relatively large placenta in the presence of low birth weight; this disproportionate growth between the fetus and placenta is a telltale sign of adverse conditions during pregnancy—such as impaired availability of nutrients or chronic stress.

New findings in this stream of fetal origins that Barker pioneered are coming to light just as this book goes to publication, with even more pointed implications for Generation Peace: it is the first research linking fetal growth conditions in the womb to the integration of left- and right-hemisphere brain activity later in life, which is central to mood and social functioning. In the new study, children who were born small and with proportionately large placentas showed more activity on the right side of their brains than the left—which has been linked with mood disorders such as depression. The study adds to a growing body of evidence showing that adverse environments experienced by fetuses can cause long-term changes in the function of the brain. "The way we grow before birth is influenced by many things including what our mothers eat during pregnancy and how much stress they are experiencing. This can have long-lasting implications for our mental and physical health in later life," explains epidemiologist Alexander Jones, who led the study at the University of Southampton.[30]

In essence, what Barker found in his initial research was that these men were living time bombs whose fuses had been lit in the earliest weeks of their physical genesis but didn't detonate for decades. There is a kind of unforgiving brutality in such findings, especially when we consider America's high number of premature and low-birth-weight babies. This research raises profoundly important questions, including, *Why?* Why has Nature conferred such power to the womb, and to the pregnant woman? And *What?* What kinds of circumstances in the womb have immutable, lifelong effects upon us? These are questions with barely conceivable implications, whose currently known answers attest to what prenatal researcher Dr. Peter Nathanielsz calls "the wonder and poetry of human development." In his book *Life in the Womb: The Origins of Health and Disease*, he writes:

> We pass more biological milestones before we are born than we do at any other time in the whole of our lives. The quality of development that occurs in the womb has long-term effects on mood, affect, disposition, cognitive abilities, as well as the basic functions of the heart, kidneys, lungs, liver, and pancreas later in life. If you don't have the right nurturing environment in the womb then you are going to develop in a different way regardless of your genes. As I like to say, anybody can louse up Shakespeare.[31]

Growth or Protection = Peace or Defense

The field of neuroendocrinology tells us that the growth axis is inhibited by stress,[32] and of course, malnutrition also has a direct growth restriction impact. Both stress and malnutrition (a particular form of stress) can be seen to figure significantly in the ongoing process of the "decision" of embryonic and fetal cells between cell division and cell specialization, a delicately balanced process meant to ensure that an adequate number of cells are produced prior to those cells becoming dedicated toward specialization within particular organs or tissues or blood.

The stress hormones (corticosteroids, including cortisol) play a critical role in this process by inhibiting cell growth and division; elevated cortisol levels seem to instruct cells to stop the growth process and to differentiate to their specific functions—as an organ, as blood, as muscle, etc., before they optimally would otherwise.[33] (Again, back to the adaptive survival scenario: organisms don't remain in growth mode under threat. They mobilize whatever resources they have on hand, and go into protection or survival mode.) The long-term effects of excess cortisol on prenatal development likely occur as the result of cells responding to cortisol's instruction to differentiate before they have finished growing and dividing, thus leading to suboptimal development of organs as well as to smaller overall size.

Many animal studies show increased sensitivity of the stress axis in the off-spring of mothers who were stressed during pregnancy; the research suggests that the protective properties of the placenta that inactivate reasonable amounts of maternal cortisol (stress hormones) crossing from mother to fetus break down in the presence of an excess of stress hormones. Many reports phrase this fact in terms that suggest this is a failure or breakdown in some part of the system. But what if that is not the case at all? What if this isn't a bug but a feature—and that the "failure" of the placenta to neutralize constant high doses of stress hormones represents the *perfect* functioning of the system? After all, what *is* the objective of the system?

The Intelligence of Adaptation

Recalling that the fundamental definition of intelligence is *the ability to respond to information for one's wellbeing and continuity*, we can look at fetal programming as Nature's intelligent plan to develop creatures who are as well-equipped as possible to survive in their world. Nature assumes that the world conveyed by the pregnant mother to the developing fetus will indeed be the world into which the baby will be born and where the individual will be expected to thrive. It is when those two worlds do *not* match that problems arise[34]—and that is typically the case in twenty-first century America.

Fetal programming theory regarding diabetes is a particularly good example: poor maternal nutrition impairs the development and function of the insulin-producing cells in the fetal pancreas, predisposing the individual to type 2 diabetes in later life. Barker's concept is that poor fetal nutrition imposes "mechanisms of nutritional thrift" on the growing individual. The mother-to-fetus "instruction" is that there isn't much food available in the environment, and fetal development adapts accordingly. And indeed, as long as meager nutritional circumstances persist for the infant into childhood and adulthood, problems do not arise, since the need for insulin is low when food is scarce. But if food becomes abundant—i.e., discordant with the maternal-fetal instruction about scarcity—impaired glucose tolerance or type 2 diabetes will result because the insulin demand exceeds the supply. So not only is the fetus prepared to survive in adverse conditions, it is *not* prepared to survive—much less thrive—in optimal conditions! As Barker himself has been quoted to say, "When a fetus adapts to conditions in the womb, that adaptation tends to be permanent."[35]

The implications of this mismatch between the world taught to the fetus as she absorbs her mother's experiences, and the actual world that she'll be expected to master, is a theme pervading this bountiful story of prenatal parenting, and the opportunities available for raising a generation of peacemakers! Michel Odent offers this prescription:

> If joy is the opposite of anxiety, depression and psychological distress, we can reasonably assume that it is associated with low levels of cortisol. We can therefore propose that the function of joy in pregnancy is to protect the unborn child against the effects of the harmful stress hormones. Since lasting effects are still detectable in adulthood, we can even understand that joy in pregnancy is *necessary* to transmit from generation to generation the capacity to be joyful. Let us anticipate that in the near future imaginative scientists will find ways to clarify the role hormones such as dopamine, serotonin and oxytocin in joyful experiences.[36]

Teaching Future Peacemakers a Peaceful World

One of my high-school cell biology students stopped me in my tracks with a question that cuts right to the marrow of the notion of consciously raising a generation hardwired for peace: "Is it fair or right for a pregnant mother—through intentionally staying calm and joyful—to convey to her growing fetus that it's a safe, peaceful world when it's so clearly not?" I thank young Thomas for putting us face to face with the staggering paradox at the heart of this entire Generation Peace proposition: it is exactly *because* our world is not a safe, secure, peaceful place that we *must* raise a generation…and then another…and then another…who are wired for peace from the very beginning!

The hyper-reactive, low-impulse-controlled, attention-deficit brain sculpted in the womb of a chronically stressed pregnant mother is more likely to survive in an atmosphere where there are physical predators lurking everywhere, but that is no longer the landscape of danger for most of the world. The greatest dangers to us are the virtually invisible, slowly evolving abstractions of climate change, world thirst, terrorist ideology, shifting economics, shimmying tectonic plates and the like. These are threats whose solutions will require brains equipped with the highest levels of cognitive and psychosocial capacities, which is conferred by robust development of particular neural structures, including the prefrontal cortexes and corpus callosum. The only way to achieve truly optimal development of these neural structures, together with the strands of psyche that attend a peaceful, well-regulated, innovative, healthily interdependent human, is to begin at the very beginning.

True enough, our daily life is filled with messages of threat—CNN alone can herd us all to anguish over the future—as well as daily hassles, annoyances and sometimes unavoidable, real-life grief and pain. As peace educator and activist Mitch Hall notes, "The paradox remains that it is adults habituated to a less than peaceful collective past who are responsible to raise peaceful children for a better future. This may be challenging, but it is possible."[37] Part of the great privilege of our evolutionary inheritance as human beings is this gift of self-reflective consciousness: we can make a thought *inside* our minds more real than anything *outside* our bodies! This is where the active work of parenting for peace comes in.

Step One's primer in bodymind principles described how much of what we experience in our environment is put through the filter of our own perceptions—the story we tell ourselves about what's happening—and how that impacts us at the cellular level. During pregnancy, the implications of perception hygiene take on higher stakes: the health of not just your own newly regenerating cells, but the healthy integrity of all of your baby's cells...and tissues...and organs...is intimately impacted by your perceptions of your daily world. Your perceptions are your baby's perceptions.

So it is critical to note that in the earlier scenario of the pregnant account executive facing a PowerPoint crisis, two mothers in the same situation could send two completely different messages to the babies in their wombs, based upon their *perceptions of* and *attitude about* the experience—their interpretation of the meaning of it, and their responses to it. (*Interpretation* is a tricky word, because we think of interpreting as a higher-order, conscious process, but here I'm referring to something that typically happens below the level of cognitive reasoning and thoughtful contemplation; this interpretation tends to be an instantaneous, emotionally driven assessment based on programming that happened when we ourselves were babies or young children.) Perhaps, rather than stressing out and yelling at the IT person, another woman in that same situation will take a few deep breaths, close her eyes, put her hands on her belly with a reassuring message to her baby, "No worries, let's figure out a good way around this," recognizing what previously unconsidered advantages there might be to making a more intimate presentation, without the distraction of PowerPoint slides.

Opportunities for this kind of perception hygiene abound in the course of daily life. Imagine two pregnant women in the same long line at the bank: one is annoyed at the delay, anxious over an appointment she's going to be late for, her dismay amplified by the fact that yet another teller just closed her window—*How* could *she?!*—while the other woman is calmly surrendering to the tide of present reality, even finding appreciation for the opportunity to slow down for a moment and tune in to her baby, introducing him or her in her imagination to the interesting array of people in line. By putting into perspective the fact that the people she has an appointment with will understand—or not—and that her wellbeing, and by extension her baby's, is paramount, this mother is helping to sculpt her baby's brain for peace.

What's a Mother-to-Be to Do?!

This may sound a little daunting. Realistically, it's hard to avoid stress and upset 24/7—and you would never want to! Healthy prenatal development relies upon the dynamics of the ebb and flow of *reasonable levels* of maternal stress levels. And, recalling that stress by definition is simply the "nonspecific response of the body to any demand," we have to recognize that just the normal movement and activities of life fall into this category. (In other words, a stress-free life doesn't exist, thank goodness.)

And when it comes to emotional, mental or psychological stress as in, "I'm stressed out," there is a helpfully simple guideline found at the heart of Zen practice: *Wanting something to be different than it is, is what causes stress.* So the goal is not to eliminate every stressor, but to reorient ourselves so as to navigate the currents of life in ways that support optimal, growth-oriented development of the embryo and fetus.

Annie Murphy Paul was pregnant when researching her book *Origins: How the Nine Months Before Birth Shape the Rest of Our Lives*, and rather than seeing it as a litany of dire warnings, she instead tapped into the scientists' "excitement of discovery—and the hope that their discoveries would make a positive difference. We're used to hearing about all the things that can go wrong during pregnancy, but as these researchers are finding out, it's frequently the intrauterine environment that makes things go right in later life."[38]

Once you know these principles of prenatal development, you hold a powerful key to your child's lifelong emotional health and wellbeing. Generation Peace parents are mindful of the unceasing question being asked by the baby in the womb—which is continually answered chemically and energetically via the mother's thoughts, feelings and behaviors: *Mommy, what kind of world am I coming into?* If they understand that this basic question—and its nine months' worth of answers—drive fundamental aspects of their baby's brain development, they can begin to comprehend how important it is for the pregnant mother to feel safe and supported, to feel loved, to feel joy—at least most of the time—so their baby can arrive ready to love and learn, not struggle and resist!

It is also helpful to keep in mind that *repeated, consistent, chronic* circumstances shape prenatal development, not necessarily one-time or occasional situations. For instance, in the scenario described above, if Mother #2—typically the easy-going one who keeps things in healthy perspective—has an uncharacteristic meltdown one day, she hasn't irreparably harmed her baby's brain development. On the contrary, if that stress gets resolved in due time, and doesn't become a protracted or chronic state of anxiety or depression, research hints that it may possibly even be constructive.[39] (The fetus learns at the most basic level—as will the toddler, preschooler and teen in similar circumstances—that distressing things can happen and the world doesn't fall apart: *repair happens, Life can be trusted!*) Of paramount importance is a pregnant mother's ongoing typical mental outlook and emotional tone: this is what becomes the baby's normal.

Joel Evans, author of *The Whole Pregnancy Handbook*, is a clinical professor of obstetrics, gynecology, and women's health—a physician whose personal growth and professional path have led him to understand that the wonder and wisdom of the universe manifest in every pregnancy. He finds that mother and baby often do best when the healthcare system gets out of the way and allows the birthing and bonding process to occur as nature intended. Dr. Evans' primary prescription? "If I was forced to reduce all of the important information I want to share with women as they think about pregnancy and motherhood to one recommendation, it would be to never lose sight of the power of intentionality. Through intention you can give your child the gift of feeling loved, desired and connected, a gift that easily overcomes whatever challenging circumstances arise that you feel prevent you from being the 'perfect' mother. The paradox is that the 'perfect mother' is the one who loves, desires and connects with her child, before, during and after pregnancy, regardless of the worldly circumstances in which mom and baby find themselves. That intention—the desire to nurture and simply do the best she can and surrender all self-doubt and criticism—is the most powerful force in the universe."[40]

Yes, remember that you are working together with the universe! You need never feel alone in this endeavor, because there are legions of collaborative energies working with your intentions to bring a peacemaker on earth. It is believed by many that one of your key teammates in this is your very child: spiritual teachings often mention how your child's soul is by your side, inspiring and strengthening you; and during pregnancy this spirit occasionally visits the baby's body in the making—much as the owner of a house visits his new house from time to time while it's under construction.

Prenatal Learning: What Is the World, Mommy, Through Your Eyes?

Woman is the artist of the imagination and the child in the womb is the canvas whereon she painteth her pictures.

PARACELSUS

Over recent decades, researchers have dispelled the archaic view of the newborn as a *tabula rasa*—"blank slate"—and updated our understanding of brand new babies: they are surprisingly sophisticated. And clearly their brilliance doesn't just appear once they emerge into the world; it comes into being while they're in the womb. Babies are born with a suite of impressive mental skills that include the ability to discern between different voices, smells, and tastes; between their parents and strangers; and even between stories they've heard in the womb and unfamiliar tales.[41] A particularly well-known study by De-Casper and Spence found that newborns whose mothers read them *The Cat in the Hat* while they were in the womb indeed recognized and preferred that story as compared to others after they were born;[42] and babies whose mothers

had watched a particular U.K. soap opera (*The Neighbours*) during their pregnancies demonstrated their remembrance of the show's theme music in a variety of ways, including giving it heightened attention, and calming down to
that specific music when fussy or upset.[43] Researchers recently discovered that
newborns can even learn—while they're asleep, no less!—to distinguish between complex vowel sounds that differ only very subtly.[44]

While still growing inside you, your baby is listening, paying attention, *and
remembering*. What you live, he learns. U.C. Berkeley biology professor Marian
Diamond—whose pioneering research proved the brain-healthy effects of enriched pregnancy on rat pups—points out that the Japanese have recognized
this for over two thousand years, with their principle of *Tykio*, which means,
"think pleasant thoughts."[45] I'm not suggesting you become a blandly re-
sponse-free Stepford mother, but rather a mother who is reorienting herself
into the posture of holding a protective, buffering space of appreciation within
which her child is unconstrained by inhibiting forces, free to blossom as robustly as possible and grow to his or her fullest potential. A mother who re-
gards the world with care toward how it would look through brand new eyes...
how it would sound through brand new ears...how it would feel to a brand
new being whose mandate is to prepare itself to match the promise of the
world she portrays.

In this complex, challenged world I realize it is a tall order to cultivate such
a becalmed outlook on life, especially as you are facing all the normal concerns
of ushering a new life into it. This is why the endeavor of raising Generation
Peace is largely frontloaded: the significant work you do in exploring and cultivating mastery of your own inner life beginning even before conception pays
untold dividends throughout the coming years of your child's early years and
lifelong experience. Fostering a fundamental peacefulness, wonder and trust
regarding the very processes of pregnancy and fetal development is an approach not only suggested by timeless wisdom traditions but by current hard
research.

Curt Sandman, whose lab has been funded for over thirty years by NIH
(National Institutes of Health) to study the effects of maternal stress on fetal
development and birth outcomes, has taught me for years that maternal stress
during pregnancy correlates with many different suboptimal outcomes that
in turn each have further associated negative downstream results, including
preterm labor. In light of the epidemic of prematurity in this country (one
baby in eight), and the cascade of lifelong challenges that comes with it—for

the parents and for the child being born—it bears noting Sandman's team's most consistent and statistically significant finding: the strongest psychosocial predictor of short gestational age (i.e., prematurity) is *pregnancy-related fears and anxieties.*[46] Not work stresses, not daily hassles, but how secure, resolved, at peace a woman is feeling *specifically in regard to her pregnancy.* But in today's world, even having navigated well through Steps One and Two, a self-possessed, joyously pregnant mother can succumb to our culture's subtle tug toward insecurity through its unending siren call: "You are not enough."

In our technocratic, information-revolutionized world, a pregnant mom simply being herself can end up feeling behind the curve and even somewhat negligent in foregoing newfangled inventions available to "optimize" her baby. We all want the best for our children, but in trying to figure out exactly what is best, parents are met with a dizzying selection of enrichment options, including prenatal stimulation programs.

> *I am floating, weightless, in my sea of dawning life, my energies being spun into cells. With you I am weaving life into the organs of my body. You are offering me your very substance, who you are, how you feel, what you think—your very perceptions of the world, of this life of yours, and of mine. I hear the sounds of your day, I feel the embrace of your womb, I delight in the undulations of your movement, your walking, your dancing, your taking a simple shower. Your heartbeat sets the rhythm of my existence. I am enthralled by everything you are. I ripen in the glow of your love, under the caress of your voice, as you share with me your songs, your imaginings, your—*
> "Tap tap tap." "Rub rub rub."
> *Now you want to teach me something. Train me. Interrupt our poetry. Don't you trust this flowering I do each day in the womb of your body, in the womb of your life? Am I not enough? Are* we *not enough?*

The growing mainstream recognition that babies, even in the womb, do learn and remember is a fantastic development, one that should inspire us toward more respectful approaches to pregnancy, birth and the early months. However, the way most of these programs and products deploy this understanding is a disheartening reflection of our culture's approach toward early education in general: bombard the child with data without concern for the relational context. It's electronic beeps and blips, or an arbitrary Vivaldi selection, or Mom or Dad "tap tap tap"-ping on the belly, summoning baby's attention. As a passionate opponent of the full-swing, counterproductive downward thrust of the first and second grade curriculum into the early education of children *outside* the womb, I have considerable reservations about harnessing our current understanding about fetal learning capacities to devise contrivances to thrust it downward even further.

Lots of prenatal stimulation and bonding programs boast developmental gains in the babies. Yes, you might be able to get your baby to roll over seventeen days earlier than average by tutoring her as a fetus, but my scientific curiosity kicks in with the question, *Is this necessarily a positive outcome?* You see, a biological tenet throughout the natural world holds that accelerated development is often a response to threat; indeed, we are biologically geared to detect threat, and attend to it for survival purposes. Further, accelerated development frequently has growth-or-protection consequences that aren't positive in the long run (often a sacrifice in robust growth), and sometimes even maladaptive (the *opposite* of useful). Everywhere in nature, when we try to skip a grade or hurry past any given developmental stage, we cause problems—like when we "help" a butterfly with the shedding of her chrysalis and the butterfly dies because she required that struggle to initiate the hydraulics inside her wings.

I propose that prenatal stimulation programs and systems veer into a similar territory of technological arrogance as does IVF—similar to the region in which obstetricians can be heard using the phrase, "an uneventful pregnancy." An *uneventful pregnancy?!* Have we grown so sophisticated, so technologically myopic, that we can speak so cavalierly about this extraordinary, barely fathomable stream of events? Is this why we feel the need to go in and tinker, tweak and, in our conquering mentality, strive to create a "New and Improved" baby? Exerting our heroic influence to orchestrate some miracle that we in our limitation cannot perceive as already there?

Every prenatal book includes detailed timeline information about all of the details of embryonic and fetal development, including the negative possibilities. Some programs direct mothers to envision in detail the intricacies of their baby's development at various stages. But whatever we can think, imagine, visualize or mentally conceive—even in the spirit of optimizing the process of fetal development—likely falls woefully short of the individualized, miraculous unfolding of each individual baby, according to the vast design of Life. When we systematically require the attention of the baby in the womb according to some structured program, are we not possibly disturbing some unfathomable growth process that is taking place perfectly well in the scheme of prenatal development? Would a wise gardener think of training the roots of a growing tree, or would she nourish the earth that sustains those new roots?

I wonder about the relational messages inherent in these very early educational experiences—that while I love him I need more from him somehow? That I want him to perform better? That there are already conditions being imposed on my relationship with him? It seems that both baby and mother suffer a kind of loss. For the baby, it is "I am not okay just being me. I have to accomplish something, maximize my potential." For the mother it is, "I am not enough, I can't provide the best for my baby by being myself—I need to enroll my baby in a Prenatal University."

The most scientifically proven prenatal education program consists of a mother's perceptions of the world, as taught to her baby through her thoughts, feelings, words and behavior. And keep in mind that each pregnant mother's daily life, her inner life—attitudes, reactions, imaginations—*is* an individualized prenatal education program, which is continually answering her unique baby's everpresent mandate: *Teach me your world, Mommy.*

Fathering a Peaceful Future

Research consistently attests to the central importance of a pregnant mother's feelings of being supported and nurtured. Does that mean that the extent of an expectant father's calling is to act as her supporter and nurturer—back-rubber, chauffeur and coach? Do these "staff support" roles reflect the monumental potential influence fathers* have in their children's lives? And do they weave the most fruitful early foundations for joyous, peaceful family life? The prevailing notion is that a father's only option is to look on with wonder (and sometimes envy) at the beautiful relationship forming between his once-doting partner and this tiny interloper. That must change for parents of peacemakers!

Fathers actually have a natural, even biological, inclination to begin forming an attachment to their babies during pregnancy, but this is largely ignored by

---

* The term *father* here refers to the mother's male husband or partner, but can also serve to refer to a pregnant woman's lesbian partner, although the hormone profile is a little different.

the scientific community and by our collective culture. When a couple announces that they are having a baby, the role of the mother is tightly defined. Her family, friends, coworkers and even strangers treat her in an unambiguous fashion: she is doted on, showered with attention (sometimes to her dismay), and regarded in a way that emphasizes her mother-to-be status. Her partner, on the other hand, has no designated, well-choreographed role to play. He is usually left to stumble along his path to fatherhood with little direction or acknowledgment of his own internal processes.

Michael Trout, director of the Infant-Parent Institute in Champaign, Illinois, points out:

> Our language and our culture clearly support the notion that it is never he, only his mate, who is expecting a baby. He is often treated as a donor, a bystander and—if he is any good at his multiple but vaguely-defined jobs—it is understood that he will be supportive of the one who is truly important, the only one who is doing any work, the truly pregnant one.[47]

Yes, pregnancy is a lot of work for a woman's body—rearranging ligaments, building blood volume and cranking out hormones. Oxytocin, the closest thing in Mother Nature's pharmacy to an elixir of love, spikes just after birth and is responsible for biologically inspiring many maternal behaviors. But guess what? A father, too, experiences a cascade of hormonal changes during pregnancy that quietly echoes that of his partner.[48] During his mate's pregnancy, a man's oxytocin level begins to rise, encouraging him to desire closeness with his mate and child. Together with vasopressin, it makes a male more protective of his family and committed to their care. (Vasopressin has been called "the monogamy hormone" because it causes males to desire the comforts of home as opposed to the thrill of the chase.)

Pregnancy, birth and parenting awaken for all of us, mothers and fathers alike, old feelings and sense-memories of our own womb and babyhood experiences, which further make parenthood a journey of unprecedented proportions. Though it is rare for a father to be considered pregnant along with his wife, why should he not be given this consideration and status? He, too, is on a profound, life-altering journey! Perhaps as a result of this early exclusion, and feeling insufficient support and opportunity for forming a prenatal attachment, fathers often feel uninitiated and awkward with their newborns. Infants are exquisitely sensitive to emotional cues, and may react with discontent to a father's insecurity. This can set off a cycle of uncomfortable and not-quite-right feelings between dad and baby. Defeated, the father may interpret this as confirmation that he is simply not good with babies and decide his efforts will be better received (and rewarded) when the kid is older.

So how can dads jump-start their fathering during pregnancy? Some find that laying their hands on the mother's abdomen and making contact is a powerful experience. Kevin recalled lying with his wife in the early evenings and placing his hands on her still-flat belly. He whispered to the baby quietly, so his wife couldn't make out what he was saying, and when she inquired, he'd grin and say, "This is a private conversation between me and my little girl."

Mothers-to-be can be encouraging and sensitive to these delicate first steps, putting forth every effort to making their baby accessible. Brett, father of eight-month-old Elissa, described the weeks when Elissa's movements were first noticeable under his touch, and the emotional tidal wave that washed through him, carrying with it the reality of his unborn child. He reminisced about times when he could scarcely attend to his work during the day because he was so anxious to get home and feel his baby moving beneath his fingertips.

> I liked to just lay with my head resting on Jae's belly so I could breathe on her skin. I thought that maybe somehow Elissa could become accustomed to the feel of my breath surrounding her and she'd know how much I couldn't wait to see her, and maybe she'd know me when she was finally born.

Fathers can be full participants during pregnancy, deeply affected by the experience of conceiving and loving a child, and processing the experience in their own profoundly personal ways. And still, of course, one of the best ways that a "pregnant father" can contribute to his baby's optimal development in the womb is to love, celebrate and cherish his baby's mother...to dream of the great and noble qualities he dreams of for his coming child...and to hold a positive outlook on daily living. Just as a mother's perception of life powerfully influences their baby's prenatal development, a father's perception of life deeply influences his baby's mother, which strongly influences her perceptions of life!

A pregnant mother particularly relishes strength, creativity and a sense of optimism in her partner at this momentous time.

Building a Healthy Baby Body

We can no longer make a clean distinction between psychological wellbeing and physiological health: the robust integrity of tissues and organs—particularly the brain—allows mental and emotional capacities to flourish. Many books are available with specific guidelines for optimal pregnancy nutrition, so rather than going into detail on dietary issues, I'll briefly mention a few points related to fostering development of the greatest possible peace potential in your developing baby.

Keep in mind that a key principle behind eating for two is that you want to maximize nutrient intake without necessarily adding that many more calories. Avoid processed foods that up your calories without upping your baby's nutrient supply. Moderation is key (sure, have that pistachio ice cream you're craving—but not the whole pint!), and organic and locally grown is ideal if you can find it. Important always, but especially in pregnancy, is a well-varied diet that includes those famous five-to-seven servings of fruits and vegetables, whole grains, and lean protein sources.

A wise precept, especially during pregnancy as well as breastfeeding, is to avoid extremes of all kinds—going for *all* raw, fat-*free*, *zero* carbs, *no* animal products. Animal fats and cholesterol are vital factors in the human diet, necessary for reproduction and normal growth, healthy immunity, and proper function of the brain and nervous system. This is never more true than when you're eating not just for you, but for your growing baby: his or her developing brain depends for its optimal health upon the essential fatty acids found in lean animal products. Fish can provide the necessary EFAs without the ethical bind posed for some by other animal products,* and once you understand the facts about mercury contamination (mentioned in Step Two) you can consume fish without undue worry.

While some experts say that it's enough to limit caffeine intake to less than 200 mg. (about two cups of coffee), the research is inconclusive and is prima-

---

* I have heard it put this way: Would you go fishing? If so, then eat fish. Would you go hunting for cows, lambs or pigs? Behead a chicken? If so, then eat meat.

rily targeted at avoiding such drastic outcomes as stillbirth and miscarriage. Far better to avoid caffeine, which is a potent central nervous system stimulant that crosses the placenta and gives baby a far more intense jolt than Mom experiences. Such stimulation—especially when repeated routinely—may impact cellular and organic structure and function in the fetus, and is also a prenatal lesson about the world (*"Being stimulated is required"*).

The same goes for alcohol, a central nervous system depressant. Though mixed messages abound out there on this topic, no amount of alcohol has been proven safe during pregnancy, and a recent study reported by March of Dimes found negative developmental effects in four- and eight-year-old children of women who had *less than one drink per week*.[49]

Tend Your Inner Knowing

In Step Five I discuss the problems that arise when we separate mothers and newborns after birth, which is routine in hospitals despite volumes of research concluding it shouldn't be done. To understand the conundrum—and to help you navigate around it—it helps to recognize that this impulse toward separation actually begins much earlier, abetted by our enchantment with technologically informed pregnancy. This features many processes that slip wedge after subtle wedge between mother and baby, making the ultimate physical separation of the mother and newborn the culmination of an inexorable erosion of connectedness and intimacy.

We no longer give a second thought, for example, to ultrasound imaging; despite the fact that routine (as opposed to medically indicated) ultrasound use does not improve maternal or infant outcomes,[50] and despite mounting data suggesting it may carry unnecessary risks,[51] it has become the ubiquitous Baby's First Photograph, and is now typically done during every prenatal visit.

Scholars who explore the "technological gaze" of fetal imaging articulate how—apart from its benefits in the small number of cases of true prenatal diagnostic need, and its possible dangers otherwise—it insidiously erodes the natural rhythms and connections of pregnancy and birth, not least by subtly deemphasizing the mother herself. Points out Steven Mentor, "…everywhere you look there are fetuses but no women (Laborie 1987.) The image on the screen vibrates inside an electronic virtual womb, kept alive not by the mother (over there) but by the on-switch, brought into view not by birth but by a turn of the probe, now appearing, now disappearing."[52]

Cultural anthropologist Robbie Davis-Floyd notes that women routinely come to see the image *as the baby*, that the murky blur on the screen becomes more real than any sensation inside her womb or her imagination.[53] Indeed, for most modern parents, their baby is somehow rendered more real by what Mentor calls "the dominant reality engine of our time"—the screen.

The ultrasound screen gives way to the electronic fetal monitor, which morphs into the radio-frequency baby monitor at home, and before long a GPS tracking app on the child's cell phone.* And all the while we let our inner knowing atrophy, and our capacity to cultivate trust diminishes. No wonder anxiety roils when our children finally begin venturing beyond our electronic surveillance net: as in the universal dream that features the I-never-went-to-class-and-today-is-the-final-exam panic, we are faced with the anguish of worrying, pacing and nagging if we have neglected year after year after year to foster and engage in a trusting collaboration with Life.

Raising Generation Peace: The Collective Endeavor

Knowing what we know—that an expectant mother's experiences and perceptions of daily life are fundamental in shaping the baby in her womb—we must recognize that we will disappoint our future if we fail to step up for pregnant women. Instead of "optimizing" a fetus through stimulation, let us uplift a mother through inspiration. As individuals and as a society, let us support her by offering her more means through which she can be at her best, her most authentic. The implications of some of the frontier findings discussed earlier—about the impact our thoughts and attitudes have on those around us—are that not only does the pregnant woman have a powerful, enduring effect upon her developing baby from the earliest moments of creation, but so too does the surrounding culture: family, community, nation, race, world. The thoughts, dreams, visions we hold for and of our children, for and of the mothers of the world, may well be as important as a pregnant woman's intake of vitamin B and her avoidance of stress for the healthy, untrammeled development of our future adult citizens and, ultimately, our world. Suggests Michel Odent:

---

* I write this facetiously: children should *not* have cell phones. See Joe Mercola's important information at products.mercola.com/blue-tube-headset.

The first duty of all those who meet pregnant women is to protect their emotional state. In the age of routine medicalized prenatal care the attitudes of health professionals can have powerful effects on the emotional states of pregnant women. Thus the main preoccupation, even the zeal, of doctors, midwives and other specialized professionals, should be to avoid the "nocebo effect" during prenatal visits. In practice, this means that they must create such interactions that a pregnant woman feels even happier after a prenatal visit than before...or at least less anxious. This will not be easy as long as the dominant style of prenatal care is to routinely offer all pregnant women a standardized battery of tests, thus turning every prenatal visit into an opportunity to realize all the risks associated with pregnancy and childbirth.[54]

Bulgarian philosopher Omraam Mikhaël Aïvanhov proposed in 1938 that rather than spending billions on hospitals, courtrooms, and prisons, governments concentrate their attention on pregnant mothers: "The cost will be far less and the results infinitely superior." Omraam suggested that prisons could be closed in two generations with such an approach.[55] Can we only imagine—or can we take the next step and discover—what might happen if we as a society dedicate ourselves to carrying every woman's pregnancy in an uplifted collective consciousness? If we commit our sociopolitical resources toward assuring that pregnant women enjoy a safe, loving, beautiful environment? Inspired by Omraam's vision, Laura Uplinger conceived of a world in which there

> reigns a true spirit of kinship with all life, and pregnant women are treated in a very special way. The arts and crafts of each community are made available to them; they admire trees, statues and fountains, as they walk through beautiful parks filled with flowers. By day, the birds' songs embrace them. By night, the stars entice them to visit distant worlds. In these parks there are houses where the mothers can take part in many activities: they sing, weave, sculpt, embroider, draw. There are also theaters, libraries and cinemas, and they can study, teach, meditate, laugh and cry.[56]

Until we manifest that world without, we can create such a world within, beginning with this simple prescription from the gifted Laura Huxley, late widow of visionary author Aldous Huxley:

If you can take even five minutes a day, to think good thoughts, listen to your favorite music, or nourish yourself in any way you want, your kindness will be multiplied a thousand-fold and become an organic part of a person's being for years to come. Five minutes of care is worth years of wellbeing.[57]

By weaving our babies from the strands of our joy, our inspiration, our vision, we will be "practicing evolution," in the manner so compellingly described by Bruce Lipton and Steve Bhaerman in *Spontaneous Evolution: Our Positive Future and a Way to Get There from Here.* Through understanding and embracing the extraordinary, paradoxical force of human joy, we "claim our right to become personally empowered co-creators and architects of a brave and loving new world."[58] Indeed, by claiming the unequaled opportunities of attuned conception and radiant pregnancy, we can tap into our true evolutionary potential through which we will indeed "change the world from the inside out."

Ahh...you are back, Mommy. Yes, I need you...for me, with me, with the gift of love, and of trust...that we are enough.

PRINCIPLES TO PRACTICE

Presence – As earlier noted, one of the best ways to cultivate the qualities of presence is to engage yourself fully—awareness, interest, attention—in whatever is going on at the moment, and pregnancy offers you so many opportunities for that. Shopping for baby is fun—all that pastel!—but consider, as you're preparing for your baby's arrival, that the most important nesting you can do is possibly the least appealing, because you can't put it on your plastic: Cultivate your ability to *just be.* One of the major causes of parental misery is our impulse to be somewhere other than where we are right now (or to wish our *kids* were somewhere else), whether right now is a colicky baby who is crying for her twenty-seventh straight evening, or a toddler who has again missed getting to the potty (recalling that bumper sticker, Shit Happens). Much of our distress lies in the very resistance to giving ourselves over to what *is.* And paradoxically, when we let go of our idea of what *should* be in this moment, and instead receive this moment as it is, any moment can become perfection. Bliss Happens.

- Take a few minutes from time to time to marvel at the miraculous processes that are taking place within you. And, when you are sweeping the floor, or slicing an apple, be there completely. Appreciating both the momentous and the mundane composes an engaged life.
- Before your baby physically arrives you still have an excellent opportunity to begin or further develop regular practice of meditation, contemplation, or prayer, a foundation that will serve you and your baby richly! A good prenatal yoga class can be a tremendous avenue for practicing presence now.
  - As the authors make clear in *Parenting from the Inside Out*, these kinds of practices that draw on the right hemisphere of the brain (which is nonlinear, holistic, visual-spacial, relational, nonlinguistic, antianalytical) help strengthen the functioning of your social brain, which in turn is a boon to your child's peaceable development.

Awareness –The key awareness for you at this step as a pregnant mother is to recognize the powerful influence of your thoughts, feelings, lifestyle, and diet upon the lifelong health of your baby: he or she is marinating in the general mood and matter of your life! The same goes for you, the father: though not connected as intimately with your baby as is your partner, your thoughts, feelings, and attitudes are a key influence on prenatal development.

- Continue to cultivate a growing fluency with your own story—childhood, infancy, your mother's pregnancy, even circumstances of conception and before. If possible, engage one or both of your parents in a conversation about your beginnings—your mother's pregnancy with you, her birth experience. Were you together right after birth? You might ask about what you were like as a baby and young child: did you have colic, were you a fussy eater, were you content or irritable, did you sleep much? The more you are able to identify where you may have tender unfinished business, the more you'll cultivate the flexibility needed to avoid the knee-jerk emotional responses we so often have when children push those buttons.
- Unfortunate but true, anger is often one of the biggest challenges in parenting. It is always helpful to keep in mind that most of the time, anger is simply a disguise for another feeling. A somewhat overly simplified slogan is nevertheless instructive: *mad is* really *sad.* I would add that mad is very often *hurt,* or some variation. Here are two excellent awareness resources for addressing your patterns of responding when angry, stressed, sad, fearful, etc., which will pave the way for much more peaceful, joy-filled parenting:

- Marshall Rosenberg's model of Nonviolent Communication (NVC) is a wonderful tool for developing awareness of what motivates us both toward violence (physical, verbal or emotional) and toward compassionate connection. NVC is particularly helpful in working with anger, proposing that anger can be transformed into more life-affirming connection when we keep our focus on what our feelings are—based on needs that either are or are not being met in any given moment—rather than turning our focus toward analyzing and judging "what he did" that "made me furious." Here is a wonderful exercise from Rosenberg to help us become more aware of the specifics of our anger buttons, which are always simply some needs of ours that are not being met: 1) List the judgments that frequently pop into your head by using the cue "I don't like people who are…" 2) Looking at what you've listed, ask yourself, "When I make that judgment of a person, what might I be needing at that moment? What unmet need might I be having that's getting expressed through that judgment?" 3) List those needs alongside the judgments, and then next to that, the feelings you may have when those needs are not met. (I suggest using the NVC needs and feelings lists for inspiration.) In this way you train yourself to frame your thinking in terms of unmet needs and the feelings they trigger—which tends to open hearts and minds—rather than in terms of judgments, which shuts down openhearted connectedness. This takes practice, which is why I've listed it before your child is born!
- *Parenting from the Inside Out* decodes the latest science of brain-and-relationship in a way that clearly outlines why we are so prone to responding to our children in ways that are automatic and negative, rather than ways that align with our intentional vision of parenting for peace. And it offers guidelines and exercises for disentangling ourselves from this auto-pilot mode in which we find ourselves—*despite our best intentions*—snapping, shaming, blaming, dismissing, and even hitting. That, together with its many illustrative stories and examples, makes this book a key resource for you.

- As I mentioned earlier, many books include timelines of specific gestational developmental details, including what can go wrong. Rather than devoting your mental energies to such an awareness, Uplinger's Womb Service imageries offer empowering—and less invasive—avenues for a pregnant mother dedicated to her baby's most vibrant development:

Lie down,
close your eyes,
Smile while breathing peacefully, deeply.
Speak in friendship to the cells of your body,
in their zillions they are you.
Thank them for composing your organs.
Encourage the harmony of their collaboration.
Ask them to excel in their functions.
They will hear you
and respond by working even more in concert,
Enhancing the quality of your health and pregnancy[59].

• Most expectant parents engage in some form of childbirth classes. I'm re-minded of a colleague's wise observation that "the best childbirth preparation begins long before puberty." So much about your birth will be influenced by your inner life and attitudes about your body and your confidence in its abil-ities—which were shaped long ago. That said, it is good to empower yourself with constructive information about the processes of labor and birth. Discern-ment is imperative when choosing a class; many hospital-based programs are understandably designed to orient you to all the technology so that you will be more comfortable using it when the time comes. Michel Odent points out that prenatal care has become "prenatal scare"—and there is some research ac-tually showing better labor outcomes without prenatal care, because the mother's confidence hasn't been eroded by listening to the litany of negative possibilities.

  - While individual teachers vary, three programs I endorse are Birthworks, Birthing From Within, and Bradley—all of which are faithful to the phys-iological requirements of Nature and her unmatched, elegant system for birthing.

  - Eisenhower once said (referring, unfortunately, to battle), "Plans are use-less, but planning is indispensable." This applies well to labor and birth: plan for privacy—who's going to be there and not be there; when you'll call the midwife or doctor; whether you want to labor in water or not; what atmosphere you'll want, etc. Beyond that, be prepared to ride the powerful waves of the emerging process, moment-by-moment. I love what Pam Eng-land writes in *Birthing from Within* about "the birth plan trap," wisely point-ing out that "birth is what's happening while you're busy writing birth plans."[60] I also think her chapter on "Babyproofing Your Marriage" is one of the most important aspects of childbirth preparation awareness to engage in.

- Tune in to unexpected insights, interests and impulses you might have; be aware of what you're drawn to, and consider indulging in it even if it seems out of the blue or "not like you." This might be your baby's influence! Many parents have reported getting messages in various ways from their babies, either in dreams, or in waking intuitions. A pregnant mother might, for example, become suddenly interested in architecture, or a father devoted to working out puzzles. Consider this a prelude to your coming apprenticeship with a Zen master designed uniquely for your advancement, otherwise known as your child.
  - One lovely way to become aware of hidden or subtle dimensions of your inner rapport with your pregnancy, anticipated birth, and future motherhood is through art, dance, and other expressive experiences. Tamara Donn, founder of Woman to Mother in the U.K., developed the Birth Art Café model in which pregnant women and new mothers gather to explore and share their journeys through drawing, painting and sculpture.

- It is important to have an awareness of the risk factors for postpartum depression (PPD): previous depressive symptoms, diagnosed depressive disorder, or other mood disorder; childhood trauma; recent "exit events" (people or opportunities have left); shame or entrapment events; current stressors (may be mild but chronic); interpersonal tensions; poor social support, especially not having a confidante.[61] If you have one or more of these, make it a priority to include preventive measures as part of preparing for baby. This can include enriching your circle of connectedness, finding a therapist or support group, making sure you're getting adequate brain nutrition (such as EFAs like omega-3s), and having honest heart-to-hearts about it with your partner. Amanda Rose's book *Rebuild from Depression* is invaluable for PPD prevention. You might consider downloading the excellent "Postpartum Pact,"* discussing it, and perhaps customizing it for your individual circumstances. (For example, one key depressive symptom doesn't appear on that list: being relentlessly focused on the negative about *everything*.)

---

* Postpartum Pact: www.postpartumny.org/media/PostpartumPactff.pdf

- In the event that you are serving as a surrogate, or if you are contemplating relinquishing your baby for adoption, it is commonly believed that your job is to remain emotionally detached while you're pregnant—that it will make it easier to separate when the time comes. This is not true! For most pregnant women—regardless of the circumstances of the pregnancy—their instincts are to embrace their babies, but there are so many messages dissuading them. You need to be supported and guided in following your instinct to connect with your baby. The unknown future of your relationship together need not—and should not!—keep you from connecting with your baby now. Despite your challenging circumstances, the most important thing for your baby is to feel your loving recognition—to feel claimed by you—and for you to know that you are everything to your baby, if only for this precious time in your womb. If and when you must later separate, your earlier connection will have laid a stronger foundation for your baby's optimal brain development and his fundamental self-esteem, and will make healing more possible for each of you. You will always know you gave your baby a blessed beginning.

Rhythm – Pregnancy offers a rich opportunity for developing a respect, appreciation and compassion for the ebbing and flowing of multiple dimensions of your body and psyche, as both travel a momentous path in preparing three new human beings: your baby, and both of you—transformed as a mother and father!

- Women, on the inevitable days when you feel really tired, or overly stretched (literally or figuratively), or like you may go crazy, it will help you to feel better if you simply acknowledge and honor that you are involved in a vigorous process that is pushing you through new doorways on all levels. It *is* taxing. And that's okay. Give yourself permission to *have* these rhythms—sometimes feeling low energy, sometimes filled with exhilaration—and the inner reassurance that this is indeed normal and healthy.
- Men, we now know that you also go through changes during your partner's pregnancy. Many fathers-to-be experience such symptoms as nausea, weight gain and moodiness, likely thanks to neurobiological responses of relatedness and empathy, mediated by such newly discovered wonders as mirror neurons. You also undergo hormonal changes toward the end of pregnancy that facilitate more tenderness and calm—Nature's biochemical leg-up for your new role as a father. So recognize that you are also in a state of change, responding to Life's rhythmic design for parenthood.

- The shaping rhythms of long ago when you were in your mother's womb may now become subtly reawakened unconsciously. It can help to know how your mother's pregnancy with you went, and possibly recognize and acknowledge that a troubling feeling you might have now is an old one being awakened—and, thanks to the vibrational quality you have invited, being healed.
- Though you are technically pregnant for a period three seasons long, most women's pregnancies span two complete seasons plus some portion of the other two. As you are emergent with the new life taking shape within, you can learn from Nature's own rhythms of creation and growth.
- A baby in the womb is subject to many extraordinary rhythms. With your imagination, travel into your baby's watery world and tune into the tidal ebb and flow of the fluid fields in the embryonic weeks…and later, the richly sonic experience of the fetus, which includes not only the lightly muffled sounds of the outside world—including voices, music, doorbells, dishwashers—but also the rhythmic whooshing of Mom's blood and digestive system, and Mom's heartbeat, the most essential organizing rhythm of your baby's existence.

Example – Your orientation to life while pregnant serves as a far-reaching template for your baby's own experience of life. The attitudes, feelings, behaviors you consistently engage in are downloaded to your baby biochemically, energetically, and aurally, as instructions for preparing for this world.

- Many wisdom traditions instruct the pregnant mother to fill her mind with thoughts and images of the splendid qualities she and her partner dream of for their child. This makes it a wonderful time to read biographies of inspiring peacemakers and innovators whom you admire. We still know so little about the how's behind the important functions of imagination and joy in pregnancy for the lifelong qualities of the individual, who is steeped in whatever his or her mother experiences during those nine months, so why not? It seemed to work for Shirley Temple's mother, who embraced these practices and gave birth to one of the most endearing actresses in our history—who went on to be a devoted humanitarian![62]
- Take some time to think about mothers you admire—famous or not—and spend time in their presence, through a biography, in person, or in writing and conversation. Ask them as many questions about their motherhood journeys as you can think of, such as *What delighted you most when you were ex-*

pecting? What did you most envision for your children when you were pregnant? If you could tell one thing to the younger woman you were when you began on your motherhood path, what would it be?

- Some wisdom traditions urge the pregnant mother to spend time each day gazing upon particularly luminous mother and child paintings, such as classical ones by DaVinci, Raphael or Reni—Klimt or Cassatt are wonderful as well, whichever move you or speak to you.

- With nutrition of such paramount importance during pregnancy, it's an opportunity for you to cultivate not just healthy eating habits, but also a healthy attitude *toward* your eating habits. Find a balance through which commitment steers clear of compulsiveness and retain a sense of ease, delight and freedom about food, which will set a wholesome example for your child from the beginning.

- One of the most nourishing pursuits is to gather with other pregnant mothers and simply be together in your ripeness! Share your fantasies, fears, intentions, delights and discoveries. In such groups you gather inspiration from the example of some, while providing that yourself for others. The term *communitas* was coined for such ways to share the experience of the *liminal*, the space between two different social statuses—the aspect of pregnancy in which a woman is "no longer who she was, and not yet who she will be."[63]
  - You can enrich the event by including a creative arts aspect—knitting, embroidering, art, weaving. Here again you can fruitfully apply the poet's law of analogy: *As I'm knitting, painting, or weaving something of beauty, may the forces in me beautifully weave the energies and tissues of my baby's being.*

Nurturance – One of the finest ways to nurture yourself and your baby during pregnancy is to steep yourself in beauty, surround yourself with what inspires you, and do what brings you joy. In a culture not particularly oriented that way, part of the process may be to simply discover what these things are for you—and that process itself is a wonderful nurturance for your baby, who wants to know you. These don't have to be grand, expensive things (and indeed, that which brings us the greatest joy is usually quite simple):

- Uplinger's Womb Service imageries are a great place to start cultivating rich avenues for nurturing yourself and your *wombmate*. For example, how lovely the simple nurturance a piece of fruit can be, as you grow your member of Generation Peace:

Take a fruit in your hands, an apple say.
See it and smell it teeming with life.
Touch it to your lips.
You are kissing whole seasons of nurturance.
This apple carries life-gifts from its tree, sunlife and rainlife,
gifts from the earth, the air and the stars.
Last year's leaves fell and gave themselves to it.
Join this procession of giving:
eat the apple as a gift for your baby
who is your fruitful gift to the world.

- The baby's father can feel a bit outside the intimate connectedness between his pregnant partner and their baby. Here's another Womb Service offering for mothers that invites the new family together to nurture their baby with communion:

  Within an intimacy, take the hands of your baby's father
  and hold them to your pregnant belly.
  With the three of you gathered together,
  have a conversation about this family.
  Talk about who you are.
  About your home, your life, ideas, hopes, dreams.
  "Your mom and I were picturing your first taste of chocolate ice cream."
  "Your dad wants to take you sailing."
  "Welcome to this tough old world. You will make a difference."
  "What a joy you are! We're honored to be yours."
  "Count on us."
  Then give all three of you a deeply felt family kiss.

- Be aware of any feelings you have regarding a preference for a boy or a girl, and strive to expand beyond the perception that one would be more desirable than the other. Your child takes in even the most subtle atmosphere arising from such mental representations, and prenatal psychology research abounds with stories of people who have carried into their lives a sense of not being quite right as they are—not loved for their boyness or girlness. When Karen and Doug were expecting their second child, they initially wanted to wait and discover the sex at birth, as they had done with their son. But not long after Karen's amnio, she became aware that despite her best efforts to be neutral, she was envisioning how lovely it would be to have a girl. She didn't want a boy to marinate all those months in that ambivalence, if that was the case, so for her the solution was obtaining the sex information from her doctor's file. She felt that if she *knew* she was expecting a second boy, she'd easily be able to reorient her fantasies to that particular joy. (It was in fact a girl.)

- I don't subscribe to the notion that once your baby's born you must keep him or her physically on you 24/7 in order to nurture your connectedness; we carry our babies with our voice, our gaze, our singing, and to suggest that touch is the only way is a limited and limiting view. There are many dimensions and senses through which to connect. Not every baby likes to be cuddled the same way, nor every mother. That said, an on-body baby carrier like a Snugglie or sling can be a wonderful nurturance tool. Now is a good time to borrow a few from friends, so you, your partner and your baby can try them out in the early weeks after her birth. Together you will know which kind to buy for yourselves.

- As a primary piece of nurturance furniture, I heartily recommend a rocking, swiveling, fully reclining lounge chair, the kind stereotypically reserved for watching football and midnight reruns of *Law & Order*. As glorious as the baby stores' glider-rockers are, wooden arms can be unforgiving, and even the upholstered ones typically have a separate, not-so-ergonomically-friendly footrest. The comfy embrace of a lounger will nurture you both through many nursing-through-the-night bouts of teething or fevers or stuffy noses— a true lifesaver, sleep-saver, and sanity-saver.

- One way to prepare beautiful nurturance for your newborn is to find some silk scarves in soft rainbow hues to drape over his cradle or bassinet.[64] They will soften the sharp contours of this brand new environment, helping him make a gentle landing into this physical body and world. Not just enchanting, but well-advised in light of brain science and the growing epidemic of sensory integration disorders—which are associated in part with the bombardment of sensations to which we routinely submit even our teeniest babies.

Trust – This is perhaps the most challenging of the principles at every step, and certainly during pregnancy, when you are bombarded from all corners with news of all the things that can go wrong. If you are following the steps and principles, as well as the health-fostering guidance of your midwife or doctor, then the beauty is, you can trust in Life's design for you and for your baby!

- Go back and read the "How We Begin" section of Step Two, about the first weeks of embryonic life. Embrace the balm of recognizing that there is some unfathomable intelligence at work behind the inscrutably intricate series of cellular events, with their miniscule error tolerances in timing, placement, and motion. When you can give yourself over as a part of that design, as an offering to Life as it composes, it brings great strength and tranquility.

- One of your most daunting Hero's Journey challenges will begin soon enough—sheltering your child from technology and screens in a culture that worships them above almost all else. You can begin flexing those muscles by questioning your obstetrician's assumption that you're automatically willing to undergo monthly ultrasounds. You also now have the opportunity to develop your trust muscle—rather than relying on an image on the screen to introduce you to your baby, month after month, cultivate your inner awareness of his flourishing inside you. Do your homework, learn how ultrasound works, how its vibration may cause *cavitation* (formation of tiny gas bubbles) in cells, and that some scientists have speculated that the fetal brain may be especially vulnerable because of the rapid growth and migration of brain cells.[65] There are certainly times when its use is called for, but we've slid way down a slippery slope of breaking it out for what seems like viewing amusement purposes. Keep in mind as you do your research that power levels for diagnostic ultrasound machines have increased eightfold (that is, *800 percent!*) since the early 1990s, so prior studies of its effects may therefore no longer be valid. Ina May Gaskin offers a wise suggestion for how to respond if your healthcare provider wants to do an ultrasound scan that you'd prefer not to have: ask him or her what specific information they are seeking; there are other, sometimes better (more trustworthy), ways to assess, for example, fetal age or pelvic dimensions.[66]

- Again, take a cue from Kahlil Gibran: "Your children are not your children; they are the sons and daughters of Life's longing for itself." As a collaborator with Life on this precious child, you have the right to ask for Life's help! Begin a conversation—even if it's pure fantasy-based imaginative play, or intellectual metaphor—with the guardian angel of your coming child. You will be lifelong colleagues, so now's the time to begin establishing a good working rapport. A verse of Rudolf Steiner's can be of wonderful help to begin cultivating a trust that will serve you and your child well; it is akin to fertilizing the soil that in turn nourishes the roots of the growing tree.

Into my will let there pour strength,
Into my feeling let there flow warmth,
Into my thinking let there shine light,
that I may nurture this child
with enlightened purpose,
caring with heart's love and bringing
wisdom into all things.

—RUDOLF STEINER[67]

- Unless you can surrender into trust that the microns and molecules forming your child are in competent charge of their own doings, you could easily go berserk. Imagine having to assemble those building blocks yourself! Trust is the only way up.

Simplicity – I find it instructive to think about this principle as it applies to certain elements, such as mercury. A single large drop of it can be forcefully split into many small spheres, which when brought close enough into proximity to one another magnetically cohere back together into a single mass. The one thing that prevents this is dust: when the surface of this quicksilver is burdened by even the tiniest particles of a substance that is not itself, it loses its central property of cohesiveness.

- Also consider the most precious of stones, the diamond. The purest and strongest of any natural occurring material, it sets the standard by which the hardness of all other minerals is measured—another example of simplicity as an agent of cohesiveness.
- Keeping in mind Leonardo da Vinci's admonition, "Simplicity is the ultimate sophistication," be mindful of what you buy in advance of baby's arrival. Most of what we think we need is an illusion conjured by our shop-happy culture, an alluring but costly response to the most natural of preparenting instincts— to nest. Radical but true, there is always time later to purchase what is needed, and in fact, waiting is a great way to begin developing the essential parenting tools of intuition, discernment and responsiveness to what's living in the moment. *You* will become the expert on your baby, discovering if she prefers sponge baths to baths in the plastic contraption, or if the sound of Velcro frightens him, or which baby sling you both like best.

- Spare yourself the pressure of believing you need the latest Quinny or Bugaboo stroller—or any other particular gadget or contraption for that matter. This materialist drive is so deeply a part of our enculturation that we slip into it without realizing it and before we know it we're more focused on baby *stuff* than on baby *building*. Let enriching your inner life take priority over refurnishing your house.

- The nursery itself can easily wait; it's time we outgrow our Victorian notion of The Baby's Room; indeed, the best place for baby in the first few years is close to you. You may choose to have a family bed; otherwise, a sidecar or a cradle by your bed will provide the closeness you both need for many months. So you have lots of time to move to a bigger place or convert the guest room. In fact, guest quarters are more important to have—along with someone to occupy them sometime in the early days or weeks. Whether it is a doula or your mother or your partner's mother or a friend, human companionship and help is invaluable—to cook, field extraneous phone calls, do laundry and fetch your water when you nurse.

- On helpers: It only qualifies as help if a helping visitor decreases anxiety, tension, and insecurity, and contributes to feelings of peacefulness, competence, and joy. This is no time to buckle under the pressure of someone else's need to feel needed and included—or worse, entertained! Nature designed the precious early postpartum weeks for slowing down to the languorous pace of new life, for falling in love with your baby, for unfolding the mother in you. Clearly discuss your needs and requests with Mom or Mom-in-Law or Jill-from-college. (And it's great practice: the ability to set authoritative, loving boundaries is going to come in handy on a daily basis for the next eighteen years.)

Resources

Michel Odent's Womb Ecology: wombecology.com.

APPPAH (Association for Prenatal & Perinatal Psychology and Health): www.birthpsychology.com

Environmental Working Group's list of cell phones: www.ewg.org/cellphone -radiation (This is an excellent site, worthy of your attention and support.)

Mercola article on EMFs in pregnancy—looks like some interesting links in there!: articles.mercola.com/sites/articles/archive/2009/04/30/Why-Where-You-Sleep-Matters-If-You-Want-a-Healthy-Baby.aspx

Aïvanhov, O. M (2000). *Golden rules for everyday life.* Fréjus, France: Prosveta.

Laura Uplinger's Wonders of the Womb website, where you'll find Womb Service: www.wondersofthewomb.com

Step Four

Empowered Birth—
The Ultimate
First Impression

Birthing for a Peaceful World

Childbirth is a decisive moment in development, a brief window of time when critical systems in the brain and body of both mother and baby organize in ways that will affect them lifelong. Of fundamental importance, as we consider birthing a generation of peacemakers, is the circuitry for oxytocin, the hormone of love and connection. Biochemical cascades triggered during an unimpeded mammalian labor and birth (and postpartum) establish in the baby enduring set points for his brain's self-regulating and social functions. These thresholds will to a great extent forecast how able this individual will be to respond to later influences—including parental, educational, and spiritual guidance—aimed at cultivating socially conscious attitudes and behaviors. How you birth matters for peace at many levels.

Each of us has had the experience of being a baby, and of being born. Birth is one of our most momentous embodied experiences. And even though we don't consciously remember this huge event in our lives, each of us carries the story of our birth etched like a pale watermark on our body and psyche—unconscious traces of somatic memory. The way you experienced your birth is how you tend to move through your life. For example, it isn't uncommon to see that the person born with the cord around his neck doesn't like tight collars or tight spots...the person pulled out with forceps resents being forced to do anything...the person born breech is always doing things backwards...the person born after an unusually fast labor has fears about things moving too quickly...the person born after an unusually slow labor has fears of getting stuck...the person born prematurely never feels quite ready for anything...the person born by cesarean can't quite finish things, or often needs to be rescued.[1]

This is an incomplete list—far too simplistic, and all focused on negative aspects of the birth experience. There are as many birth imprints as there are births and individuals: each of us comes into physical existence with our own uniqueness, and our own indiosyncratic ways in which the events of our birth inscribe patterns and tendencies. For example, some people born after their mother's labor was artificially induced are stubborn and will do things only on their own time, while others born after being induced just can't seem to get going on their own, and constantly need that nudging from the outside. Indeed, birth experiences often leave a trace of something that we both fear *and* gravitate to, since it's so familiar at such a fundamental, intangible level.

Who Starts Labor?

In the course of researching the onset of parturition (childbirth), endocrinologist Roger Smith and his team made a fascinating observation: pregnant Jewish women observing the fast of Yom Kippur, and thus (albeit temporarily) reducing the nutrient supply to their fetuses, show a peak in delivery rates that is not observed on Yom Kippur in nonfasting Bedouin women living in the same region.[2] Smith's team was studying the role of corticotropin-releasing hormone (CRH), a stress-related chemical, in starting labor; he posits that the stress of inadequate nutrition—even for that brief time—activates the fetal stress system, which involves production of CRH by the fetal brain. (Fetuses aren't always skilled at interpreting information, so the baby of a fasting Jewish mother wouldn't know that nutrition would resume after just one day—unless she made a conscious effort to communicate safety to him, which could have a protective effect.)

Pregnancy involves maintaining a balanced tension between estrogen (which tends to cause uterine contractions) and progesterone (which tends to relax the uterus), to maintain uterine quiescence until term. Even as they came to understand estrogen's role in the onset of parturition, researchers remained baffled by the nature of the switch—and whether it is in the fetus or in the mother—activating the placental estrogen secretion that ultimately tips the scales and kicks off labor. Studies have unraveled the involvement of CRH and fetal cortisol in the intricate parturition dynamic.

One finding of particular significance to parenting for peace is that researchers can predict likely preterm labor from looking at CRH levels *as early as sixteen weeks gestation.*[3] This reaches back to our discussion of inordinate stress, and the association between stress even in the earliest weeks of pregnancy and a greater likelihood of preterm labor. If we look at it from an adaptive perspective, we see a system perfectly designed to respond to environmental information about famine or danger in such a way as to optimize the outcome for the baby—in other words, to get the baby out of a suboptimal womb sooner rather than later. In the absence of an adaptive orientation to the maternal-fetal parturition dynamic, we are left with the prevailing mechanistic perspective that views preterm labor as something inexplicably malfunctioning in the mechanisms of late pregnancy and labor signaling, "a short-circuiting or overwhelming of the normal parturition cascade"[4] as one researcher calls it—a glitch at the end of the assembly line.

But data is pointing to a much more process-oriented model, which recognizes labor as an inherent element in the complexly interwoven tapestry of pregnancy—a long view that recognizes there are indications as early as four months gestation that forecast the timetable of parturition and the likelihood of preterm delivery.

Birth from Baby's Point of View

Almost without exception, books about birth are written to address the point of view of the mother, the midwife or doctor, and others involved in the process. Within the overflowing Labor & Birth shelves at the bookstore, the *baby's* experience of birth is mostly overlooked, with one notable exception— *Birth Without Violence*, which *Utne Reader* called "one of the twenty books that changed the world." Referring to the first impressions left by our birth experience, author and obstetrician Frederick Leboyer writes, "What futility to believe that so great a cataclysm will not leave its mark. Its traces are every-where—in the skin, in the bones, in the stomach, in the back. In our human folly. In our madness, our tortures, our prisons."[5]

Obstetrician David Cheek, a pioneer in the field of bodymind research, made a fascinating discovery when doing interviews under hypnosis with adults whom he had delivered: when he asked them to notice any sensations of head position in relation to the shoulders as they were being born, each ac-curately demonstrated the postural pattern of movement (e.g., neck and shoul-der rotation) they had enacted during delivery—as confirmed by the detailed notes Cheek had taken on their deliveries decades earlier![6] Our bodies remem-ber. And this body-borne memory is intimately entwined with our psyche.

A bleak demonstration of this reality comes from the extensive Scandina-vian research of Bertil Jacobson on teen suicide, revealing a strong association between the type of distressing birth event a person experienced and the method that person later used in suicide or suicide attempts. For instance, oxygen deprivation, such as having the cord tightly around the neck, correlated with suffocation or strangulation; "mechanical trauma," such as the use of for-ceps, was associated with attempts to self-destruct with instruments such as guns; drug addiction or overdose was associated with opiate or barbiturate medication given to the mother during labor.[7]

Leboyer vividly describes what the newborn experiences as she crosses the fateful threshold from the watery, weightless world of the womb into the world of gravity, air and embodiment. Referring to the epic internal transition that takes place in the newborn's respiratory and circulatory systems at birth, he writes, "Depending on whether this transition occurs slowly, gently—or bru-tally, in panic and terror—birth becomes a peaceful awakening…or a tragic one."

> Nature, they say, doesn't move forward in sudden leaps.
>
> Yet birth is just such a leap forward. An exchange of worlds, of levels.
>
> How can we resolve this contradiction? How does Nature make smooth a transition whose very essence is so violent?
>
> Very simply.
>
> Nature is a strict mother, but a loving one. We misunderstand her intentions; then we blame her for what follows.[8]

Disturbing Birth

Indeed, we humans with our fancy monkey wrenches often thwart Nature's elegant plan for birthing our babies. We've applied our Western brilliance toward vainly trying to foolproof a process that through centuries of human collective thought has terrified us. Nestled deep in our shared cultural psyche is the fear of the mother dying in childbirth, and right behind it is the fear of giving birth to a dead baby—both of which do occur, but extremely rarely. Nonetheless, childbirth and death have been unjustifiably entwined in our collective unconscious for many centuries; just think of all the legends, fairy tales, and movies featuring "The mother died in childbirth."

This fear of dead mothers and dead babies has been conflated into vague and not-so-vague fears of the birth experience itself. Every aspect of our cultural experience, including scenes from movies and television shows, bows to this fear, and then soothes us with the promise of salvation through technology—epidurals, Pitocin drips, fetal monitors, episiotomies, and c-sections. Yet our U.S. infant and maternal mortality rates are some of the highest in the developed world.[9]

The field of obstetrics rests on a younger foundation of research evidence than do other medical specialties. History has witnessed that with the rise of monotheistic, patriarchal religious and moral systems came the systematic devaluation and disavowal of all functions having to do with a woman's body and life cycle. So not only did the gynecological territory of the female anatomy in general become the poor stepchild in the world of medical research, obstetrics was particularly neglected, since pregnancy was the awkwardly prominent evidence that a woman had (gasp!) engaged in sex, which was taboo. We painted ourselves into a medically ignorant corner with our cultural sanitization of pregnancy (as in, "She's *expecting*").

In the mid-twentieth century, atop our relatively meager understanding of birth physiology arose—in admirable industrial fashion—the desire of hospital administrators for cost efficiency in tending to laboring patients. Thus was born in 1955 the notion of active management of labor, when Emmanuel Friedman developed the *partograph*—a chart that allowed obstetrical attendants to determine whether the progress of their patients' labor conformed to an ideal mathematical curve. Labors that lagged behind the ideal could be made to keep the prescribed pace with the use of oxytocic drugs (such as

Pitocin, a synthetic form of the body's own oxytocin, the hormone of human connection and contractions). The Friedman curve is designed to help physicians keep labor advancing along a "normal" route. A woman who fails to fall in step is considered to be having an "abnormal" labor, which can be made "normal" again with Pitocin. Feminist author Alice Adams suggests that sociologist Michel Foucault's analysis of "disciplined and docile bodies" that have been subjected to "anatomo-chronological schema of behavior," bears important implications for the principle of active management of labor: "First, the active management paradigm emphasizes physiological conformity, enforced by continuous monitoring and regulation of women's behavior and progress in labor. Active management is a practical expression of the profession's conviction that unregulated childbearing leads to social chaos."[10]

Electronic fetal monitoring (EFM), Pitocin induction, and cesarean section were designed for use in a very small number of cases, when extraordinary measures were called for (and they are indeed a blessing in a small percentage of anomalous cases). But once the equipment was bought, paid for and sitting in relative disuse, there came the inexorable impulse to begin using it routinely, for all pregnant women and in all births, which is where the trouble began. Complications from any of these interventions range from annoying (itching) to life-threatening (high blood pressure, blood clot, heart attack) in the mother, and include disturbances in fetal heart rate as well as a variety of complications in the newborn. A third of women who receive epidurals early in labor, *along with their babies*, develop a fever of up to 103-104. Because the physician cannot be sure the baby's fever isn't evidence of an infection—rather than simply an artifact of the epidural—invasive diagnostic tests are required for the newborn (septic workup, including a spinal tap and blood draw) and—most insidious of all, in light of our overarching theme of connection or disconnection—the newborn is placed in an isolette in the nursery, away from Mom. He will stay there, receiving preventative intravenous antibiotic treatment, until his or her cultures (i.e., a repeat spinal tap and blood draw) show no infection, usually three days.[11]

It bears noting here, given our thematic focus on fostering the capacities of peace, that a team from UCLA who followed 4,269 men born in the same Copenhagen hospital found that the most potent risk factor combination predicting violent criminality eighteen years later was birth complications (including invasive medical procedures) together with maternal rejection[12]—

which is how a newborn would primitively experience the trauma of separation from her, regardless of the medical circumstances requiring it.

Routine use of EFM was widely instituted in the 1970s in the absence of proof of clinical effectiveness. EFM has in fact never been shown to do what it set out to do, which was to improve birth outcomes. In 1987 the prestigious medical journal *Lancet* reported that the routine use of EFM "had no measurable effect on death or illness of infants or mothers" and even worse, that it "was associated with a higher rate of Cesarean deliveries, which increases surgical risks to mothers."[13] Yet twenty-three years later, in the absence of evidence to contradict this damning conclusion, the vast majority of births in America involve electronic fetal monitoring. In our current climate of malpractice litigiousness the presumed medical groupthink is that if practitioners use all the available technology it protects them from accusations of negligence—even when much of the available technology has proved ineffective or even counterproductive in normal births. And in response to the glaring question, "If EFM doesn't work, why haven't obstetricians abandoned it?" birth educator and author Henci Goer notes that doctors and hospital administrators aren't exempt from our cultural fascination with high tech equipment, and are as susceptible to slick marketing of the latest innovations as any other gadgetry enthusiast: "EFM is expensive, scientific, and complicated. It simply *had* to be better than putting a stethoscope or even a Doptone—the little hand-held ultrasonic device—to the tummy."

And the consumers—parents bringing their children into the world—are just as enthusiastic. (I have to wonder how many of them—like myself when our son was born—realize that the internal form of EFM requires that an electrode, in the form of a tiny screw, be stuck into their baby's scalp.) It has been suggested that our wholesale embrace of EFM taps into our delight over anything we can see on a screen or a monitor, on which in this case, writes anthropologist Elizabeth Cartwright, "the intimate world of life in the womb is transcribed into a visible form....The hidden is revealed."[14] Rather than attending to the laboring woman, all eyes are on the monitor and the heart rate strip it churns out. Cartwright points out that the mother's movement is restricted to produce the clearest and most interpretable strip; her natural motions are not allowed—"it is 'interference,' it is 'noise.' If the mother should try to move, the strip will show that motion and a nurse or physician will look into the room [from their usual position at the bank of EFM monitors at the nurses' station] to make sure the unwarranted movement is stopped." The doctors and nurses talk not about the experiences or conditions of the laboring mother, but rather, "the quality of the strip: *We need to see some accelerations* [of fetal heart tones], or *If this strip doesn't start to look better we're going to need to consider a c-section.* It is the strip, at least in part, that needs to be cured."[15]

(Could it be that we still harbor, deep in the shadows of our collective unconscious, a distaste for and avoidance of direct contact with a woman's body—especially one ripe to bursting with a child—and that the allure of machines that allow doctors and nurses to keep their distance is more compelling than the reams of data declaring those machines a failure?)

If the EFM strip pronounces that things aren't progressing apace, Pitocin is dripped into the woman's bloodstream, eliciting contractions so powerful, so seizing, that an epidural virtually always follows. Ironically, epidurals slow labor, and increase the likelihood of instrumental delivery (forceps, vacuum) and can also increase the likelihood of a surgical (cesarean) delivery, especially in first-time mothers.[16] One of the reasons is simply that after an epidural, a laboring woman is usually confined to bed—cannot stand or walk, both of which are gravity-leveraging ways to unite Nature and the woman's body in their cooperative birthing task. (Also, 25 percent of babies born with epidurals have difficulty in quickly, easily and smoothly latching on for breastfeeding; and epidurals partially interfere with the release of oxytocin that normally occurs at birth, which can affect bonding and the mother's falling-in-love feelings toward her baby.)[17]

This is what cultural anthropologist Robbie Davis-Floyd refers to as the One-Two Punch of the cultural management of American birth, as "biomedicine mutilates the natural rhythms of birth by multiple interventions in every phase" (Punch One)—withholding food and drink from laboring women, which weakens them; administering pain-relieving drugs that slow labor; making the woman lie flat on her back (compressing her aorta) during labor and birth and thereby reducing the flow of blood and oxygen to the baby—and then (Punch Two) introduces "solutions" to the problems they have caused—inserting IVs to administer the fluids the woman is not allowed to drink; injecting into the IV drugs to speed up labors slowed by drugs that relieve pain, which further inhibit blood and oxygen to the baby; electronic fetal monitoring of the baby's level of distress, which will rise as its blood and oxygen supply drops with the mother restrained flat on her back, culminating in the delivery of a medically distressed baby by forceps or cesarean section, and a vaguely bitter feeling of incompetence and ineptitude within the mother.[18] This in turn carries further consequences for her mothering: the shadow of feeling unfit and worthless is an impediment when setting out to parent for peace.

The steadily rising rate of c-sections is due in part to the perception of control, predictability, and even convenience conferred by the technology of surgical birth. And what chance do mainstream women have to make informed decisions to the contrary, when the president himself of the American Academy of Obstetrics and Gynecology stated repeatedly that elective c-sections are safer for the baby and "nearly as safe" for the mother?[19] First used as a means of saving the fetus of a dead mother, cesarean is childbirth by major abdominal surgery. For those women who consider it as the easy way around labor and delivery, Davis-Floyd shares the notes from her own medical chart describing the c-section she had:

> A transverse skin incision was made sharply with a knife and carried down through the subcutaneous layers until the fascia was reached. The fascia was sharply incised with the knife and the incision carried laterally. The rectus muscles were separated in the middle and retracted. The parietal peritoneum was grasped with clamps and incised, exposing the abdominal cavity. The visceral peritoneum overlying the lower uterine segment was then grasped, incised, and dissected sharply and bluntly creating a bladder flap over the lower uterine segment. The lower uterine segment was then incised sharply with a knife and the incision extended bluntly. The infant was delivered from the cephalic position as pressure was exerted on the uterine fundus. The infant was briefly placed on the mother's upper chest and then handed to the father to be taken to the nursery for further care. The placenta was manually extracted and appeared intact. The uterus was then externalized from the abdominal cavity and explored for any remaining placental fragments. The uterus was then replaced in the abdominal cavity and the defect was repaired in a single layer closure.[20]

Nancy Wainer Cohen's classic exposé of the cesarean epidemic, *Silent Knife*, included an eleven-year-long study that found the rate of death from c-section was twenty-six times higher than from vaginal delivery.[21] Other studies have put the risk of death after cesarean at two to four times greater than that of vaginal birth. Nonlethal risks to the mother following a cesarean include negative psychological and emotional impacts, higher rate of secondary infertility, infection, excessive bleeding requiring a transfusion, injuries to surrounding organs, and abnormal blood clotting.[22] Cesarean birth also poses a statistically higher mortality risk to the baby,[23] as well as surgical cuts, respiratory problems, breastfeeding impairment, and a significantly elevated risk of developing asthma by the age of eight.[24] Author Andrea Henkart, in anonymous personal conversations with three obstetricians, was told of horror stories about colleagues accidentally amputating fingers from a newborn's hand, or accidentally breaking bones while surgically removing the infant.[25]

Preliminary research suggests that babies born by planned cesarean may experience changes to the DNA pool in their white blood cells, possibly related to altered stress levels during this method of delivery. The findings would help explain why c-section babies are more susceptible to immunological diseases such as diabetes, asthma or leukemia than those born by normal vaginal deliveries. "Our results provide the first pieces of evidence that early so-called epigenetic programming of the immune system during birth may have a role to play," says researcher Mikael Norman at Sweden's Karolinska Institute.[26]

What's rarely mentioned as a negative consequence of surgical childbirth is the interruption it inserts into the securely connected relationship between an infant and a mother who is coping with post-surgical recovery that is at best uncomfortable and at worst debilitating and even sometimes requiring hospitalization—together with the fact that c-section babies often have more trouble breastfeeding.

In the face of all these backlashing technologies—including reproductive ones like IVF—I find it difficult not to think of Aldous Huxley's dystopian portrait (*Brave New World*) of an era in which we can bypass the messy business of women and wombs altogether. (From screen-based pablum entertainment to ubiquitous mood medications to asexual human reproduction, how eerily prescient Huxley was, writing in 1932!) What is happening to the valuation of our own intricately calibrated fetal monitor—our inner knowing? Davis-Floyd observes that our unquestioned embrace of technology—and the myth that technology will improve every aspect of our lives, and confer a sense of order and control over processes that quite normally and healthily *are chaotic*— has rendered us unable to trust our own resources. "Normal" reproduction is seen as a sort of "traditional throwback—dangerous, risky, random... Because we so deeply trust technology, we cannot trust nature anymore. Natural reproduction, when successful, becomes a special category: lucky."[27]

With machinery handling the jobs of imaging, assessing and predicting fetal wellbeing and labor progress, the clinical exam that features human hands connected to a human brain and heart has been rendered quaintly obsolete. We've now graduated a generation's worth of medical students groomed not to examine, engage and encourage laboring women, but to survey the strip, tighten the strap and adjust the drip. That the leading American and Canadian obstetrical organizations decreed that intermittent listening for fetal heart sounds with the Dopler is equivalent to or even preferred over continuous electronic monitoring[28] may be moot: today's doctors don't really know how to do that, because machines took over those duties for them around the time when they themselves were born!

The incongruity between the collected evidence and the practices persisting in hospitals across the country is one of the stark realities of an obstetrical industry that is as market-driven as other for-profit industries. The preceding litany of complicating birth interventions make sense, suggests somatic psychotherapist Robert Leverant, "only if you 'follow the money' and not the baby."[29]

Or the mother. While the early twenty-first century finds the U.S. crowned with the mightiest of technological achievements, and the rate of innovations soaring, we have failed on two fundamental measures of a society's wellbeing: in 2011, our infant mortality rate soars above that of 45 other countries in the developed world, and American women die from childbirth in the U.S. at a rate that puts us 39th in that ranking, behind countries where cesarean rates are lower and vaginal births after previous cesareans are the norm rather than the exception. When one looks at that sorrowful list of countries and their maternal mortality rates (MMR), something even bleaker jumps off the page: while most developed countries' MMR has dropped over the past generation, ours has increased—*by more than any other of them.* The percentage rise in the rate of birthing mothers who die in the U.S. is comparable to that of only a handful of other countries—those that fall way down the list on MMR rates, such as South Africa (125th), Namibia (156th), Malawi (179th) and Afghanistan (181st and last).[30] In a similarly bleak indicator of American maternal-fetal wellbeing, the March of Dimes in 2010 again awarded the U.S. a D on its prematurity report card;[31] one in eight babies is premature, a rate higher than for most developed countries.

Research data overwhelmingly confirms what five countries with some of the lowest infant mortality rates know: in Japan, Finland, Sweden, Norway and Denmark, midwives provide the primary health care in over 70 percent of births.[32]

Joining Forces with Birth

The hallmark of midwifery care is its orientation to birth as a normal, healthy process that happens for each woman differently and according to her—and her baby's—unique bodily rhythms. Modern obstetrics frames birth (as well as pregnancy) as a medical event calling for routine interventions and a standardization of the mode and timetable of labor. In *Pushed: The Painful Truth About Childbirth and Modern Maternity Care*, which provides a compellingly vivid portrait of each model, investigative journalist Jennifer Block writes:

> The old debate over "natural childbirth" seems quaint at this point. I don't have much use for the term, which has become synonymous with vaginal birth. What's happened to normal birth—what *is* normal birth? Not simply nonsurgical birth…. Not simply unmedicated, either. It is natural, after all, to want to alleviate pain. The term I find most useful to describe normal birth is *physiological* birth: labor begins and progresses spontaneously, the woman is free to move about for the duration, and she pushes in advantageous, intuitive positions.
>
> We know that if we take our otherwise healthy patient in LDRP [Labor, Delivery, Recovery and Postpartum], release her cuffs and bands, unplug the probes and sensors, and turn off the Pitocin and morphine, 9 times out of 10 her body will birth a baby with minimal interference or injury, especially if she has the one-on-one support of a skilled caregiver. We know this from the experience of other countries, but also from studies of American women who choose to birth with certified midwives in birthing centers or in their own homes.[33]

In a recent study of five thousand low-risk women who experienced planned home births, only 2.7 percent received Pitocin, 2.1 percent had episiotomies, and 3.7 percent had cesareans. Low-risk women giving birth in hospitals have far higher rates of intervention and surgery, yet the same number of neonatal deaths.[34] The World Health Organization is pointed in its conclusion: "Midwives are the most appropriate primary health care provider to be assigned to the care of normal birth."[35] Unhampered by the tethering belt of an electronic fetal monitor, the laboring mother within a midwifery model at home or a birthing center can move as her body's impulses call her to move. Without the metronomic electronic *beeps* of her baby's amplified heartbeat piercing the peacefulness of the tranquil room, the only sound may be her wide-open breathing and the tones of her own primal, interior voice.

During an unmedicated birth, natural opiates are released by the laboring mother, which not only help facilitate a kind of transcendent alliance with the momentous physical processes of birthing, but which also mediate important fetal and newborn neurodevelopment—a process inhibited by the use of anesthesia. Stress during pregnancy (many months earlier) hinders the effectiveness of natural opiate production during labor: Curt Sandman's prenatal research team found that chronic pregnancy stress led to a disregulation of pleasure- and stress-hormone responses and reduced sensitivity of opiate receptors— meaning, a laboring woman's own internal pain-relief system would not be up to par. Thus, Sandman's team found that a pregnant woman's stress levels months earlier could actually *predict* her use of anesthesia during labor![36]

Obstetrician and researcher Michel Odent suggests that the best way to join forces with birth is to remember that we are mammals, and the need of all mammals to birth smoothly and successfully is the same threefold need we (like other mammals) require to fall sleep: safe privacy, quiet, and low light. The higher thinking centers need to be excused from the laboring woman's experience, and she needs to be allowed to go to that inner space of her deepest primitive callings, where her bodymind's instinctive knowing can do what it knows how to do. The most common way to disturb birth is to do *too much talking* (even the most supportive coaching affirmations). When the neocortex (the area of the brain that processes language) becomes engaged, many aspects of the physiologically brilliant birthing process are impeded; thinking requires adrenaline, which prevents the necessary levels of oxytocin required to dilate the cervix. How many cases of failure to progress are caused simply by too much talking, even the most well-meaning of inquiries such as "How are you doing?" Ever try falling asleep while someone is asking you questions? ("Are you almost asleep, sweetheart?") Risking the wrath of many in the natural birth movement, Odent points out that sometimes our best intentions can be counterproductive to a smooth birthing process:

> It may not always be best for a woman to have her partner there. Certain men have a beneficial presence, while others only slow labor

down....I think of one incident, when a woman couldn't seem to get beyond eight centimeters' dilation; when her husband left the room for a short time to rest, their baby was born. Though this woman had told us that she wanted her husband present, her body was saying the reverse....Men sometimes find it hard to observe, accept, and understand a woman's instinctive behavior during childbirth. Instead, they often try to keep her from slipping out of a rational, self-controlled state. It is not mere coincidence that in all traditional societies, women in labor are assisted not by men, but by other women who have had children themselves.[37]

Birthing at home with a midwife (the choice of about 2 percent of Americans) affords a woman and her partner the greatest freedom to choose the atmosphere they find most secure, nurturing and conducive to the birth they want. But many of us have been so irretrievably enculturated to believe in the need for hospital technology nearby that being at home could actually work against that biological imperative to feel completely safe. With some research, it is possible to find doctors who subscribe to the nonintrusive baby-catcher aspect of their role, allowing a mother the space and time to labor as her body instructs her, push as her impulses mandate, and open as her body will naturally (all of which do lead in the vast majority of cases to a safer, shorter, less complicated, more satisfying labor and birth).

Birth facilities that are committed to this kind of mother-baby-centered approach have far lower levels of complications at all levels, including cesareans: at The Farm Midwifery Center in Tennessee, led by world-renowned midwife Ina May Gaskin, the rate is 2-3 percent; at France's Pitiviers Clinic when Michel Odent was the resident surgeon, it was 6-7 percent—compared to the average rate in American hospitals, 30 percent and rising; and in private hospitals in Venezuela and Brazil, where the c-section rate is upwards of 95 percent.

Birth from the Mother's Point of View

Childbirth anthropologist Robbie Davis-Floyd set out to solve an important puzzle as she came to recognize that there had to be something other than rational logic at work in the vast majority of Americans who trust and believe in the relatively higher degree of safety and effectiveness provided by a hospital birth, despite all evidence to the contrary.[38] For example, take the counter-productive yet standard lithotomy birthing position:

> Despite years of effort on the part of childbirth activists, including many obstetricians, the majority of American women still give birth lying flat on their backs. This position is physiologically dysfunctional. It compresses major blood vessels, lowering the mother's circulation and thus the baby's oxygen supply. It increases the need for forceps because it both narrows the pelvic outlet and ensures that the baby, who must follow the curve of the birth canal, quite literally will be born heading upward, against gravity.[39]

In Davis-Floyd's landmark book *Birth as an American Rite of Passage*, she offers a compelling explanation for the seemingly counterrational embrace of our copious interventions in birth, which bears profound relevance for a generation of peacemakers geared toward healing culture and fostering a sustainable status quo. She explains how all societies mark major life transitions by putting on display their core values and beliefs in the form of a ritual. Any such ritual that moves participants from one social status or stage—think bar mitzvahs, confirmations, graduations, weddings, and of course, birth—is called a *rite of passage*. Through these rites of passage, the society makes sure that the symbols and meanings experienced by the participants reinforce the core beliefs and values of their society.[40]

Participants in such rituals are frequently in an altered state of mind, whether through music, dance, chanting, patterned breathing, meditation, mind-altering substances or, as in the case of labor and birth, the potent bio-chemicals flowing through mother and baby—and even father. The altered state makes participants highly receptive to symbols, which are prominently featured during ritual and which are imprinted on the image-oriented right brain. Once she understood all this, Davis-Floyd got it: "Could this explain the standardization of American birth? I believe the answer is yes."

> By making the naturally transformative process of birth into a cultural rite of passage, a society can ensure that its basic values will be transmitted to the three new members born out of the birth process: the new baby, the woman reborn into the new social role of mother, and the man reborn as father. The new mother especially must be very

clear about these values, as she is generally the one primarily responsible for teaching them to her children, who will be society's new
members and the guarantors of its future.[41]

Davis-Floyd identifies various ways the values of our modern technocracy
are enacted and reinforced in standardized hospital birth. (The term *technocracy*
refers to a society driven by an ideology of technological progress. In a technocracy, we constantly seek to improve upon nature by altering and controlling
it through technology.) She writes, referring to standard hospital protocol and
interventions, "These procedures are profoundly symbolic, communicating
messages concerning our culture's deepest beliefs about the necessity for control
of natural processes." She refers to how a laboring woman has a similar psychophysiological profile as those involved in religious ecstatic ritual, and how
this neuroreceptive state typically functions to impress and reinforce the importance of technology, order and precision in our lives as Americans.

> Consider the visual and kinesthetic images that the laboring woman
> experiences—herself in bed, in a hospital gown, staring up at an IV
> pole, bag and cord, staring down at a steel bed and huge belts encir-
> cling her waist and staring sideways at moving displays on a large ma-
> chine. Her entire sensory field conveys one overwhelming message
> about our culture's deepest values and beliefs: technology is supreme,
> and you are utterly dependent upon it.[42]

There is a strong sense of symbiosis, Davis-Floyd finds, between the woman
and the technology, in large part due to how it "removes the chaos and fear
from women's perceptions of birth." And pain, let's not forget the removal of
pain. There is a widespread assumption on the part of today's technomodern
woman that unmedicated childbirth is a form of senseless suffering, as outmoded as shoulder pads, best banished with a blithe wave of the epidural
wand. Three out of four American women elect to receive epidural anesthesia,
perhaps unaware of what many scholars recognize as the cascade of interventions that this can set in motion.

Since epidurals typically slow down labor, it leads to the use of Pitocin to
augment it (thus the standard order heard in maternity ward nursing stations
every hour across the nation, "Let's Pit her"—one of many disquieting facets

of hospital births revealed in Ricki Lake's eye-opening film, *The Business of Being Born*). And this cascade often happens in reverse: if the woman's labor isn't progressing to the Friedman norm, she'll be given Pitocin to "get things going." Unlike the body's natural contraction-stimulating hormone oxytocin, Pitocin is infamous for bringing on contractions far more intense and frequent than would be natural—*slamming* and *relentless* are words commonly used by women to describe them. Even women who had initially desired to birth without anesthesia buckle under the onslaught and (understandably) ask for an epidural. And as we saw above, this significantly increases the likelihood of forceps, suction or even a c-section. Not long before this is going to print, the respected Cochrane Library reports findings from eight randomized studies of over a thousand low-risk women that while Pitocin shortened labor by an average of two hours, it did not achieve its stated purpose—note the irony here, please—of reducing c-sections or increasing the number of unassisted vaginal deliveries (i.e., without forceps or vacuum).[43]

One birth intervention that seems virtually taken for granted is the episiotomy, in which the vaginal opening is enlarged by cutting the perineum with scissors. It is the most common surgical procedure in the U.S., performed in 96 percent of U.S. births, compared, for example, to just 5 percent of Scandinavian births.[44] Its purported benefit is to make delivery easier and prevent tearing, although many experts agree that a) any small, jagged tearing that occurs naturally in the perineum heals more effectively than the artificially cut episiotomy site, and b) episiotomies can actually *cause* tearing.[45] Routinizing the episiotomy fits neatly into Davis-Floyd's technoritualized model: it displays our culture's tendency toward impatience while also expressing "the value and importance of one of the technocracy's most fundamental markers—the straight line."[46] Henkart quotes the opinion of a Dutch midwife who sees episiotomy as "the last word by doctors that 'you really cannot do this without our help'."[47]

Davis-Floyd frames all this as the "cyborgification" of childbirth (with cyborgs being symbiotic fusions of organic life and technological systems), and suggests that in the name of this progress, "women and fetuses are endangered and a primal, intrinsically embodied act that women themselves used to perform is turned into a series of technological procedures performed on them."[48] And the sad irony is that although most American women are raised on the belief in the greater safety of a hospital birth, and put implicit trust in the body-as-machine principles of modern obstetrics, it is not uncommon for a woman, following a technologically managed birth that she welcomed, to feel a kind of pall…of some vague…sense of…*having been cheated*? Alice Adams offers an intensely personal exploration of this critical conundrum:

> I knew that I had lost something essential to my survival, but it was an unnamable loss….If anything had gone wrong with my labor or the baby's vital signs, all the proper equipment and expertise would have been immediately available.
>
> And yet something *had* gone terribly wrong. My absorption into the ordinary medical machinery marked the moment when I began to lose the sensation of being inside my body, a sensation I recognized only when it was gone. The progressive merging of my body with the machinery meant that, whenever and wherever the body-machine overlap occurred, I lost perception and control. Amniotomy, fetal monitor, I.V., anesthetic, episiotomy, forceps: I retreated from my body more with every intervention, until I could no longer connect my consciousness to the abject body that contained it.[49]

Could this unnamable loss—having to do with an essential disconnection of self from self during this momentous experience called birth—have contributed to the postpartum depression Adams suffered? I believe so, absolutely. With all sense of the sacredness of birth eclipsed by the intensely secular, mechanized efficiency of medicalized obstetrics, we suffer losses of many intangible kinds at the level of soul. Childbirth at its optimum is a profound initiation, a rite of passage, a sacred doorway into a new level of experience.[50] I believe that all women, consciously or not, participate in a collective knowing about the stunning, transformative potential that childbirth offers us, a faint and haunting collective memory of the empowerment and profound initiation we might claim in the birthing of our babies. But instead, as Davis-Floyd has so thoroughly researched, the majority of women have a birth experience that is demoralizing and dispiriting—not an ideal milestone in parenting for peace.

> When I see the entire obstetrical staff of a given unit hanging out in the hall staring at the computerized monitor banks, instead of hanging in with the women in labor, rubbing their backs and holding their

hands, I want to scream that this is wrong, this is a distortion, a per-version, of what we could have become.[51]

What we could have become. Let us not be saying those words fifty years from now, or twenty years from now! Let us embrace the unequaled opportu-nity offered us at birth to allow our children to continue on their upward spi-raling course of wellbeing. Let us claim with determination and clarity that window of experience through which lifelong neurophysiological potentials are shaped. Quiet confidence in one's unique convictions, the will to chart an original course, the strength to challenge the status quo—all this will be re-quired of Generation Peace, and the imprinting first impression of birth is an auspicious moment to actively demonstrate these qualities for your newly ar-riving child.

When Cesarean Is the Way You Birth

It may be that despite all of your enlightened intentions, your self-inquiry, your loving preparations for a natural birth, you do end up having a cesarean. It is helpful to maintain enough flexibility in your consciousness to allow for this possibility, lest it deal a disempowering blow to your soul. Midwife Pam England, author of the excellent book *Birthing from Within*, wrestled for years toward an answer to the question people continually asked her (maven of conscious childbirth!), "Why did you have a cesarean?" She finally came to believe, "In the moment a Cesarean birth (or any event) happens, no one can know all the forces which converged to create that event."[52] (One very prac-tical way to exercise your continued empowered involvement in how you give birth in this circumstance—and ideally you have this conversation with your care provider well in advance—is a recommendation that comes from Ina May Gaskin: specify that you want your uterus to be sutured closed in two layers.[53])

There may be some grieving to do, some making sense of it—or not—and just allowing yourself to authentically feel whatever you feel about it. And while it's a reflexively human impulse to place blame when we're feeling loss or pain, it's not a healing place to go with the energy of a birth that didn't unfold as you'd envisioned or wished. Within her important chapter "How to Give *Birth* if You Need a Cesarean," England wisely counsels, "It's over-simplified to blame or praise any individual or isolated event for how a birth turns out. Our challenge is to live with ambiguity, embrace the birth that happened, and move on with our family into the future."[54]

If your future leads you to a subsequent pregnancy, however, you do have more choice than our current medical climate would suggest, regarding whether to automatically have another cesarean. The VBAC (vaginal birth after cesarean) movement began in 1970 and peaked in1996, when 28 percent of women with prior c-sections gave birth vaginally. The research comparing VBACs with repeat cesarean continued to mount and it all agreed: VBAC trials (meaning attempting a normal vaginal labor, whether or not a cesarean is ultimately performed) were safer for mothers (with transverse lower-uterine incisions) and equally safe for babies; and nearly 80 percent of women who tried VBAC were able to give birth vaginally.[55]

A 1995 position statement—supported by extensive published research evidence—from the American College of Obstetricians and Gynecologists (ACOG) encouraging VBAC and recommending limiting repeat cesareans to those that were medically necessary seemed to ensure that VBAC would remain an option for women. But in a classic retrogressive, maintain-the-status-quo backlash, it took only a few intervening years for medico-legal and economic forces to swoop in and slam the door shut on this choice for women. (Hmmm, that's a frightening thematic specter…) The evidence didn't change (and indeed was largely omitted from later ACOG position statements) but the recommendations did, and according to Ina May Gaskin—whose chapter on VBAC is a must-read if you are hoping for one—"Sadly, the newest ACOG recommendations effectively close the door to VBAC to most women. For them it might as well be 1970, when few U.S. physicians conceded that women facing repeat cesareans ought to have a choice in the matter."[56] (ACOG issued a new position statement in July of 2010 backpedaling on its former restrictive VBAC guidelines, but many birth advocates feel it will do little to change a decade of entrenched physician and hospital policy, or to reopen VBAC access to most women.)[57]

Ironically enough, given this retrogressive effacement of VBAC, the woman who had the first successful cesarean, in 1500—successful because both mother and baby survived—went on to deliver six more babies vaginally, including twins! Gaskin outlines the impressive VBAC rates at her Farm Midwifery Center, and also mentions the Amish women she knows who've had a cesarean for their first baby and gone on to have twelve, thirteen VBACs without complication. She also offers practical advice for those women wanting to pursue VBAC—a richly viable path to take when you understand the territory: 1) choose a caregiver who has a VBAC rate of 70 percent or more* (who will be knowledgeable enough to make sure, for example, that your placenta is not overlying your existing uterine scar); 2) do not use synthetic oxytocin, Cytotec, or other prostoglandins to induce or augment labor, since the collected evidence strongly suggests it is *these* that increase the risk of uterine rupture; 3) keep vaginal exams to a minimum, which is possible with skilled practitioners who can closely estimate dilation by observing your breathing and body language; and 4) avoid an epidural, especially early in a VBAC labor. Last but definitely not least, counsels Gaskin, "spend your pregnancy loving your uterus and your baby. I mean this literally. Positive energy makes a good birth outcome more likely, so go for it."[58]

Birth on the Brain

As with sex, the brain, not the vagina, is command central for a successful birthing experience. As I mentioned above, during an unmedicated birth, a woman's brain is designed to pour out natural opiates. But you'll recall that the robust pain-relieving action of these natural opiates is blunted if a woman has been under consistent stress during her pregnancy, making pregnancy stress a double whammy for the baby: bad for fetal brain development during pregnancy *and* during birth, since it increases the likelihood of anesthetic drug use.

Contrary to what most women in labor are told by doctors, drugs injected into the spine do cross the placenta: epidural effects on the baby revolve primarily around maternal hypotension and can result in reduced circulation, which may lead to fetal depression or a "sleepy" baby, just one of the myriad effects in the early-mentioned cascade of interventions and complications that often follows epidurals.[59]

Among the many unintended effects of birth interventions on children, a new study has identified Pitocin as a "significant risk factor" for developing

---

* Meaning, of all his or her patients with previous cesareans, at least 70 percent of them attempt VBAC with subsequent pregnancies.

later ADHD,[60] and researchers are currently exploring Pitocin induction and epidural as possible factors in the complex causal tapestry involved in autism.[61] Physician and primal health researcher Michel Odent has adopted a revealing new lens by looking at the central feature of conditions such as autism—what he terms "an impaired capacity to love." When he used this novel perspective from which to survey a wide range of supposedly disparate research—on juvenile violent criminality, teen suicide, and autism—he found something striking: "[W]hen researchers explored the background of people who have expressed some sort of impaired capacity to love—either love of oneself or love of others—they always detected risk factors in the period surrounding birth."[62]

Odent suggests that up until now in our human history, it has been evolutionarily advantageous to develop the capacity for aggression. How best to do that? Make birth more difficult! He points out that this was well known in such warrior cultures as Sparta, where they made it a point to disturb the natural birth and postpartum process, knowing it would result in more aggression later in life. Given the violent demands of their world, they deliberately cultivated in their new citizens an "impaired capacity to love."

But today's world poses very different demands: its sophisticated complexities call for a robust capacity to love. Whatever evolutionary survival advantages difficult birth might have conferred in the past are not only no longer useful, they may be our undoing. The challenges faced by coming generations will require a level of cooperative interdependence never yet seen on a large population scale in human history. Just as the paleontologist and priest Teilhard de Chardin predicted about our techno-united world, now is the moment when we need to cultivate and harness the energies of love. The lasting first impressions at birth play a fundamental part in that cultivation.

"Birth's Epilogue": A Secret Key to Peace and Joy!

We tend to consider birth finished once the baby has emerged, but during the third stage of labor—between when the baby is born and the baby's placenta is delivered—mother and baby undergo massive, life-shaping transitions that have major implications for Generation Peace. A full discussion of the hormonal complexities of the third stage of labor is beyond the scope of this book, but here's one factoid that should get your attention: today's typical "active management of the third stage"—in which the cord is clamped directly after the baby's birth—can deprive a newborn of up to *one half* of his rightful blood volume![63] Rather that being redistributed as needed to the baby's newly functioning lungs and internal organs, this elixir of life—impeded by the cord clamp from its intended purpose as a gentle transfusion to the baby—ends up discarded along with the placenta. Once again, our medical good intentions have yielded suboptimal yet widely accepted outcomes. Family physician Sarah Buckley—whose book *Gentle Birth, Gentle Mothering* beautifully outlines the hormonal complexities of labor and birth, including the third stage—says that during this important time, "when mother and baby meet for the first time, the gap between our instincts and genetic code, and our culture's usual birthing practices, is especially wide."

She tells the story of a woman whose homebirth featured respectfully quiet attendants, low light, plenty of warmth—all those factors needed by the mammalian brain to labor and birth smoothly. But as soon as the baby was born, everyone went back to their normal ways of interacting, including the mother. As the room came alive and bustled with congratulations and festivity, the mother's neurohormones abruptly changed course, and she went "out of labor": her uterus didn't expel the placenta, and she had to be transported to the hospital.

Even in the most natural, nonintervention births, there is the tendency to forget that even after the baby has been delivered, the mother *is still in labor*! As Buckley points out about the third stage:

> From a hormonal perspective, we could say that mother and baby are more "in labor" than ever at this time. The hormonal peaks enjoyed by mother and baby after birth reflect ongoing labor processes and adaptations that are crucial for the survival of both. Further, this hormonal situation is unique, and will never again occur for this mother and her baby, representing our best (and most evolved) opportunity to ensure successful attachment and breastfeeding and therefore species survival.[64]

Birth as an Ecstatic Rite of Passage

The natural potential for birth to encompass ecstatic experience can be harnessed, through the principle of presence, to invite a true rite of passage into

new levels of empowerment for both mother and baby. Davis-Floyd writes a
vivid description of such an experience with the birth of her own second child,
her daughter:

> Without any pre-plan, I simply gave up and surrendered to the over-
> whelming force of the contractions. Until that moment, I had been
> struggling to maintain myself as separate from the pain, to back away
> from it somehow, or at least to do something about it—to chant with
> it, dance with it, breathe with it—*anything* but let it be. Suddenly I
> just let that effort go. I completely gave up, and I said to the pain,
> "Take me, I'm yours." Then a miracle happened. I felt that I, body
> and soul, *became* the pain, and once there was no more separation be-
> tween me and the pain, there was no more pain! I lay there on the
> bed, utterly relaxed, breathing softly, in total peace. I could hear the
> midwives whispering, "Good, that's really good." And that was, for
> me, one of the most important life-lessons of this birth—the value of
> yielding, of complete surrender.…As Elizabeth Noble puts it, "Resis-
> tance to the pain is the pain."[65]

As described by renowned birth educator Sheila Kitzinger:

> One is swept away like a little boat at sea in a great storm of exultant
> emotions and a tremendous sweep of physical energy. The body takes
> over in what seems a wholly marvelous way. It kneads and squeezes;
> contraction follows contraction powerfully and with precision. In-
> deed, in spite of the strength and the relentless force of its action there
> is a delicate accuracy about its workings at this time. We can only be
> in awe and deliver ourselves over, in faith, to this wonderful thing—
> the female body at the work of creation.[66]

Let us indeed "deliver ourselves"—and our coming generation—over not just
to the female body in its wisdom, but to Life itself and its elegantly efficient
birthing system. Yes, most of us have been baptized in technology, so let us embrace the blessings of our modern brilliance, which was originally meant to bring
freedom. Nothing has the power to control us once we can name the players
and the game, once we can free ourselves from the prevailing fear-based group

think and become capable of making choices that are in the best peacemaking interests of ourselves, our children, and the vibrant future of humanity.

──────── PRINCIPLES TO PRACTICE ────────

Presence – I can think of few more potent opportunities to discover and practice advanced dimensions of this principle than during labor and birth. Robbie Davis-Floyd, in describing how she charted a new rapport with presence during her second labor (a home VBAC), compares it to swimming a marathon, noting that the champions "don't count the distance. They enter a timeless dimension, where this stroke is all there is. This stroke, and this one, and then this one. I am in that timeless world. I quit wondering eons ago when the baby will come out. There is only this contraction, and this push, and this pause, and then this contraction, and this push, and— Then the midwife's Voice, summoning forth my consciousness from its burial in the depths of sensation."[67]

- Let yourself go to that deeply interior space within yourself, steeped in pure sensation and raw instinct—beyond words, beyond self-consciousness, beyond propriety, beyond rationality—where you may commune with your most essential nature, knowing, and power.
- To the laboring woman and her partner: know that through the power of presence, you can bring *any* place or situation under your dominion. Even if you end up headed to the OR for a c-section, there is a component of surrender you can engage in that is eminently powerful: forget who you "are"— the collection of thoughts, plans, and what some call *ego*. Open up a silence within; tell yourself this is *your* place and *your* moment. Own it, and go inside. You know how it is when you're engrossed in a fabulous book while sitting in a bustling crowd at an airport, and everything else falls away because your attention is so firmly focused inside the story? It can be like that, no matter what's going on around you. Focus inside your story of graceful surrender, and of welcoming your child into the world. This is so empowering: women, you know your strength, and partners, you're assured that even if you cannot protect her, she can protect herself.
- Fathers, see if you can find the space within yourself to be present with your laboring partner in a way that resonates with where she is. Find the aspect of

you that *allows* without doing or fixing (those wonderfully masculine impulses without which we wouldn't have skyscrapers or spaceships). Let your strength be devoted toward simply sheltering your partner's authentic process, which may be intense and raw, and may include pain, noise, and general upheaval. She needs you to shelter her, not save her.

- While you're laboring you can be present to your new little one through your welcoming, encouraging thoughts: *Baby, we're here working together—we're almost in each other's arms! Let the anticipation of our togetherness be for joy— this adventure is about to come to fruition. Sweet baby, this is a crazy world, but let's make it better together.* Remember that this is a love story that began when sperm met egg, and now you long to meet this beloved in a new way. Your longing for the gaze of your baby can bring a mixture of excitement and peace.

Awareness – Perhaps the most important awareness to hold during this step is that a woman's body is elegantly and intricately designed to birth on its own, providing that a few basic mammalian environmental requirements are met: safety, privacy, lack of verbal and mental stimulation.

- Know that if you're hungry during labor, you're not yet in active labor, and you *should* eat. Eating lowers the adrenaline, for one thing, which helps labor to proceed. Birth is physiologically programmed to happen in an oxytocin-saturated state, and oxytocin accompanies digestion, so eating a little helps coax this along. So yes, eat a bit if you like, but not for the commonly ac-cepted reason that you're preparing for a marathon and will need so many calories for energy. It's actually the reverse—you are preparing for an extended series of episodes of deep relaxation, in which, ideally, you even fall asleep between contractions.
- The use of water during labor has become popular, perhaps most lyrically portrayed in Elena Tonetti's beautiful film *Birth As We Know It* (which itself, aside from the water birth aspect, comprises some excellent childbirth prepa-ration). Water immersion can work seeming miracles for labor, but it is im-portant to be aware of the role of *timing*: women who enter the pool too soon can hinder rather than ease their labor. Obstetrics physician Michel Odent explains that "a laboring woman shouldn't enter the water before her cervix has dilated to five centimeters, as the common response to immersion is a redistribution of blood volume that stimulates the release by specialized

heart cells of the atrial natriuretic peptide (ANP). The inhibitory effect of this peptide on the activity of the posterior pituitary gland is slow—in the region of one to two hours." What this means is that nature offers us a window of time—one to two hours—during which the water provides relaxation and pain relief, and the synergy between oxytocin production and blood distribution produces a spectacular progress in cervical dilation. But if the woman remains in the pool for more than two hours, exceeding this ideal window, labor is likely to stall. Essentially, the body's intelligence says, "We've now been in water long enough and other aspects of physiology require attention; we cannot keep producing oxytocin any longer!" In fact, in light of sheer birth physiology principles and his almost fifty years of attending births, Odent suggests such immersion can be seen as a reliable test of whether a cesarean is called for: "If the already well-advanced [five centimeters or more] dilation remains stable in spite of water immersion, privacy (no cameras!), and dim light, one can conclude that there is a major obstacle. There is no reason for procrastination. It is wiser to perform an *in-labor non-emergency caesarean* immediately."[68]

- Before your baby's birth, if it's a boy, you need to become fully aware about circumcision. Most conventional wisdom on the subject is misinformation and conjecture. The good news is that the U.S. circumcision rate has dropped to 32 percent due to changing attitudes and understandings of this significant genital surgery; the bad news is that 68 percent of baby boys still have their penises cut in the first hours of life. First, the pain issue: anesthesia is almost never used (and when used, it's not very effective), even though circumcision has been described as among the most painful procedures in neonatal medicine. And it isn't just the ablation procedure that is excruciating; the post-op days are also very painful for the circumcised baby boy. But the larger issue for our purposes of parenting in collaboration with Nature's elegant design is that of respecting the body's integrity; once again our human arrogance has deemed the foreskin a mistake, when in truth it is an exceedingly sensible part of the functional male anatomy. You need to ask yourself if you want to subject your son to a procedure first instituted medically in the 1800's as a deterrent to masturbation, which was then mistakenly believed to cause disease. It is now correctly known that circumcision does indeed diminish sexual pleasure in adulthood. Of particularly poignant relevance to our intentions of parenting for peace, it has been said that circumcision is where sex and violence first meet. As with certain issues you may confront later (piercings, tattoos), my guideline for circumcision is to shelter a child's bodily integrity until adulthood, when he can make his own truly informed choice.

Rhythm – During birth, rhythm reigns—or at least it should. Women, to the extent that you are willing to give yourself over to the mighty rhythms of your body's birthing wisdom—to surrender to the mystery—you will have an empowering experience.

- Early labor offers you the opportunity to acquaint yourself more directly with your body's gathering birthing rhythms, and to befriend them. One is the time-honored way of noting the time between contractions (or what uber-midwife Ina May Gaskin prefers to call "rushes"). Honor the relaxed rhythm of these early hours. A commonly endorsed calculus for determining the onset of true labor is: one contraction lasting for one minute occurring every five minutes.

- One of the many reasons intravenously administered synthetic oxytocin is an assault to the natural rhythms of labor is that the body's natural delivery format for oxytocin—as with most of her brilliantly orchestrated chemical messengers—is *pulsatile* rather than continuous, marked by a rhythmic rather than linear flow. Immerse yourself in the powerful tides of life moving in and through you, allowing yourself to be carried upon the rivers you yourself are creating! Oxytocin peaks for a mother in the first hour following birth; she will never in her life (aside from other births) have as much of this bonding hormone as she does then. Biology installed it there—along with the newborn's high oxytocin levels—as a sort of Super Glue to ensure their naturally designed connection.

- Dad is also subject to some transformative rhythms of pregnancy and birth. In the three weeks prior to his partner giving birth, an expectant father will experience a 20 percent rise in his levels of prolactin, named for its role in promoting lactation in women, but also related to parental behavior in some animals and even birds. Following birth his testosterone levels will drop by one-third, and although they return to their former levels within a month or two, scientists have found that the effects of this dip endure lifelong; this ebbing of testosterone together with a brief rise in (don't freak out) estrogen levels allows a man's nurturing side to come forward, and may actually induce the process of family bonding.[69]

Example – Realize that you are joining a sacred living history, a stream of women who through the eons have made this journey and charted the way for you. In the wake of this noble lineage of birthing women, you're able to enrich their past knowledge with new resources and perhaps even have a better birthing experience. This brings healing and joy to the lineage.

- It is always good to have a woman in the room with you who has birthed in a way that you consider successful. She serves as a subliminal guiding model, through body-to-body, brain-to-brain resonance—in the same way that it is easier to meditate in a room with another who is meditating, or how we find we're suddenly more intelligent in proximity to a brilliant person.
- My friend who needed fire near her during her labor used it as an example of what she knew she needed to be: mystery in action. One never knows where the flame is going next, so she used fire as a remedy for her overly Cartesian, linear mind.
- Made popular by the Lamaze method, the use of a focal point can be seen as harnessing the example principle: *as I gaze on this singular point, I echo within me its symmetry, organization, and simplicity.* You can also use sound in this way, by choosing music, chant, or kirtan that is repetitive, like a mantra. It must be monotonous so as to not stimulate your brain's cortical sensors for novelty; it should be something you're very familiar with, that feels like home to you. I found all that in Robbie Gass's beautiful, meditative "Om Namaha Shivaya"; it was only years later that I learned that the mantra itself is steeped in many layers of powerful meaning with profound effects. I just found it a soothing river of sound to ride.

Nurturance – Fathers and partners, this is the golden hour for you to express this principle magnificently!

- Make sure that your laboring partner is as relaxed as can be. Sleeping between contractions is the best indicator that there's sufficient oxytocin flowing, and optimally low levels of adrenaline that would undermine her body's work of cervical dilation.
- You now act as her womb: it's up to you to cocoon her from phone calls, texts, tweets, visitors, and all other contact—anything characteristic of the modern human, especially lights and language. All such stimulation brings adrenaline

to her system. You yourself should use the very minimum of softly spoken words with her—again, so as not to call forth the labor-slowing adrenaline.

- Rather than humanizing birth, as some reformers call for, Michel Odent suggests we need to *de*humanize birth, or rather, *mammalian*ize it—by taking away everything that distinguishes humans: rationality, speech and technology. Cameras are big culprits; the camera-face a woman feels she must put on will right there interfere with the process! Odent confidently declares, "Go ahead, let everyone into the room, chat, watch TV, run the cameras—and she'll give birth after thirty or thirty-six hours of labor. If you respect the physiology, that same baby will be born in less than five hours."[70]

- Be aware that during labor, every sound, every light, every scent is amplified and more intense, so try to minimize all such incoming sensations.

- Advocate for your laboring partner to remain free in her movements and position. Ina May Gaskin writes about the importance of moving freely and letting gravity work for you. She also graphically illustrates how a woman's pelvic bones can open far more flexibly in positions other than lying on her back.[71]

- If your woman enters the hospital for birth, she will greatly benefit from you softly but confidently crooning a little mantra of mastery to her (such as, "You are the owner of your moment, right here and now"). As labor has been steadily progressing in the comfort of your home, once in the unfamiliar environment of the hospital, neurophysiologically speaking, she has a short window of time in which to feel at home there. See that you transform this foreign place into *your* place in short order—not more than fifteen minutes. Hospital intake forms can wait; her hormonal profile for an effective labor should not.

- The latest, hottest technology for midwives (or anyone else attending a birth) is... wait for it... *knitting!* A midwife (or doula, or partner) sitting serenely in a corner knitting is considered state of the art in progressive labor care. Knitting reduces adrenaline (in the knitter and by extension in the laboring woman) and cultivates the perfect atmosphere: monotonous, repetitive and beautiful. (A fringe benefit is that knitting is also known to facilitate hemispheric integration in the brain, readying a caregiver for optimally effective responsiveness when he or she is needed).

- If, as suggested, you have a woman attending you who herself has successfully birthed, she has a knowing within her of how to nurture you during labor.

She stays calm, collected; she does not massage you (unless you ask her to); she does not give verbal affirmations and praise—which wake up your rational mind and bring adrenaline. She understands that this is a matter of sheer, mammalian physiology: just as you don't mess with the laws of gravity when skydiving, you don't mess with laws of physiology when birthing!

- Men, the prerequisites for you being there in a way that truly nurtures your partner and your soon-to-arrive child are: a) can you keep your adrenaline level low; b) can you keep your natural impulse to fix things in check; and c) in your honest heart of hearts, can you feel confident that witnessing your partner birthing will not carry negative consequences for you in your future sexual relationship with her? This is *so* politically incorrect, *so* countercultural—the great unmentionable. But those who are profoundly familiar with the process have seen it time and time again—the woman giving birth *just* when the father has left to buy a paper or get some coffee. Along with the welcomed opportunity for men to attend the birth of their children came, it seems, the automatic *expectation* for them to do so. We have to remember that up until a nanosecond ago in human history, birth has always been strictly women's business, and many men may feel utterly out of their element with it. An excellent discussion of these issues can be found at womantowomancbe.word press.com/2008/04/28/should-men-attend-the-birth-of-their-baby.

- For some men, however, their natural impulses toward protection and mastery become beautifully channeled for birth. A midwife friend tells of the father whose wife was in labor at home, when his family (who lives in the same apartment building) came pounding on their door to rail in outrage about their choice for homebirth (which they'd only just found out about). The father calmly yet determinedly posted a note on the door: "We need your silence and your prayers." Strong. Silent. Gets it.

- Patrick Houser, author of the *Fathers-to-Be-Handbook*, offers the sage guidance (ideally used well before your partner is in hard labor), "Remind your partner to say *Yes*, in every part of her being, no matter what her body is feeling. '*Yes*' encourages the body to open, relax and work with the process. '*No*' will do just the opposite. Yes and Thank You with a contraction will support her to stay focused on what she is doing, in that instant. It can work miracles for both of you."[72]

- Remember, after the baby is born, the mother is still in labor. Don't disturb the atmosphere or *do* anything! Let the cord continue to give the baby all his or her rightful blood. Don't wash the baby. Let the silence, the darkness, the reverence continue. This ensures the healthy delivery of the placenta and the peaceful beginnings of the bonding process.

- If you have birthed a baby whom you are relinquishing for adoption, or have been contracted as a surrogate, it is in the best interests of the baby—and his or her parents—that you have the opportunity to engage in Nature's physiological bonding process in the hours following birth. Through your skin-to-skin togetherness the stress hormones activated during the birth process give way to the pleasure hormones of oxytocin and natural opiates; the baby's first impression of the world is a welcoming one in which he feels safe, secure, and connected. The alternative—which is far more common, sadly—is that the baby is separated from everything familiar (thus, safe), so that the stress biochemistry of birth not only doesn't resolve, it is compounded by the loss of his bioregulatory "mother ship," which further overwhelms his nervous system with adrenaline, cortisol and other stress hormones.

- This is such a basic rule of Nature that even the youngest child instinctively understands it. After hearing the story of the day she was born—for the nth time—my own daughter, only three at the time, startled me by asking me about the day that *I* was born. I hadn't really given any thought to how I would convey the idea of adoption to my children, so I was on the spot. I did a decent enough job of answering her in story form at her level of understanding—"The mommy whose tummy I grew in didn't have what she needed to be a mommy...she didn't know a lot of the things mommies need to know...she didn't have a room for me...she didn't even have a daddy for me." Eve was spellbound, her gaze locked onto me. I continued: "But there was another lady who really wanted to have a baby, and who couldn't grow one in her belly, so they decided that she would take me home and be my mommy." After a long pause, her eyes glistening with tears, Eve's question came: "Did you get to say goodbye?"

Trust – The primary application of this principle at this step is perhaps best summed up in the title of one of my favorite books on the subject, Andrea Henkart's *Trust Your Body! Trust Your Baby!*—a collection of chapters designed to cultivate your faith in the wisdom of the multitude of processes within you that are designed to birth a baby safely and with relative ease. It points out, "The uterus already knows how to birth a baby. The mother takes classes only to 'learn' to accept the process and trust her body."[73] Rather than a lifelong learning of such trust via routine exposure to birth, as in other cultures, we spend decades gathering antitrust beliefs and attitudes promulgated by our technomedical model, particularly regarding our bodies as machines prone to malfunction.

- Various modalities for clearing counterproductive emotional imprints and implicit beliefs can be helpful in cultivating trust in birth; Emotional Freedom Technique (EFT) is a particularly user-friendly such tool.
- Mantras are wonderful for recalling ourselves to our trusting nature. A helpful one is "I surrender to Life, to my body and my baby."
- As in the Jewish tradition, any certainty you have should be accompanied by a question mark (thus avoiding arrogance)—and the trust that the information will make itself known.
- Trust that the baby has chosen the correct time to be born.
- Often a woman's apprehension about birth has less to do with labor and more to do with what comes after: when we say "Trust your body," some women say, "Sure, but I won't know what to do with a baby!" Relax—you'll learn, you'll teach each other.

Simplicity – The requirements for a successful birth could not be simpler. Anyone who's been present at the birth of a colt, calf or kitten has witnessed the needs of a mammalian mother (which we are): safe privacy, period. What could be simpler than a farm? Find a farmer and *un*learn what you know about birth! For animals, it's like real estate—location, location, location: their favorite barn stall or dresser drawer, because familiar is safe. The more familiar we are with the territory where we birth, the more at peace we are and the fewer interventions we'll need; indeed, what we need *is* less—less language, fewer questions, lower light: simplicity. If we could just remember and connect with our mammalian nature, birthing would be so much simpler.

- Remember that childbirth is not a performance. It is an act of utmost sacred intimacy. No superficialities allowed, only gravitas—the dignified simplicity of authentic being.
- If you find yourself leaning into the siren call of technology, remember that the principle of simplicity presides over birth in a way that is statistically sound: remember that the governing bodies of the professional obstetrical societies in both the U.S. and Canada have found that intermittent listening

with a handheld device is as effective, or even more so, than electronic fetal monitoring.[74]

- The lasting joy of simplicity is astonishing; just as the residue of a disempowering birth can stay with you forever, so too does the empowerment of a simple birth. Here again, it sets into motion a fractal wave that continues in the inner life of the mother and thus enriches the child—auspicious for a peacemaker generation.

Resources

National Organization of Circumcision Information Resource Centers: www.nocirc.org.

Doctors Opposing Circumcision Policy Statement: www.doctorsopposing circumcision.org/DOC/statement0.html

Pushed Birth: www.pushedbirth.com. The sister site to the important 2008 book *Pushed*, "to provide women with uncensored, unsweetened information about U.S. childbirth care. Author and journalist Jennifer Block spent years researching why so many labors are begun by induction, why so many births end in cesarean section, and how modern maternity care is impacting women and their families. This site provides key findings — a quick read for a better birth."

Create Your Own Partograph: partograph.com/tools/partograph.

Step Five

NATURE'S PEACE PLAN—
INSTALLING PEACEMAKER
HARDWARE IN YEAR ONE

*If you want one year of prosperity, grow grain. If you want
ten years of prosperity, grow trees. If you want a hundred years
of prosperity, grow people.*

CHINESE PROVERB

The Best Investment for Peace

The first hours after birth, followed by an infant's early weeks and months,
offer us the most fruitful opportunities in life to shelter and nurture all kinds
of inner processes—in both mother and baby—that are designed to weave
and shape the capacities required of Generation Peace. A colleague of mine
likes to put it this way: if parenting stages were stocks on Wall Street, those
who invest in the first hours of life would get the biggest return for their
money!

Instructions for the New Mother

Give up your calendar and clock,
start flowing with milk time.

Hunt for the frayed scraps
and threads of your fears.
Wrap your child's cries around
the skein of your days.

Stop racing to meet your familiar ways—
know change
will always beat you.

Lower that small fist of resistance
still struggling to rise within you—start now—
unclench your life.

ANDREA POTOS[1]

The quality of those first hours, days, and weeks is to a great degree a culmination and reflection of aspects of the mother's history—immediate (labor and birth), medium-term (her pregnancy and marriage or partnership), and long-term (her childhood and development as a woman)—which coalesce to express ease or apprehension, receptivity or anxiety, joy or melancholia at this pivotal moment of transition to new motherhood. These qualities in turn permeate her baby's first impression of the world, of life, and of his very self.

Two Postpartum Portraits

Claire* – A successful freelance casting director, Claire had gradually tapered off work during her first trimester. The high-pressure entertainment atmosphere didn't accommodate morning sickness well. Claire greatly enjoyed her pregnancy; she felt regal as her belly blossomed, and she reveled in the process of sharing her substance with her developing baby. She and her husband, Rob,

---

* Names in this story were changed

had consciously chosen to conceive, and over the months Claire read *The Secret Life of the Unborn Child* and studied Joseph Chilton Pearce's ideas about the natural unfolding of intelligence in *Magical Child*. She skillfully pulled together the baby's room in a comfy, "not too done" style that featured light pine furniture and sweet touches of country warmth and whimsy. The one piece she was frustrated by not finding by her due date was the vintage chest of drawers in her mind's eye, tall enough to double as a changing table.

Claire and Rob took childbirth preparation classes with a Dutch-born maternity nurse whose approach was more like Bradley than Lamaze: she didn't focus on teaching techniques to avoid pain, but rather on deeply understanding and working with the powerful processes of the mother's body during labor and birth. Well before her due date Claire had shared her desires and concerns about labor with her OB, who patiently listened, endorsed her commitment to a drug-free birth, empathized with her determination to avoid a c-section, and then explained that while that was all well and good, ultimately whatever it took to bring her baby into the world healthy and whole was the important thing. "Once your baby's here, everything else will seem far less important."

In what Claire only half-jokingly took as an indication of her son's brilliance, he did what only 5 percent of babies do: he arrived on his due date. Her labor was straightforward and unusually brisk for a first birth, just four and a half hours from the onset of active labor to Josh's entrance into the world. Due to the sheer speed of things Claire felt like her ideal scenario had gotten away from her in many respects. There were the little things—like how during early labor at home she didn't feel free to express her needs to Rob, including her annoyance at his decision to grill up some burgers for lunch so the meat wouldn't spoil while they were away at the hospital. The smell nauseated her, but asserting herself had never come easy, especially in the vulnerable posture of labor, so she grazed the issue with a halfhearted attempt at a joke and then let it go.

Once at the hospital, her labor in full swing, the birth scene she had envisioned—Rob soothing her with his steadying voice, rubbing her back and stroking her hair, while the kindly labor nurse murmured reassuring encouragement—never materialized. Instead, Claire was briskly assisted out of her clothes and into a hospital gown, installed on her back in bed, and hooked up to an IV before she really was aware of it. Dr. Weiss inserted an internal electronic fetal monitor up through her vagina and into her baby's scalp. While Rob was downstairs filling out admittance paperwork and the doctor was at the nurses' station, Claire felt a powerful contraction come on. As she rode it out with a plaintive, crooning moan, the labor nurse didn't budge from her spot at the table in the corner of the room where she was charting notes. It seemed to Claire that she barely even looked up. She was relieved when Rob returned, but when Weiss came back, he authoritatively directed Rob to step aside ("You can take pictures") and to leave Claire alone in the short lulls between contractions.

The beeps of the EFM sang out the story that with each contraction Josh's heart rate dropped precipitously. On several occasions Dr. Weiss literally rocked Claire's belly back and forth between contractions: "C'mon, wake up, baby." The beeps resumed their normal quick rhythm each time. The cord was around Josh's neck, and with each contraction—during which the baby also works, pushing himself further down the birth canal—it would tighten and staunch the blood flow to his heart and his brain. Had there been more time for Claire's mind to catch up with the events speeding by, with her merely along for the ride, she'd have recognized a likely approaching c-section scenario. As it was, she was just barely able to hang in and hang on in her own body—so she was at least spared that worry. The next thing she knew, Weiss became an Olympic coach exhorting her to push with everything she had. ("No, don't make any noise when you push, you lose power that way!" he claimed, although it felt natural for her to do so.) Claire didn't yet have the urge to push that she had read so much about, so when she pushed she didn't experience that deep relief she had also read so much about. Just pressure— from Josh inside, and from Weiss outside. And the growing burning tightness between her legs that she felt would split her open. With only her vague awareness, Dr. Weiss gave her "just a touch of something [Nicentil, a narcotic pain reliever no longer on the market] to take the edge off."

Claire had long since lost her sense of anything like center when Weiss announced he was doing an episiotomy, and by that point, frankly, all Claire wanted was relief from the pressure. To this day she regrets yelling in what by then felt like equal parts rage and panic, "Get it *out of me!*" Weiss instructed her to reach down and indeed she did have the primally satisfying experience of lifting Josh from between her legs up to her chest. Suddenly the storm had passed and contentment filled her. Where moments ago she was raging, now she was crooning to this new little alien life form nestled on her chest, as Rob leaned in close to complete the new family tableau.

Dr. Weiss, known for being more progressive than most obstetricians in their area, waited for Josh's umbilical cord to stop pulsing before he clamped it and let Rob do the honors of cutting it. (Memorably, blood spurted onto Rob's glasses.) Weiss gave the new family lots of time for quiet, dimly lit nuzzling, bonding and early breastfeeding—which helped with the delivery of the placenta. After stepping in as photographer, Weiss went to work stitching up Claire's episiotomy site and then packing her vaginal area with standard gauze pads called four by fours (and which Claire, her sense of humor back, said felt like actual wooden 4x4s he was cramming up there).

There came the moment, however, when hospital policy deemed it necessary for Josh to be taken away to have the standard battery of newborn treatments. Rob went along with the nurse for that, Dr. Weiss went out to confer with the nursing staff, and there was Claire, feeling solo and adrift on the desert island of her delivery bed. Out of many months of habit, she began to talk to Josh—and then remembered with a pang of nostalgic longing that he was no longer there inside her. She wonders looking back if she'd ever felt so alone before, so bereft. The fact was, she had. Her own primal history, a history she had never explored despite years of therapy, was now catching up with her and would soon complicate this delicately rhythmic process of newly forming connections: after her own birth, she had been held just once, briefly, by her biological mother before spending five days in the newborn nursery. Her adoptive parents waited until her sixth day of life to pick her up and take her home. Connectedness and disconnectedness were processes equally fraught with terror for Claire. But what made it worse is that she had no idea that was so. She just knew she should be feeling so... happy.

Soon the new little family was reunited in their private room. Josh seemed to be getting the hang of nursing already, but Claire's nipples didn't know what hit them. There soon developed the routine of Claire digging her fingernails into Rob's forearm as Josh latched on, and when the hospital delivered them the traditional candlelight first dinner, she was relieved to take several deep sips of the wine that Rob had smuggled in. It took the edge off the breastfeeding pain, and off the other, vaguer distress bubbling up at her center. Certainly all of the prolactin and oxytocin flowing through her was soothing, but anytime Josh began to fuss or squirm, Claire tensed: *What does he want? What do I do? How do I do this?* Even though her pediatrician—well known for his holistic, baby-centered approach—had entreated them to exercise their rooming-in privilege and keep Josh with her at all times, Claire relented when the night nurse, who was so skilled at swaddling Josh so his fussing stopped, suggested she take Josh to the nursery so that Claire could get a good night's sleep—"maybe one of your last for awhile." Claire was a little scared to go home and leave all these experts behind.

Claire's childhood friend Shari came to stay for a week in the role of postpartum doula. She was an experienced mother, so she not only handled household chores and cooked nutritious food, but also helped Claire learn to do such basic yet alien tasks as bathing Josh and clipping his surprisingly long newborn nails. On her surface Claire was beaming, but she found herself crying easily. They all watched a Barbra Streisand special one evening and the song *Somewhere* ("there's a place for us") just took her away to some deeply melancholic place. Her first escape from Josh was on their second day home from the hospital. While Rob was leaning comfortably into the postpartum slow-down, the sweet haze of new life, Claire was driving all over town looking for that chest of drawers of the right height to serve as a changing table. She had to sit down every few minutes because her episiotomy site throbbed. (Despite this vivid demonstration of it, many years would pass before Claire began to understand the painful toll of her perfectionism.) Just about the time her engorged breasts felt ready to burst, she called home to see if Josh was hungry yet.

"Yep, he's getting pretty hungry, and I don't think the pacifier is doing it for him anymore, Claire," Rob told her over the phone. Those words turned her into a menacing mother on the road. She zagged frantically through traffic, yelling at pussyfoot drivers, "I've got to get home to feed my baby!" Thus began Claire's postpartum mothering experience—a treadmill of unease, marked by a vague conviction of her incompetence and the thin but steady pressure to prove herself worthy of her role as a mother.

Megan – As a therapist specializing in the issues of gifted, hyperachieving young women, Megan was able to continue working well into her pregnancy. Like Claire and Rob, Megan and her husband, Charles, were conscious and deliberate about conceiving, and even sought counseling for approaching prenatal parenting in the healthiest way. But unlike Claire, Megan was beset by ambivalence and feelings of insecurity once she knew she was pregnant; many tears would flow as she contemplated the momentous road of motherhood she was embarking on. In particular, the aspect of the *unknown* terrified her.

Over the months, she gently explored the roots of her fears, and realized that as a child she couldn't show vulnerability or weakness, feeling she had to always be in control and in the know. She was smart enough to understand "it takes a village to raise a child," and yet asking for help felt foreign to her. One of her counselor's ongoing homework assignments was that Megan practice asking for help in a number of ways. Over the weeks she became more fluent with her own early story, and Charles also participated in this exploration, taking the opportunity to consider his own beginnings as an adopted person and how that impacted his attitudes about connection, family, etc.

It became customary for Megan to begin crying as soon as she came into their counselor's office, which they saw as part of a softening process Megan was inviting: consciously leaning into the unknown adventure of parenting had initiated a healing process. Her early experiences of having needs that didn't get met, and of not feeling supported, were gently uncovered and addressed, so they could be retired rather than replayed in her own parenting, as so often happens. Over the months Megan assembled a team of helpers: in addition to her counselor she sought out a chiropractor specializing in pregnancy and women's health, a prenatal yoga master, and an acupuncturist, all of whose involvement helped weave in Megan an inner fabric of flexible, flowing confidence and openness to the unknown. Aware of her own risk factors for postpartum depression, she was particularly vigilant about that, proactively resourcing herself with the help of all of these supports she had assembled.

Because Megan's pregnancy ran a week past her due date, labor was induced with Pitocin, and after enduring the intense contractions for eight hours she finally asked for an epidural, which allowed her to get some sleep. Megan doesn't look back on her labor as at all ideal ("The nurse didn't like my doula, which made for tension..." "The doula ended up going out to sleep in her van..." "The nurse told me after I finally got my epidural, 'You're just not crunchy enough to do it naturally,' which was obnoxious..."). Although she experienced a bit of the same dazed and confused "Now what?" feelings as Claire regarding how exactly to care for the new little creature in her arms, she was anxious to get out of the unsupportive atmosphere of the hospital and back home with her new daughter, Katherine.

Megan is one of the only mothers I've heard say that the postpartum period was "easier than I thought it would be." I have no doubt it's because she and Charles were so intentional about setting it up to be that way: they made a staggered schedule of visiting helpers over the first two months, arranged so that the tasks people felt they were good at coordinated well ("My mom hates to cook but Dad loves it—but my mom was a night nurse, so that was great"). Megan and Charles had agreed early on that the only visitors would be those who contributed to a sense of calm: "We didn't let anybody in who was going to be drama." When they first got home, friends pitched in to get them a fabulous basket of delicious food that fed them for three days, which for Megan felt very nurturing. Megan had come a long way in her inability to ask for help; she not only asked for it now, but gratefully, graciously soaked it up.

They cocooned at home for almost six weeks, cultivating a no-stress atmosphere of beauty and calm. Megan thinks she felt up to it that first week because she was able to get sleep and good food. As the weeks unspooled, Megan knew herself enough to know she had to focus on the here and now in a very simple way with her baby: "If I thought I had to figure it all out, it was too much, so I'd just stay basic: keep things as stress-free as possible, for her and for me. Beginning even when she was tiny, when we'd walk her around the house pointing out all the pictures of family, naming everyone, that would sooth her. That and Bob Marley. We had Katherine's chart done when she was born, and it said dance would be a big part of her life. So we danced a lot."

Megan went to a half-day workshop her counselor presented when Katherine was a few months old—so, roughly a year from when she had first stepped into the counselor's office. The transformation was exquisite: where Megan had once sat weeping with insecurity over whether she had what it takes to be a mother, now she exuded a calm, loving centeredness that in turn helped her baby daughter regulate her own infant states of upset or discomfort. Nothing seemed to faze Megan. She had come a long way.

Nurturing Connection: Weaving Peace as Your Child's Foundation

A baby's need to be physically close to a predictable, caring adult is rooted in the biological drive for survival: millennia ago an infant too far away from an adult risked starving or being devoured by predators. But the survival function of attachment has evolved, along with our human consciousness, technologies and lifestyles, away from a focus on physical safety to a more complex requirement: to develop a suite of psychosocial competencies fundamental to the survival of not just each individual, but of our human family and our shared home, the planet earth.

Immediately after birth a complex hormonal cocktail orchestrates biochemical exchanges between a mother and her newborn, offering never-to-be-repeated opportunities to set the stage for optimally healthy psychosocial development. Levels of oxytocin—our hormone of love and affiliation, peace and healing—peak during this time, potentiating important brain circuitry for the baby's social and emotional centers, and fostering the mother's urge toward maternal behavior. Oxytocin is a primary peacemaker hormone in the body: it elicits a relaxation and growth response, which in turn reduces activity in the stress (fight, flight or freeze) system. (Remember the central peace-related question continually being asked by the organism: is it safe to grow, or do I need to protect and defend?) We're all familiar with the idea that love conquers fear, and thanks primarily to oxytocin, it's not just a worthy ideal, it's a basic feature of our physiological design. Along with its ability to moderate a person's tendency to switch into stress-response mode, oxytocin is involved in such basic Gen Peace capacities as empathy, adaptation, tolerance, cognition, and interdependence. Impairment of the oxytocin system has been implicated in autism, as well as schizophrenia, drug addiction and even cardiovascular disease.[2]

Beta-endorphins, the brain's own powerful pleasure chemicals, also flow in abundance in the first hours following birth. Essentially, the newborn's brain is primed to imprint *Connecting with Mom feels good*. This biologically mediated process between mother and baby is called bonding, and it is organized around their face-to-face, skin-to-skin togetherness. Yet American hospital protocols typically disturb this momentous, complex weaving in the first hours of life through routine separation of mothers and newborns. Too many newborns end up in plastic isolettes, receiving a distorted relational imprint (*I connect with things, not people*), that can impair development of their capacity for healthy human rapport, social intelligence, and the foundations for peace.

This is the evidence-contraindicated portion of the hospital ritual whereby, says Robbie Davis-Floyd, "society demonstrates conceptual ownership of its product."[3] The four- to twelve-hour ritual separation of mother and child after birth and bonding, still common in many hospitals, powerfully reminds the mother that her baby belongs to society first. Sending the mother this message now interrupts the powerful feelings that holding her newborn baby generates in her, working to ensure that she will be willing to give her baby over to society's institutions (hospitals for medical care, schools for socialization) for the rest of its life.[4] By way of baby's ongoing indoctrination into the technocracy,

Davis-Floyd poses the idea that the plastic isolette in which the newborn is placed "metamorphoses into the crib, the playpen, the plastic carrier, and the television-set-as-babysitter—and a baby who bonds strongly to technology as she learns that comfort and entertainment come primarily from technological artifacts. That baby grows up to be the consummate consumer, and thus the technocracy perpetuates itself."[5]

New research from the Karolinska Institute vividly demonstrates that there is a highly sensitive period during the first one to two hours after birth that lays the long-term foundation for myriad Generation Peace conditions. Researchers studying the long-term effects of hospital delivery and maternity practices on mother-infant interaction found that close contact (skin-to-skin and suckling) during the first two hours after birth, when compared with separation of the mothers and their infants, led to increased levels of maternal sensitivity, infant self-regulation, and "dyadic mutuality and reciprocity" one year after birth. The most striking aspect of their findings was that the negative effect of a two-hour separation after birth *was not compensated for by the practice of rooming-in.*[6] There is something unique and irreplaceable about those first hours following birth—and we want to use them to their fullest peaceable potential!

We want to maintain an atmosphere of sheltered tranquility during these hormonally primed *falling in love* hours following birth. Oxytocin is a shy hormone: it doesn't like to be observed. Just as in labor, low lights, privacy and quiet optimize the action of this powerful hormone of connection during the immediate postpartum hours. The closer the contact between mother and baby, involving all five senses, the more primed for peaceful joy both will be. So skin-to-skin togetherness, eye contact, gentle crooning, taking in the scent of one another, baby nuzzling at mother's breast—these are all potent ways to chart an auspicious Gen Peace course.

Nature has designed the system so that when a baby's stress system is ignited by hunger, pain, overstimulation, or indeed, separation, her cries summon the timely attention of her mother, whose soothing touch, loving voice, familiar scent (and often, milk) turns down the volume of the baby's stress response and fires up the reward system circuits in her brain, resulting in pleasurable feelings of contentment. The baby's brain over time associates that voice, scent, touch—all her mother's qualities—with the safety and security needed for her optimal growing to happen. In his book *Born For Love: Why Empathy is Essential—and Endangered*, child psychiatrist Bruce Perry points out, "These crucial associations between positive human interactions, reward systems, and the stress response networks are the neurobiological glue for all future healthy relationships. They are at the core of why empathy matters."[7] When this system is thwarted, the circuitry of the baby's social brain wires up differently—to suit the individual to more brutal, uncaring circumstances in which empathy is not only unnecessary but likely a handicap.

A Poignant Glimpse of Attachment Research History

Being separated from one's mother as a baby is solidly associated with impaired lifelong experience on many levels. Harry Harlow's pioneering work with rhesus monkeys at Cornell in the 1950s and 1960s yielded an achingly poignant, undeniable understanding of how deeply a baby needs not just nourishment from a mother, but also warmth and touch, in order to mature into a healthy adult. The rhesus monkeys he removed from their mothers clung desperately to the nearest thing they could find to a mother, preferring some measure of comfort and security to mere nourishment; the babies chose to cling mostly to cloth-covered surrogate "mother machines," as Harlow called them, over the stark wire contraptions that could give them formula.[8]

Cambridge ethologist Robert Hinde did similar research in which infant macaque monkeys whose mothers were temporarily removed sequentially exhibited "protest, despair"—marked by endless wailing—followed by "detachment" and then "an apparent return to normality," as the infants began to reorganize their behavior in light of their loss of security. (Mothers, too, called piteously, and for hours—the unpublished side of the macaque studies.)[9] For them, protection mode quickly became the norm, and any hopes of being a deeply peaceful, interdependent creature, were lost. The reorganization of our children's behavior in light of their loss of security is one of the most central processes we aim to prevent when raising peacemakers.

Of central importance to our aims is what happened to Harlow's monkeys as they matured—even those whose mothers had only been *temporarily* removed and were later reunited: their social behavior became bizarre. They engaged in stereotyped behavior patterns such as clutching themselves and rocking constantly back and forth, they were excessively aggressive, and their sexual behavior was severely distorted. It was as if their inner compass for *how to be a monkey with other monkeys* had been fundamentally corrupted. And most devastating of all, the behavior of these monkeys as mothers—the "motherless mothers" as Harlow called them—proved to be disastrous. They were either indifferent or abusive toward their babies. The indifferent mothers did not harm their babies, but neither did they nurse, comfort, or protect them. The abusive mothers violently bit or otherwise injured their infants, in many cases until they died. Humans, too, are frequently "Harlow mothers," displaying the same kinds of feeble, fragile, and often distorted maternal instincts as did those piteous, indifferent monkeys.

Chapter Two of Perry's book relates a modern-day, human version of this horror story. Out of nothing more evil than simple ignorance—together most likely with their own early lack of close nurturance—a wealthy, successful couple hired a nanny to care for their son since the father worked full-time and the mother wanted to continue with her full schedule of social and philanthropic activities. That fact alone wouldn't have necessarily posed a problem for baby Ryan's development, since that first young nanny provided him with the soothing, closeness and responsiveness he needed for his social brain to wire up well, and for empathy to flourish. Ryan's parents believed in quality time with their boy, and spent about an hour or so with him each day. When Ryan was eight weeks old his mother was distressed to notice that he fretted when she held him, but smiled and cooed at the nanny. The nanny was fired for being "over-involved" and a new one was hired. Ryan had eighteen nannies by the time he was three. As a decorated high-school athlete already accepted to an Ivy League college, he lured a developmentally disabled neighbor girl to his eighteenth birthday party at his house, gang raped her with his friends, made her "put on a show" for them, and never flinched. With sangfroid he related his story with indignant conviction—that he didn't "know what the problem was, really," and that "she never would have gotten laid by anyone as good as us."[10] Ryan had no inner compass for how to be a human with other humans.

Separation as Trauma: Baby's POV

In many studies of prenatal learning and newborn cognitive capacity, newborns have demonstrated their recognition of and preference for their mothers over anyone else.[11] Myron Hofer has spent decades studying what happens when that preference is not respected; in researching the biology of loss, Hofer has relentlessly pursued the question, "In maternal separation, what exactly is lost?" His work with orphaned rat pups has led to specific, nuanced findings about the effects of separation on infant physiology. His team found that the bond between mother and infant is woven from many physiological strands, each a distinct regulatory pathway in the body: "The elements of the lost interaction…that we had sought…turned out to be *regulators* of the infant's developing neural systems."[12]

Simply through her presence, a mother continuously adjusts her infant's physiology in countless healthy ways, including moderating nervous system arousal, which can interfere with his sleep duration.[13] The enigma of sudden infant death syndrome (SIDS)—of which the U.S. has the highest incidence, despite our medical technologies and sophisticated pediatric care—has been theorized to involve the lack of the critical bioregulating influence of the parent on the young infant sleeping alone in his crib, and in broad terms,* human societies with the lowest incidence of SIDS are also the ones with widespread infant co-sleeping.[14] New research shows that the rate of SIDS rises on occasions when parents of infants drink more,[15] suggesting that this bioregulating effect may be impaired by alcohol.

As psychiatrist Thomas Lewis and colleagues put it—referring to all mammals, including humans—"When the mother is absent, an infant loses all his organizing channels at once. Like a marionette with its strings cut, his physiology collapses into the huddled heap of despair….Once separated from their attachment figures, mammals spiral down into a somatic disarray that can be measured from the outside and painfully felt on the inside."[16] Indeed, the early loss of, or separation from, one's biological mother is associated through an extensive research literature with impaired lifelong physical and neuropsychological wellbeing.[17]

A baby without her mother nearby loses her ability to regulate her physiological states, early maternal-infant separation qualifies as trauma, since by its very definition trauma is *overwhelming experience*: experience that overwhelms the nervous system's capacity to effectively respond in a way that preserves the bodymind's homeostasis—and leaves the individual unable to regain internal balance, in other words, to perform one of the most basic tasks required of

---

* The co-sleeping safety issue is layered with complexities and must be regarded within multiple contexts—family, cultural, ethnic—and in light of such behaviors (smoking, drinking, drug use) that are often associated with co-sleeping infant deaths. I highly recommend reading the article cited here, available in its entirety online.

Generation Peace, to self-regulate.[18] And, early maternal separation leaves the individual forever more highly vulnerable to losses, both real and perceived.[19] The brain and psyche become wired to recognize the atmosphere of that early experience of loss, and any later experience that even vaguely resembles that early loss will fire up the same emotional responses. Psychoanalyst Lynda Share suggests that trauma forms "meaning networks": trauma becomes an "organizer of experience," whereby "all later developmental events, conflicts, and experiences are drawn into it."[20]

We also tend to react to such awakened, ancient memories at the cognitive level we were at when the painful experience happened. This can lead a grown adult, in response to a seemingly benign event that happens to "vibe like" his infant abandonment, to suddenly find himself with primitive capacities of judgment, rationality, and self-regulation. So if a baby's first impression of the world includes the trauma of separation, it's very possible that his later capacity to deal with challenges or conflicts will be severely compromised—not our best offering for a generation of peacemakers.

Separation: Mother's POV

When mother and baby, in accordance with most hospital protocols, miss their undisturbed bonding dance of eye-to-eye, skin-to-skin contact in the hours after birth, or are separated by a well-meaning night nurse to "give Mom a well-deserved rest," a mother is deprived of Nature's powerful biochemical leg up to her extraordinary new role. The potent hormonal cocktail of oxytocin, prolactin, and natural opiates that flow when mother and baby remain together has, as mentioned earlier, been called Nature's Super Glue in its ability to ensure successful bonding and the beginnings of healthy attachment.

The most fundamental separation for a new mother without her baby involves a basic separation from herself—from her own deepest instincts and perceptions of herself *as a mother*—and has typically begun long before the baby is in (or out of) her arms, during the kinds of birth interferences described in the previous chapter. This insidious, subtle, and devastating undercurrent of disempowerment paves the way for her to go along with being separated from her baby: *They must know best.* A woman in her full and glorious maternal empowerment doesn't let anyone take her baby from her! We can't blame the mothers; it is our culture that has veered off course.

Postpartum Parenting for Peace

The consensus among social scientists is that the ongoing rise in youth suicide rates is one of the more tragic social developments of our time; neuropsychologist James Prescott calls it the worst possible indictment of a society.[21] Not only is it without historical precedent, it is impossible to explain within the framework of a materialistic value system; conventional predictions would expect to see a corresponding rise in poverty over those periods in which there was such a drastic rise in youth suicide. Rather, points out researcher Mary Eberstadt, it is "quite the opposite—and little in the way of any other external evidence suggests why the materially best-off adolescents on earth are killing themselves at such shocking rates."[22]

Anthropologist Sarah Hrdy points out that no monkey or ape mother in the wild has ever been observed to deliberately harm her own baby.[23] Prescott thus poses the questions, How did the human become the most violent primate on the planet when our closest genetic relative (the bonobo chimpanzee, who shares 99 percent of our genes) is the most peaceful primate on the planet? And what happened along the evolutionary trail that led to the sudden appearance of infanticide and injury to the young in the Great Ape *homo sapiens*? The answers, he believes, lie in the same sad place where Harry Harlow found them: in the complex of physiological, neurological and psychological developmental curtailments suffered by infants and young children deprived of sufficient and adequate nurturing connectedness with their mothers.[24] Verified throughout three decades of research in diverse cultures, Prescott's findings are a cautionary tale that is ever more relevant to our own culture's growing epidemics of psychosocial disorders. And they are ripe with Generation Peace potential.

> Extensive scientific research in animals and humans have documented, without question, that mother-infant/child separations (loss of bonding/mother love) induces a variety of developmental brain disorders that mediate depression, impulse dyscontrol, chronic stimulus-seeking behaviors that include self-mutilation, and the violence of homicide and suicide.
>
> Children are now killing children; children are raping children; and the massive psychiatric medication of our children and youth that

was unheard of a generation ago all indicate the disintegration of America from within.[25]

This then becomes a generational legacy, from motherless mother to motherless mother. Generation Peace finds its wellspring within mothers.*

Sheltering the Tender Beginnings of Peace

When I was pregnant with our daughter, I took prenatal yoga with Gurmukh.[†] We closed each class by singing a Kundalini farewell blessing (originally lyrics from an Incredible String Band song):

> May the longtime sun shine upon you,
> all love surround you,
> and the pure light within you
> guide your way on.

Isn't this perhaps the highest aspiration we can hold as parents—to nourish, protect and support that pure light within our children, as it guides them on their singular life paths? Call that light what you will: spirit, soul, singular personality and temperament, unique intelligences. It is indeed all of these things plus infinite others that weave the human mystery. Gurmukh also taught me the concept of The Forty Days. For many reasons, including the immature development of his brain and the fact that the energy field of his body is not yet fully formed and intact, a newborn is extremely sensitive to incoming energies and sensations—especially sound and touch. I love how the late poet John O'Donohue described babies as "fresh from the eternal."[26] Partly to protect the integrity of their newly arrived babies, cultures around the world have postpartum rituals with a common theme: a new baby remains sheltered at home, with just family around her, for forty days. This is equivalent to the six weeks that pediatricians once routinely prescribed as the length of time to wait before exposing the new baby to the wider world. (Any trip to the mall, where

---

* *Three Cups of Tea* author Greg Mortenson has discovered that the most powerful dissuading influence on a Muslim man contemplating radical extremism is his mother's unwillingness to give her blessing to violence.
† Gurmukh is so famous in California that she only needs one name, like Oprah or Cher.

you're sure to see a few brand new humans being toted around, is enough to show you how outmoded that prescription is.)

I see the practice of The Forty Days as intimately related to a child's "pure light within": It is one of the first ways in which parents can concretely demonstrate active love of their baby, safeguarding for him a gentle landing into this world, so all that makes him uniquely him can remain unadulterated, strong, and pure. In case it sounds a little airy-fairy, this concept fully lines up with the latest science of brain development: a steady diet of too many incoming sensations—like one would encounter, say, at the mall!—can overwhelm immature brain systems and may contribute to later disorders. The rates of sensory processing disorders—complex, under-researched neurological conditions in which children's brains can't adequately integrate (make coherent, meaningful sense of) sensory stimuli such as touch, sound, or movement—appear to be skyrocketing, joining the epidemic of ADD and ADHD.[27]

From the perspective of Rudolf Steiner's* threefold nature model of development, birth is the birth of only the physical body, with several others yet to be born—which happens, interestingly, in precise timeline correspondence with when the three aspects of our triune brain develop. This gradual incarnation of the child means that there are other aspects of your child still gestating and thus requiring close shelter and care. Right now it is his *etheric body* that is still as if in a womb—until around age seven. Called *chi* in China and *ki* in Japan, and harnessed in East Asian medicine and martial arts, the etheric body is the source of all health and vitality. Its forces build up and shape the human body, cause it to grow, and repair it when it is injured or sick. Historically dismissed as superstition by Western science, the etheric body is gradually coming to be recognized as a real part of the human being; therapies such

---

* Steiner was a student of mathematics, physics, and chemistry, and ultimately took his doctorate in philosophy. Close to what we might call a celebrity in his day, Steiner enjoyed "a considerable reputation among those who knew him as an original, if unacademic, thinker." [Easton, Stewart C. *New Vistas in Psychology: An Anthroposophical Contribution.* Whitstable, Kent: Whitstable Litho Ltd., 1984, pg. 40]. For example, lines of people seeking just a few moments of his counsel would form around the block of his hotel when he visited New York. His practical advice was sought by doctors, therapists, farmers, businessmen, academics and scientists, theologians and pastors, and of course by teachers. His *anthroposophy* (a science of the spirit of man) included a medical aspect, which does not regard illness as a chance occurrence or mechanical breakdown, but as something intimately connected to the biography of a human being.

as acupuncture and Reiki utilize the life-bearing etheric forces in the service of healing.

The mother's etheric body also needs attention now, as it has just expended a tremendous amount of energy building and birthing a new human! The etheric body thrives on warmth and rhythm above all. So indeed, for the mother, too, postpartum is a time of unprecedented transformation and reorientation, with many new inner peace possibilities to be tenderly protected and nurtured. The profound, mysterious connectedness between mother and baby that began in the womb continues to be woven between them in this face-to-face, skin-to-skin setting. Nature's plan (and the Peaceful Parenting Prescription) for this time is to give yourself over to the unfamiliar rhythms, slow down to the languorous pace of new life, and allow the mother in you to unfold.

This prescription tends to clash with our culture's "have a baby but don't miss a beat" mentality: *I am woman, see me birth…and then plan a party and land that important client.* Yes, slowing down during the early weeks and months is typically the biggest challenge for the woman who is intelligent, capable and used to "doing." This is especially true if she had a great birth: she feels on top of the world and may have the tendency to perform, to organize, to accomplish. But here's a central piece of the transformation process: when a mother chooses instead to enter a primarily *receptive* mode during this time…to freefall into the hazy, uncharted territory of her baby's subtle (and sometimes not so subtle) signals and rhythms…to slip into Nature's intended entrainment with his breathing, his moods, his sleep…to let his soul imprint itself upon hers…she casts a shimmering net of secure connectedness far into the future of her relationship with that child, and his relationship with Life.

Think of the animal kingdom, of which we're a part: mothers won't let you near their babies! A tenderly protected, connected postpartum time brings countless blessings, all of them related to the unfolding of peace, joy and multiple intelligences in both baby and mother. Not only is it a potent preventative for postpartum depression,[28] it can also bring about deep healing within the mother, infusing the baby she once was—who may have suffered hurts, losses, her own newborn separation—with more ease and harmony. This can result in an influx of new energy over the coming months for the new mother (when she most needs it!): when we experience inner healing, the energy formerly needed to contain the wound is freed to be used elsewhere—often as joy.

Breastfeeding is also much easier when there is no separation and distractions are few.

Of Love and Milk

Mother's milk. The term is synonymous with everything nurturing, nourishing, loving. Indeed, a slogan writer bottom-lined it succinctly: *Breast is Best.* Of course most parents know it's the best nourishment for their babies, but they may not know how really miraculous the biochemistry of breast milk is. Nature has prepared it as a most exquisite elixir, to perfect and complete our journey from one fertilized cell to a young human being. Like so many other women, I felt that to not participate in this natural continuum that nature devised seemed somehow awkward, an abrupt interruption of an elegantly choreographed process.

Given the conclusive evidence about the comprehensive benefits of nursing our babies, why is there so much ambivalence about breastfeeding? Why do mothers wrestle with the choice of *will I or won't I breastfeed?* This inner tug-of-war about breastfeeding is not a modern burden: a Byzantine legend about the life of Hercules tells that Zeus wanted his bastard son Hercules to nurse from his wife, the goddess Hera, and thus become immortal. He slipped the baby to Hera's breast while she slept, but when she awoke, Hera shoved the foundling away. The force of the baby's Herculean sucking sent a spray of *gala* (Greek for "milk") into the heavens. Thus was our *gala*xy christened, producing a term for humankind's universe that is, appropriately enough, derived from mother's milk.

Henri Nestlé's invention of formula in 1869 initially saved countless babies in foundling homes, but the later widespread use of formula as a "new and improved" system seriously undermined breastfeeding. Yet long before Nestlé, humans devised ways to disrupt the process of mother-infant connectedness by circumventing breastfeeding. It is often the most privileged classes who first embrace disconnecting innovations and technologies, and such was certainly the case in the widespread use of wet-nurses in ancient times as well as in seventeenth- and eighteenth-century England and France. The practice of hiring out the job of breastfeeding infants of the noble class left a wake of illness and death—for either the nursed infants or the children of the wet-nurses, who often went without adequate nutrition. Wet-nurses were called "angelmakers" in England, so risky (yet popular) was the choice not to breastfeed. Indeed, one of the little-discussed reasons mothers of that era sometimes chose not to breastfeed their babies themselves (aside from the desire to get pregnant again quickly, or that it was seen as lower-class, or that they would be "bad wives," as it was believed that sex spoiled breastmilk) was that the child had been unwanted and there was a good chance that the child would not return from the country wet-nurse's home alive.[29]

Today, our internal conflicts about breastfeeding aren't so Dickensian, but they still pluck chords within our unconscious having to do with modesty and propriety. Rather than the amount of bare breast revealed (usually not much), it is the startling intimacy of breastfeeding that can stir discomfort when a mother nurses in public (even when that "public" is family and friends within a home!). Mother and baby respond to each other physically and emotionally while in direct skin-to-skin contact, which in the minds of many is unconsciously associated with sexual activity—something that should happen in total privacy.

Another obstacle is the sense of imprisonment some women sense in the breastfeeding relationship. True, the seemingly incessant demands by an infant for mother's milk can sometimes feel like a kind of assault. Our sleep suffers, our capacity to function normally suffers, our ability to accomplish even the most basic tasks suffers. This is when we have the opportunity to develop what people seek at the feet of spiritual masters: the power to respond to what Life is asking of us, in this moment, right now. *Presence.* Poet Andrea Potos sums it up in the opening of her poem: *Give up your calendar and clock, start flowing with milk time.* (And, get thee to a La Leche League meeting ASAP.)

If you sometimes find the day-in and day-out tasks of mothering to be tedious, you needn't feel guilty—join the club! It can help enliven our minds to learn more about the subtle complexities and extraordinary implications of what we do every day as mothers, and this is certainly the case with breastfeeding. Here are some ideas to kindle your imagination and inspiration toward embracing breastfeeding with extra delight:

- Powerful immune and growth factors are present in your breast milk in a dynamic way that cannot be duplicated in a laboratory: from colostrum to milk, from night feeding to day feeding, for a healthy baby or an ailing one, a mother's milk varies its composition in an intricate response to her baby's immediate needs. A mother produces a different milk for a premature baby than for a term newborn; different milk for an infant than for a toddler; and even different milk for a boy than for a girl![30]
- One of the main hormones of breastfeeding (together with oxytocin, of course) is prolactin, known as the "mothering hormone"; prolactin is also

found in the bloodstream during deep relaxation, meditation or hypnosis. Think of it as a natural coping agent that helps us deal with fatigue and focus on the essential—the baby. It even blurs our short-term memory to help keep us wholly in the present, the only place where our child can meet us. Nature is so clever in her strategic hormonal planning!

- Breastfeeding during the hour following birth—in addition to reducing the risk of postpartum hemorrhaging—is suspected to protect against postpartum depression, as it supports the gaze-to-gaze falling in love process that releases a nurturing flow of oxytocin, serotonin and dopamine. This in turn engages the mother's brain in the delight of breastfeeding, while beginning to build the oh-so-magnificent and important scaffold for all development and learning in the baby—secure connection. In the process, both mother and baby are enjoying oxytocin's haze of love—a recipe for bliss! If a mother is struggling in her new role, as I did and so many others do, nursing can go a long way in helping smooth the way; it is a safety net of sorts.

- A powerful soothing element in a newborn's life is something that has been a constant sensory presence—his mother's heartbeat. When a baby can look at his mother's face—his very favorite landscape, a primary stimulus for his brain development—and feel her heartbeat—that comforting, regulating constant he knows so well from the womb—together with the familiar containment of her heart's energy field*, he is in what we would call an optimal learning state.[31] Joseph Chilton Pearce charts nature's perfect plan for supporting the earliest unfolding of our children's intelligence: by making human breast milk the weakest and wateriest mother's milk in the animal kingdom (the lowest in fat and protein) nature ensures that nursing will be very frequent. And thus, the infant's two critical needs (the face and the heartbeat/heart field) will be

---

* In the last decade the new field of neurocardiology has amassed much evidence that Rudolf Steiner was right in his prediction of one hundred years ago: the heart is much more than a pump. Not only has research found that heart rate variability and heart rhythms stand out from all other physiological and psychological measures as the most dynamic and reflective of our inner emotional states, notably including stress, but that due to the heart's powerful electromagnetic component, when people touch or are in close proximity, one person's heartbeat signal is registered in the other person's brainwaves. [McCraty, Rollin, Mike Atkinson, and Dana Tomasino. *Science of the Heart: Exploring the Role of the Heart in Human Performance.* Boulder Creek, CA: Institute of HeartMath, 2001.]

met consistently and often, and learning (which for now means developing a secure connection) will unfold according to nature's brilliant plan!

- Further amplifying the brain-building aspects of breastfeeding, nursing automatically puts the infant into a lateral or cross-crawl position: her outside eye crosses the midline of her body as she gazes at you. This laterality nourishes important neural connections (a positioning good to remember if bottle-feeding).

- The composition of breast milk changes in the course of a single feeding. One way to avoid colic is to empty one breast before offering the other, so that your baby gets the rich hind-milk containing digestion-enhancing agents.

All else aside, one of breast milk's most appealing benefits is a practical one for the tired mom: it's always the right brand, always ready, always at the right temperature, and you never have to stumble around in a dark kitchen to find it.

Of course there are circumstances in which nursing isn't available to the new mother and baby—adoption, medical conditions contraindicating breastfeeding, and the rare cases in which certain obstacles just cannot be overcome. In such cases, it is important that mothers process the feelings that go along with this if it represents a loss—often including guilt, anger, grief—so that they can bring the same depth of uncomplicated presence to bottle feeding as they had hoped to bring to breastfeeding. The peace-nourishing elements are not just in the flow of milk, but in the flow of connectedness.

Nursing Generation Peace

Leading-edge brain development science explains that our attunement, our engaged emotional availability to our baby during those close connection times such as breastfeeding, is as critically important for her growing brain as calories—even more so![32] Breastfeeding—or bottle-feeding—isn't a time to exit energetically and put mothering on autopilot while watching TV, talking on the phone, or chatting with guests. Imagine you and your partner are in a most intimate moment together, and he or she switches on the TV or invites a friend in to sit and chat while you're engaged in this intimacy! In short, it's no longer intimacy, and rapport erodes rather than deepens (not to mention that resentment gradually seeps in). Feeding time is an exquisite opportunity for you and your baby to learn each other, which is at the heart of true intimacy.

At nighttime, many a mother has discovered the saving grace of nursing her new baby in bed while co-sleeping: it's so much less sleep-disruptive to just turn over, nurse, then go back to sleep, rather than having to fully awaken, walk to the bassinet (or—hopefully not—the crib in the baby's room down the hall), and then most likely spend extra time soothing your very agitated infant, who by then is more frantically hungry for milk and for skin-to-skin contact. Research has even found that co-sleeping nursing mothers get more sleep![33] A new mother typically feels like she's breaking every rule when bringing her baby into her bed; it violates all the guidelines in most parenting manuals, and all the well-meaning advice from Mom and the pediatrician and the busybody next door—but it saves her (and her partner's) sleep and sanity. (Remember prolactin—the coping chemical.) Nursing freely during the night also helps the baby learn the all-hallowed lesson of the difference between day and night, because the milk's biochemistry differs predictably from day to night. Perhaps the biggest benefit of co-sleeping is an eminently practical one: it results in a less tired mother, which improves everything in the home!

Not only is sleeping close together a protective measure against SIDS, but it provides a potent nightly dose of the skin-to-skin connectivity, entrainment of physiological rhythms and energetic rapport that is the foundation of robustly secure connectedness. When a mother nurses without being completely awake, her neocortex remains largely unaroused, keeping adrenaline flow to a minimum, which in turn increases the flow of nature's love potion, oxytocin. I wish I had known back then that I could perfectly well skip the diaper changes in the middle of the night, and instead of making those night feedings major waking productions, I could have luxuriated... *relaxed*...in the sleepy comfort of embracing my nursing babies. (For a thorough discussion of the history and benefits of, research about, and safe ways to practice, co-sleeping, I recommend Sarah Buckley's *Gentle Birth, Gentle Mothering*.)

As an adopted baby it was a given that I would be bottle-fed. But I knew nothing of such social arrangements; babies arrive with breast milk, this elixir of life, as their birthright. Thus, I found nursing my son and daughter especially precious. And though they are now adults, I still enjoy a certain abiding confidence gained by breastfeeding them. Deep connection and trust were established through the joy of our nursing relationship that helped very much once the teen years arrived with their tender challenges—in a manner that was out of their conscious awareness but very much in mine.

We cannot overestimate the effects of breastfeeding in helping create a foundation of peaceful security, joyful comfort and enhanced brainpower for the child—effects that endure lifelong. It is a mighty component of healthy, flourishing social intelligence.

Special Circumstances: Adoption, the NICU and Other Separations

What about when a newborn is separated from his or her mother because of unavoidable medical necessity, or in the case of adoption or surrogacy? Here again, Nature is a strict taskmaster: neither the best intentions nor the noblest justifications can rewrite her laws of neurophysiology. The above realities about the trauma of maternal separation don't yield to accommodate our cultural arrangements. The only recourse available to us in these cases—as whenever Life throws us a curve ball—is the consciousness with which we perceive and engage with the events we encounter.

When Nancy Verrier began writing about the topic that made her a household name in the world of adoption, she brought three important credentials to the table: she was a psychotherapist who had worked with many adopted people wrestling with a similar constellation of social and emotional difficulties; she was a scholar who had extensively studied the literature on attachment, separation and loss; and she was the mother of two daughters—one biological and one adopted. The insights she found at the intersection of those learning streams comprised her landmark 1993 book *The Primal Wound: Understanding the Adopted Child,* in which she wrote, "Many doctors and psychologists now understand that bonding doesn't begin at birth, but is a continuum of physiological, psychological, and spiritual events which begin in utero and continue throughout the postnatal bonding period. When this natural evolution is interrupted by a postnatal separation from the biological mother, the resultant experience of abandonment and loss is indelibly imprinted upon the unconscious minds of these children, causing that which I call the *primal wound.*"[34]

Verrier points out that the primal wound doesn't affect only adopted babies; varying degrees of this type of trauma can occur under other circumstances, such as neonatal intensive care unit (NICU) stays for premature or ill babies—

which involve not only separation, but such things as painful medical procedures, isolation, and harsh, invasive surroundings.

Rather than deeply question whether the experience of relinquishment and separation in adoption or surrogacy is traumatic, we as a society tend to believe that enough love and care can make everything right. But ever since Freud, psychologists have taught us that the first stage of psychological growth includes the development of trust as a foundation for secure relationships with others. Babies separated from the only connection they've ever known—their first biological and psychological home—have had their nascent sense of trust violated. And so all that love and care we give to the adoptee can have a hard time getting in. As Verrier says of her relationship to her own adopted daughter, "I discovered that it was easier for us to give her love than it was for her to accept it." On very deep levels, adoptees may unconsciously feel that it's too dangerous to love and be loved, authentically and deeply; how can they trust that they won't be hurt or abandoned again?[35]

Most of my previous body of work has been on adoption, particularly such primal issues as separation at birth and even before—the psychosocial impact of having been carried in an ambivalent or outright rejecting womb, perhaps by a mother contemplating abortion; and having been conceived without being intended by one's parents.[36] The experience of adopted people has so much to teach us about the impact of these early processes; reciprocally, researchers could mine prenatal psychology for important insights into what has for decades been a persistent social science riddle: *What that we've yet to identify contributes so saliently to consistently higher levels of psychosocial vulnerability in adopted people?*

Adoptees are consistently overrepresented in clinical, therapeutic, and correctional settings. Although they make up only 2 to 3 percent of the general population, over 7 percent of special education students identified as emotionally disturbed are adopted,[37] and adopted adolescents comprise anywhere from 5 to 20 percent and higher of caseloads of mental healthcare professionals.[38] In the gripping book *In the Realm of Hungry Ghosts*, which illuminates the associations between disrupted attachment and addictions, author Gabor Maté details several ways in which the prenatal and perinatal experiences of adoptees renders them neurophysiologically more vulnerable to various disorders—such as ADHD, which is indeed more prevalent in adopted youth—which in turn heightens their risk for addiction.[39] He points out that many adults who were adopted as infants "harbor a powerful and lifelong sense of rejection" and includes the sobering statistic that the suicide risk for adopted adolescents is double that of their nonadopted peers.[40]

Researchers who use the reports of adoptees (or others who were separated from their mothers at birth for a substantial length of time) find they use terms like "alien," "rootless," "flotsam," and "in limbo" to describe themselves. One study found the three salient themes of the narratives of adopted adolescents to be "a) a sense of 'homelessness,' b) an experience of being different, not belonging, or of having fallen 'out of everydayness,' and c) a profound estrangement from generally taken-for-granted realities such as the security of parental relationships. As a result of these themes or issues, participants, particularly those involved in treatment, often felt anxious, ungrounded, and unworthy…."[41]

I don't embrace a hand-wringing, doomsday attitude that pathologizes adoptees and adoption; when we can expand our perspective and apply an *adaptive* lens to adoptees' behaviors and "disorders," we can see them as brilliant adaptation strategies that have gotten stuck and are no longer adaptive, but disruptive. An adaptive lens interprets a child's behaviors and expressions *in light of what they have experienced*. Participating in a panel presentation on ADD at an adoption conference years ago, I proposed a new label to use for children who had suffered through maternal separation—which essentially engraves the threat of annihilation in their nervous system—and who years later could not gather their attention and focus on a given task: Natural Organismic Response to Massive Abandonment or Loss—acronym, NORMAL.

Contrary to the breezy, overly simplistic characterization of adoption (and now, increasingly, surrogacy) as "just another way to build a family," adoption is a somewhat more complicated way to build a family than nature intended and calls for extra consideration and care. When we overlook complications we risk missing rich opportunities for building family intimacy, which pulses at the heart of peaceful parenting. Tremendous blessings can be experienced by all the participants in adoption, but we must never forget that most often, those blessings are born of loss—the loss for the birthparents of a child they will not parent; the loss of their dreamed-of biological child the adoptive parents won't have; and the loss for the adopted child of his or her biological, genealogical, and possibly cultural, connections. When we deny adoption's losses, we also deny ourselves—and our children—its greatest blessings.

There are a handful of progressive folks around the country—such as Bryan Post, Daniel Hughes, Deborah Gray, Scott Abbott, and Michael Trout—offering excellent work with adoptees and their families based on this enlightened recognition of the neurobiological and attachment complexities of adoption and the etiology of adoptees' constellations of experiences and challenges. But compassionate care for the separation trauma, loss and grief suffered by a newborn under any circumstance—adoption, surrogacy, NICU care—needn't wait a moment: it can and should begin immediately.

In her book *Talking to Babies,* Myriam Szejer, a child psychiatrist and psychoanalyst, tells of her work in a huge maternity hospital in Paris, using words in the psychoanalytic tradition to help newborns in distress. Her book jacket reads, "In the very first days of a baby's life, the newborn, still struggling between birth and its entry into our world, already needs words. By 'needing words,' Szejer means that infants need to be talked to about the specific situations into which they are born. They need to hear about their mothers, fathers, siblings, and caretakers, but they also need to hear about problematic aspects of their histories, such as the death of a twin sibling or the death of a baby before them."[42]

Countless of Szejer's astonishing stories illustrate the power of meaningful words to reorient a suffering newborn in seemingly miraculous ways. One tells of a twin who was constipated—had not pooped yet in his one week of life—and was feeding listlessly; his condition was becoming critical. His twin meanwhile was thriving. The mother told Dr. Szejer that when she first found out she was carrying twins, she had been overwhelmed and terrified; she herself was a twin—who receded into the shadows while her sister stood in the spotlight. The idea of history repeating itself in her own children was too much, and she requested an abortion. She then changed her mind and accepted the twin pregnancy, then hesitated again. She continued to waffle until well into the pregnancy, when she settled into an oddly familiar contradictory mode of being: declaring all was fine despite her tears.

Szejer reflected to this newborn baby his true experience, in words that were straightforward and unclouded by sentiment or emotionality: he may have thought he was not supposed to live, that he needed to efface himself while his brother took center stage. She explained, "Your mother was afraid at the start of her pregnancy to have two children and not one. For a time, she considered not keeping both of you. But that didn't last, she changed her mind. That's why you were born, you don't need to efface yourself." She interpreted the effect of this on his relationship with his mother: "You ask nothing of her when you're hungry, you give her nothing when you're full."[43]

The baby had his first bowel movement within one hour and began to feed with more gusto. Szejer admits that even when one has seen many such clear results of reflecting for a child his or her truth, "they always leave you flabbergasted." Newborns being relinquished for adoption always receive a visit from Dr. Szejer. "In such cases, the child at birth is completely severed from all her prenatal perceptions; someone has to be there to name these perceptions, give them meaning, bridge the gap between the intrauterine past, the present, and the child's future."[44]

How we as the child's parents and other important adults meet, perceive and reflect an infant's hurts and losses is what can help him begin to live them in a healing way. If on the other hand we are so overly attached to a particular scenario we have dreamed of that we cannot hold our child's full, unvarnished truth, we drastically hinder his nervous system's natural inclination to self-correct. The child's greatest need is to be understood, in his most buoyant, delightful times as well as his darkest, most hurting times. When we are sincerely open in our willingness to see, hold and accept our children's sadness, it's astonishing how quickly that sadness moves through and morphs into life energy.

Our consciousness is our hero's shield with which we protect, defend and champion our children—including when they have endured difficult or painful experiences.

Attuned Connection: The Neurobiology of Transformative Possibilities

When our first child was born, long before I learned most of what I'm writing about here, I was determined to do everything I could to maximize his development. My devotion to Ian's betterment had begun during pregnancy, when I listened to my favorite classical music, took lots of walks, thought lots of good thoughts. This was a good start, mainly because these were all activities that inspired *me*. But once he was here, a certain frenzied insecurity set in, about making sure I was doing enough to stimulate his development. I promptly bought a book on baby exercise—*yes, baby exercise!* I dutifully followed the prescribed twice-a-day regimen of moving his various tiny limbs around and about, folding and stretching his new little body this way and that. It was supposed to get his sensory-motor development off to a head start, which sounded good to me. As luck and fate would have it, just a couple weeks into our training plan, I attended my first R.I.E. class—Resources for Infant Educarers—and what I heard there that very first day carried the blessed ring of truth. Actually, more like the booming clang of truth. And I *got* it.

I could relax—I didn't have to improve upon or optimize anything! My child had an innate intelligence that knew exactly how to unfold the unique body that was his. It didn't need me to pose it, bend it, or prop it into positions that were not yet natural for him. A basic tenet of the R.I.E. approach is "non-interference in gross motor development"—we allow the innate intelligence of the baby's developing body to determine when he first rolls over, sits up, stands, walks, and so on. (This autonomy of movement fosters important integrative development between various brain areas that end up impacting later capacities for far more than just movement.)

However, it isn't so much their child's *body* that parents today are looking to optimize in the early years—it's their child's *mind*. It was about twenty-five years ago when neuroscientists began to realize that the potential of an infant's brain is not genetically predetermined by a DNA blueprint, but is instead designed to be shaped by the environment, which can either enhance or inhibit its development. The huge spurts in brain growth from the last trimester of pregnancy through the first two years of life invite *experience-dependent maturation* of the brain: the environment a baby encounters teaches him about the world he has been born into, so his brain can adapt itself to work best in that world. Different environments inspire the development of different kinds of brains.

This finding—enrich the environment, enrich the baby's brain—set off a riptide of infant stimulation gadgetry into the consumer market in the late '80s; black-and-white mobiles and whiz-bang activity centers were snapped up by well-meaning parents anxious to give their children every possible foothold toward a successful future. But a decade later, attachment theorists and neuroscientists joined forces to identify the most critically important environmental variable involved in infant brain development, which turned out not to be mobiles decorated with high-contrast black-and-white images, or Baby Einstein* info-tainment,[45] or data on the screens of lapware computers designed for babies.

---

* The Baby Einstein juggernaut bears commenting on, just in case you feel like the mom who said, "You want to make sure you're doing everything you can for your child, and you know everyone else uses Baby Einstein, so you feel guilty if you don't." In case you missed it, in 2007 Baby Einstein, along with all other so-called educational screened programming, was found to be associated with *delayed* language development; television or video watching at this age, said an American Academy of Pediatrics spokesperson, "probably interferes with the crucial wiring being laid down in their brains during early development."

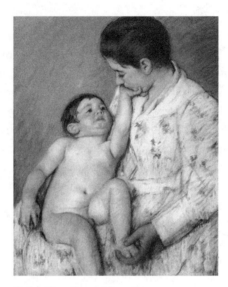

Baby's First Caress, Mary Cassatt

So, what *did* emerge in the research to be the single effective neurodevelopment optimization system? The technology is quite advanced, so try not to be intimidated by the complicated engineering as you behold this illustration of it. Impressionist Mary Cassatt couldn't have begun to fathom in 1891 the neuroscientific sophistication of the attachment interactions she cataloged so exquisitely.

Indeed, the technology of human evolutionary transformation is nothing more fancy or less humble than the secure, attuned relationship between an infant and his mother. (When I use the term *mother* or *father* or *parents,* please understand that aside from the earliest weeks, this also implies the inclusion of the phrase "or other consistently available adult caregiver." I don't want to be redundant about it, but I also don't want to leave out, say, a primary caregiving grandmother.) Once again, Nature designed it in elegant fashion. A newborn's brain circuitry is wired and primed at birth for interacting with and interpreting one thing: the human face. Take it away, and the newborn's consciousness, brain, and body functions start to stall out; return it, and everything hums back into action. Her vision system is optimal at twelve to sixteen inches focal length—that is, breastfeeding, in-arms or lap position—and is programmed to attend to and process specific types of patterns: she prefers curves to straight lines, strong contrasts of light and dark, and acute angles to obtuse angles. She is captivated by movement that occurs inside a distinct frame. "When you add up all these innate preferences," writes infant psychologist Daniel Stern in *Diary of a Baby*, "they almost spell F-A-C-E."[46]

A mother holds her infant on her lap facing her and smiles at him. He smiles and kicks with delight. She coos, and he squeals. She bends toward him making an outboard motor noise, and he pumps his legs and his arms and squeals more loudly. Then he turns his head away. The mother makes a calm "Ohhhh," sound, and the intensity of their "conversation" begins to de-escalate. When the baby looks back at her, she giggles again, and away they go, mind-to-mind delight rising again. This scene of a mother engaging her infant in a kind of reciprocal series of cooing, giggling, sighing and squealing can be found everywhere around the world, across all divides of race, religion, socioeconomic or technological circumstance.

Scientists have discovered that these playful mother-baby encounters are actually highly organized, sophisticated dialogues: mothers and infants synchronize the emotional intensity of their behavior within lags of split seconds, making it an interaction in which both partners match states and then simultaneously adjust their social attention, stimulation, and accelerating arousal in response to the partner's signals.[47] This microregulation continues until the baby averts his gaze to regulate the potentially disorganizing effect of the intensity of positive emotion. The mother takes her cue and backs off, reducing her stimulation. She then waits for her baby's signal for reengagement. It is an intimate dance between them that is designed to be immediate, instinctive, effortless. (But it isn't always so effortless, and I'll get to that in a moment.)

Sharing States

These interactions involve another, more hidden "conversation": when infants and parents engage in this kind of mutually attuned, face-to-face, gaze-to-gaze, I-laugh-then-you-laugh encounter, the baby's immature areas of the brain that regulate her fluctuating *affect* (distress, arousal, hunger, etc.—the primitive precursors to emotions)[48] fall into step, or link up—with the regulating structures of the adult's brain. The baby essentially uses the regulating capacity of the adult to manage her own affective states. What science has uncovered about this process is nothing less fantastic than the most elegant science fiction:

a currently proposed open-loop model of interpersonal neurophysiology suggests that the process of close, connected communications within a closely connected relationship is used by social mammals to tune each other's neurophysiological steadiness.[49]

While the researchers use such terms as *biological synchronicity*[50] and *limbic resonance*,[51] the sci-fi image of *mind-melding* isn't far off the mark. Writes one researcher, in evident awe, "It is a biologically based communication system that involves individual organisms directly with one another: the individuals in spontaneous communication constitute *literally a biological unit.*"[52] Here we see a major recurrence of the fundamental developmental motif that premiered during early embryonic growth: *projection of function outside before internalizing the capacity.* During these regulating interactions, the child relies upon the more organized regulatory mechanisms of the parent's limbic structures to regulate her own internal states and external behavioral responses— i.e., her emotions. Her developmental task over the early months and years is to internalize the capacity to regulate her own inner states. And how is this task jump-started?

Do be sure you're sitting down, because this is wild: Over time, and the hundreds and thousands of repeated encounters between parents and baby, the infant's own affect-regulating neural circuitry wires up *to echo that of his "partner."* One of the godfathers of attachment neurobiology, Allan Schore, puts it quite bluntly: "The mother is downloading emotion programs into the infant's right brain. The child is using the output of the mother's right hemisphere as a template for the imprinting, the hard wiring, of circuits in his own right hemisphere that will come to mediate his expanding affective capacities, an essential element of his emerging personality."[53]

What that means in plain English is that engaged, attuned, playful interactions with us are a basic and essential form of nourishment for our babies. And further, it is *we ourselves* that our children are wiring up to be, from the very beginning; this foundation then serves as their launching pad, at the most basic level of brain structure, for surpassing us into higher realms of accomplishment, social intelligence, and joyous self-mastery.

Why This Bit of Neuroscience Matters for Peace

The particular area of the brain that depends most fundamentally upon secure, predictable relationship for its most robust development is called the *or-*

bitofrontal cortex (OFC for short), which sits just behind the right eye socket in the brain's right hemisphere and quietly goes about the business of orchestrating the capacities that determine a child's lifelong prospects for healthy social and emotional functioning. Because of its unique placement and function in the brain, the OFC is fundamental to fostering skills and affinities for peace and sustainability at every level.

The OFC is the seat of common sense thinking; the ability to read other people's signals and recognize their intentions; to sense their emotions, and have empathy; to make sense of our own autobiographical histories; to imbue intellectual thought with feeling, and vice versa, to moderate emotion with rational thought. "Such neural capacities matter immensely," writes Daniel Goleman in *Social Intelligence*, not just for the richness of our interpersonal life but for the wellbeing of our children, for our ability to love well, and for our very health."[54] The OFC is indeed the brain center for social and emotional intelligence—*the skills of how to be a human with other humans.*

The OFC is the fundamental *regulating* and *integrating* structure of the brain. It allows all of the information from other parts of the brain—facts, sensations, internal feelings—to be put together in a way that makes sense, that has meaning, that fits, and that allows *us* to fit into our social surroundings in a comfortable, satisfying way. It is what allows us to *self-regulate*—to modulate our moods and emotions, our reactions, our internal sense of order. (It makes perfect sense that the OFC is suspected to be intimately involved in disorders like ADD/ADHD and OCD, which are about neural regulation, and in sensory processing disorders, which are about neural integration.)[55]

In the 1960s, attachment researchers noticed the strong connection between children whose attachment style fell into the "secure" category, and parents who had the ability to tell clear, articulate, coherent stories about their own childhood experiences. Even though they did not then understand why, researchers followed the data to form the axiom, "The most robust predictor of secure attachment in a child is the ability of that child's parent to tell a coherent narrative of his or her own childhood." Decades later, neural imaging technology finally provided a new generation of attachment scientists with the explanation to such a seemingly puzzling connection: the nature of development of the adult's orbitofrontal cortex (OFC) determines how well that adult can provide the child with the basic ingredients (the gaze, the presence, the completeness of self) necessary to foster secure attachment. Because the OFC is the seat of autobiographical memory and narrative recall, the ability to coherently* tell one's childhood story is a reliable marker for healthy OFC functioning.[56]

Lifelong Lessons

Perhaps you thought back to Ryan when I mentioned that the OFC is related to the skills of being a human with other humans. In that case Bruce Perry discovered that Ryan's parents simply weren't aware that their one hour per day with him was drastically insufficient to a baby's needs. "They didn't realize that frequently repeated routines—almost endless repetitions and specific daily rhythms—are the heart of parenting."[57] The supposedly unremarkable, daily interactions between a mother and her baby—in the nursing chair, on the changing table, in the bath, in her arms—actually comprise an intricate and complicated learning process: over the course of repeated experiences, the right hemisphere of the infant's brain—which is primarily nonverbal, noncognitive, outside conscious awareness—automatically extracts and remembers the constants that underlie those experiences. It is this kind of silent learning, taking place over the days, weeks, and months of a child's life—certainly until the age of five—that engraves upon her psyche *patterns of relating*, via the unforgiving, all-encompassing encoding process of neural memory.

"Such knowledge develops with languorous ease and inevitability, stubbornly inexpressible, never destined for translation into words," writes psychiatrist Thomas Lewis with his coauthors of the enchanting interpersonal neurobiology primer *A General Theory of Love*.[58] These patterns accumulate over the early years of a child's life into a suite of powerful—but unconscious—basic beliefs about herself, and models of and rules for expectations of others: *I am worthy of love. Others care for me. I can trust. My needs are attended to. Love feels good. Connection is safe. There is enough. All is pretty much right with the world.* Or not.

Here again we encounter the growth-or-protection theme so fundamental to parenting for peace: just as a cell or an organ "perceives" environmental circumstances that either support optimal growth or call for diverting energy to-

---

* This means the ability to make relatively ordered, sequential narrative sense of what for many people is a tangle of vague memory fragments, amorphous impressions and second-hand stories passed down through the family over the years.

ward protection, a baby perceives through his early relationships information about the world so he can best prepare himself to excel in that world. He learns through these early experiences that it is safe to grow toward his full evolutionary potential—connected to self and others, capable of empathy, vision, and enlightened action—or that he needs to protect, defend, and remain fundamentally separate from others.

Dubbed by attachment research founder John Bowlby *internal working models*, these early relational lessons act like templates to shape an individual's future, as the person seeks out situations and relationships in which those beliefs, models and rules feel familiar, feel like home—be it a happy home, an angry home or an empty home. In the bittersweet fashion so often found in nature's cyclic evolutionary urging, we will gravitate over and over and over to exactly the kinds of relationships that originally shaped us. Positive thinking, diligent goal-setting, affirmations and visualizations aside, our default is to seek the familiar, the habitual—even over what we *think* we want. The boon for Generation Peace is that we can do much to ensure that loving responsiveness, empathy, joy and delight feel neurologically familiar to our children, and that they will naturally gravitate to these qualities as they grow into the fullness of adult life!

The Takeaway Message for Parents-for-Peace

The science is indeed astonishing, but what does it mean on the ground, at home, for new parents? That it is all about the gaze, the presence, the completeness of yourself that you offer your baby, again and again and again and again and…well, you get the idea.

The Gaze – Twentieth-century poet Rainier Maria Rilke said it so perfectly, you'd think he had a degree in twenty-first century developmental neurobiology: "Face to face with you, I am born in the eye." That, in a nutshell, is what happens in the parent-child connection. The baby needs us to *really* see her, for it is within that gaze that truly miraculous things happen.

First and foremost, the baby is mirrored. It was famed pediatrician and psychiatrist D. W. Winnicott who said, "The baby's first mirror is the mother's face." It's from the expressions on his mother's face that a baby experiences, "Ah, I'm delightful, I'm wonderful, I'm worthy of love"—not at first in words, of course, but in the elixir of pleasure hormones that flows when Mama responds in an attuned way to his cues. This is how he begins to put together a "self" for himself. When the intimacy of the attuned, adoring gaze is missing, a person can go through life unceasingly seeking that missing mirroring—in eliciting admiring looks or praise from others, in being perfect, in being a people pleaser, in countless fruitless ways of attempting to fill up the space left by not having been "sufficiently adored at the proper time," as Nancy Friday so aptly put it.[59] Psychologist John Breeding invites parents to embrace their children with "eyes of delight."[60]

The depth of seeing that takes place in a securely connected interaction goes beyond what the eyes exchange. When a parent is responsively attuned, he or she communicates to the child, "I see *all of you*, even on the inside." And more than that, "I share what you're experiencing." One of the new wave of attachment neurobiology researchers distills it into the rather lyrical notion of *feeling felt*.[61] The early experience of feeling felt by an attachment figure is a foundation for the child's developing capacities for empathy, compassion and true intimacy.

The Presence – As much as your baby needs protein and fat for building her body and brain, she also needs slices of your undistracted presence (meaning, you are all here, right now). Throughout her childhood and into adolescence, she will need regular doses of you in this way, but as an infant, her brain development depends as much upon your engaged, attuned interaction for its growth as it does on calories. It isn't too far-fetched to say that she feeds off of your very "beingness" when you are present with her. Just as the infant uses the nourishment of his mother's milk to build his tissue and bones, he uses the relationship with his primary caregiver to build areas of his brain that are critical to his future social-emotional functioning, particularly the orbitofrontal cortex. Thus, what researchers have discovered is that attachment (secure relational connection) is a basic kind of developmental nourishment. (Therefore, its disruption—through neglect, abuse, or other forms of relational wounding or persistent lack of attuned presence—I have termed *malattachment.*)[62]

Together with the mirroring gaze, the quality of her mother's presence is an important series of lessons for the baby, which follows on the heels of the lessons from the womb and from birth: imagine day after day after day of a baby experiencing the cycle of "I'm in distress because I'm hungry"*—with the accompanying flood of fight-or-flight hormones firing up a global, bodily stress response—followed by "Ahh, Mama's soft body and warm milk"—triggering a flow of endorphins that fire up a global, bodily pleasure response. As this happens over and over and over, the baby's brain wires the association between Mama—her scent, heartbeat, voice—and the experience of extreme pleasure and the relief of stress. Over time this association between Mama and pleasure is elasticized to include ever more people, which is the basis of civilized behavior.[63]

And when we're thinking of raising joyful peacemakers, we need to watch our collective tendency to focus primarily on just soothing a baby's *negative* affect—his upset, his crying, his distress. Along with helping him manage his negative states, it is just as important for the optimal health of a baby's developing social brain that we also attune to, delight in, mirror and amplify his *positive* affective states, like excitement, laughter and above all, simple contentment.

The Completeness of Yourself – Raising Generation Peace is all about recognizing and leveraging the power of evolution—particularly the astonishing transformative opportunity offered us through this intricate connection process. It is available to every parent for every baby. But there is one little catch: we are not merely conduits of learning for our children—we *are* the lesson! Recall that this remarkable process of the baby piggybacking on his parents' neural regulating structures to help manage his own internal balance comes with the rather staggering twist: his social brain is wiring itself up to match his parent's brain. Face-to-face engagement within the relationship serves as *mind-to-mind training*, whereby the circuitry of the orbitofrontal portion of the infant's brain is being laid down according to the model provided

---

* The infant doesn't experience it in this verbal, cognitive way, but in an endless stream of bodily sensations, as so beautifully described in Daniel Stern's landmark book, *Diary of a Baby*. Stern's take on the primal experience of hunger: "The wind and the sounds and the pieces of sky are all pulled back into the center. There they find one another again, are reunited. Only to be thrown outward and away, then sucked back in to form the next wave—darker and stronger. The pulsing waves swell to dominate the whole weatherscape. The world is howling. Everything explodes and is blown out and then collapses and rushes back toward a knot of agony that cannot last—but does." [Stern, Daniel N. *Diary of a Baby*. New York: Basic Books, 1998, pg. 32]

by the attachment figure. Over the course of the thousands of connection en-counters that occur in the early months and years of a child's life, she essentially "copies and pastes" into her own brain key features of her caregiver's neuro-logical circuitry for emotional and social functioning.

So an infant with an emotionally available, attuned, self-possessed caregiver develops different neural templates—*patterns of relating*—than an infant whose caregiver is emotionally absent, volatile, insecure, anxious, depressed, etc. There are countless reasons why a mother (like a father) might not have the ability to be instinctively present in the attuned way that healthy relationship seeks, and the seeds usually lie in her own developmental history. Maybe *her* mother wasn't present for her, maybe *she* wasn't seen, maybe *she* did not receive the intimate mirroring of delight and ease. She may have been neglected, she may have been abused, or most likely of all, she may have suffered malattach-ment through no ill will or conscious mistreatment by her parents. She may have internalized imprints—internal working models—that feature shame, distrust, loss, or the experience that human connection is not pleasurable.

It's somewhat easier for us to fake our way around these templates when dealing with other adults in our adult world—in the workplace, the dating scene, or even within a marriage—than it is when faced with our own exceed-ingly dependent babies, fresh and new and looking to us for everything. Noth-ing calls us to our (sometimes painful) truthful selves like those newborn eyes, pooling with so much potential and expectation. That is, as they say, where the rubber hits the road, the poo hits the fan, and we either go all in or we find a way to sidestep the sometimes terrifying toll of intimacy that our chil-dren innocently exact.

The good news is that with determination and awareness, we can renego-tiate our own stories, and nurture our own OFC development in the process.[64] One of the most exciting, revolutionary scientific discoveries of the past cen-tury involves *neuroplasticity*—the fact that the brain never stops revising and remodeling itself, into middle age and beyond. Neuroplasticity simply means the ability of the brain to be changed by experience—that is, to learn. So it is possible after all to teach old dogs—and people—new tricks. As parents, not only is it possible to foster further development of our own social brain's health, but doing so is perhaps the most important investment we can make in our children's lifelong success.

Whoever wrote that bumper sticker "It's never too late to have a happy child-hood" was actually onto something. While we cannot change history, or what happened in our lives, we *can* change our inner orientation to it, how we make sense of our stories. One of the most powerful ways to foster OFC health is to engage in self-reflection, exploring your inner life with an attitude of compassionate curiosity. Consciously working on making sense of your own early story can rewire your OFC circuitry toward greater health and resiliency.[65]

Writing in a journal, speaking into a voice recorder, creating art, writing poems or songs, dancing—these are all wonderful ways to encourage further development of your social brain, when done with the dedicated intention of becoming more fluent and friendly with your own early story. (It's also possible to engage in these things as a way to… well… wallow; wallowing can be one stage of the process of self-inquiry, but becomes a dead end if one isn't mindful about keeping the process moving.) If your childhood story is particularly troubled or marked by intense malattachment, it's usually wise to seek the guidance and support of a trained therapist or counselor. When we're pursuing the goal of raising a peaceful, thriving generation, the importance of tending to our own nourishment and ongoing development as a person cannot be overstated.

One important pathway for cultivating your own OFC development is the practice of Parenting for Peace Principle #1, mindful presence. Meditation, yoga, contemplative prayer—these are all stellar examples of daily practices that foster the health of your social brain. But that can be daunting to some folks who've never ventured into that territory of spiritual practice. If you were to simply set aside just five minutes each day—*five minutes!*—to quiet your mind, and do steady, calm, deep breathing,* you would be investing wisely in your own OFC health and in the optimally successful development of your child. (I know that in a home with a baby or young child(ren), it can be difficult to find even such a small window of time, but naptime or before everyone else wakes up in the morning are good places to look.)

An important aspect of "completeness of yourself" is tending to exactly that—making sure you are a complete person: it is of utmost nourishing importance to your child that you maintain a strong relationship with the aspects of your life that exist outside of and beyond your role as a parent. Naturally,

---

* One way to still your mind is to simply count your breaths. Visualizing each number during its breath can help quiet the noise inside: when a thought creeps in, gently uninvite it and return your attention to the huge number in your mind's eye. Over time, your mind will quiet more easily, a sure sign of increased self-regulation capacity—and proof of enhanced OFC health!

in the normal upheaval of the early weeks and months with a new baby, outward engagement with these aspects will recede to a great degree, but to the extent that they were well established *prior* to baby's arrival, they will still blossom in your consciousness and the atmosphere of you. It is essential that you are a complete adult *around whom your child revolves*—like a sun. This aspect right here undermines the efforts of so many well-meaning, loving, earnestly striving parents these days: simply put, their child becomes their primary focus, the central pole *around whom they, the adults, revolve.*

While it is understood that in the early weeks you are completely preoccupied with the baby, it is nourishing to everyone for you to keep in mind that your primary connection and orientation is to Life, not to this one child. Rudolf Steiner taught that children should constellate around adults, not the other way around. Jean Liedloff, famous for her observations of parenting practices among the indigenous Yequana Indians of South America, reports that only after several extended stays with the tribe did she notice something missing from typical family life with children:

> Where were the "terrible twos"? Where were the tantrums, the struggle to "get their own way," the selfishness, the destructiveness and carelessness of their own safety that we call normal? Where was the nagging, the discipline, the "boundaries" needed to curb their contrariness? Where, indeed, was the adversarial relationship we take for granted between parent and child? Where was the blaming, the punishing, or for that matter, where was any sign of permissiveness?[66]

Liedloff's conclusion was that the Yequana are (gasp!) not child-centered. Yes, they keep the baby in constant physical contact until he's crawling, and yes, Yequana parents breastfeed according to the baby's cues, and they will often nuzzle their babies affectionately, play a little game of peek-a-boo now and then, or sing to them; however, as Liedloff emphasizes, "the great majority of the caretaker's time is spent paying attention to something else...not the baby!"

> Thus, Yequana babies find themselves in the midst of activities they will later join as they proceed through the stages of creeping, crawling, walking, and talking. The panoramic view of their future life's experiences, behavior, pace, and language provides a rich basis for their

developing participation. Being played with, talked to, or admired all day deprives the babe of this in-arms spectator phase that would feel right to him. Unable to say what he needs, he will act out his discontentment. He is trying to get his caretaker's attention, yet—and here is the cause of the understandable confusion—his purpose is to get the caretaker to change his unsatisfactory experience, to go about her own business with confidence and without seeming to ask his permission. Once the situation is corrected, the attention-getting behavior we mistake for a permanent impulse can subside. The same principle applies in the stages following the in-arms phase.[67]

This raises what can seem like a puzzling conundrum, requiring distinctions that are in some ways subtle, paradoxical even, with respect to Principle #1, presence. As we go along, I will do my best to articulate, illuminate and ease this glaring parenting paradox—the need for a parent's presence to a child without her unduly weighty preoccupation with the child. Children need to know that although they are important and in utmost need of our care, the world does not revolve around them. It is nourishing to them to know that we listen to our own inspiration and have other sources of inner fulfillment in life—and that even the joy of having a child isn't a joy as high as the connection we feel with Life. That's why we invited someone into our life—to share in, but not *be*, the joy of our connection to Life!

Nine Months In, Nine Months Out…and Then…

Unlike all other animals, humans are born long before we're ready to function precisely *because* of our vast difference from all other animals at the level of brain growth. Were we born with brains close to their mature or even childhood size, as Joseph Chilton Pearce points out with a wink, our skulls would be so big, "We'd never get outta there!" Humans are necessarily born as essentially premature creatures, and for us to develop to our fullest potential, we need the close, near-constant connection with our mothers for the better part of the first year. Many people even refer to the early months as The Fourth Trimester.

Pearce reminds us of the implications of Nature's specificity with respect to her plan for peace-oriented development: between the ninth and twelfth months in the life of a child who has been in close contact with his mother and enjoyed attuned, responsive, loving care from her, together with adjunct relationships with a select few (one or two) other close adults,* the *orbitofrontal loop* develops. This is part of the upgrade described in Step One, which brings the area of the brain currently on line in the baby—the sensing-doing brain—into more harmonious, seamless coordination with the higher-ordered pre-frontal lobes. It routes through the OFC, which acts as a sort of clutch mechanism to help the gears of the various brain circuitries to engage together and synergize effectively.[68]

At this same time, the cerebellum has a massive growth spurt, equipping the baby to stand up and begin moving out—to continue building what child psychologist Jean Piaget called *structures of knowledge*. By virtue of healthy, connected development during his first nine months, this child is primed to discover a welcoming, nurturing world…but…what is he likely to find instead? Research shows that the typical child of this age, newly toddling about to discover her world, is met with an emphatic "No!" every nine minutes.[69] Just one such "inhibiting directive" that so naturally rolls off parents' tongues can raise a child's level of the stress hormone cortisol for twelve hours. Pearce points out that cortisol is one of the most neurotoxic substances known to man: it kills brain cells. It also drastically suppresses immune function, as most of us know all too well from falling ill after a bout of stress, especially some severe disappointment. Cortisol is one of the primary information substances that instruct the bodymind to shift from growth mode into protection mode.[†]

So then what happens to the peace-oriented, upgraded development that had begun so beautifully in the first nine to twelve months of this baby's life? Assuming he continues to receive the standard series of prohibitions and other well-meaning yet inhibiting directives, between his twelfth and eighteenth months Nature will call for a drastic course correction in his brain develop-

---

* This doesn't mean that having lots more helping hands around—as in an extended family or communal situations—isn't also a boon to children; as long as the child has a close, connected, consistent and predictable relationship with one or two *primary* caregivers, having more (healthy) adults around is actually a good thing: the primary caregiver has social and practical support and his or her own nourishing web of relationship. But this is not the same as the tag team, pass-the-baby-around approach some people consider cooperative child-rearing.

† As with most hormones, this is too simplistic a characterization; its function can vary depending on the target organ, the developmental phase, and many other variables, and sometimes it is associated with healthy, necessary functions. For instance, cortisol plays a key role in fetal lung maturation prior to birth.

ment, in response to the consistently thwarting environment: the pathway integrating his OFC with the primitive and higher brain centers—central to empathy and the process we might call "conscience"—will be rerouted to instead link the reptilian and the limbic structures—to equip him with the hyperalertness, impulsivity and hair-trigger emotions needed to survive in a hostile world. Why? Because when he began moving out, he found a hostile world!

So we need to keep in mind with our infants and young toddlers that scolding makes no sense and, worse, does this kind of fundamental damage. We redirect, not reprimand. Show the way, not shout it. Demonstrate, not debate. And thus we retain something that is all-important through each of these steps: connection with our child, and by virtue of that, her own inner connectedness. A mantra that will serve you well—and the sliver of Generation Peace you are raising—is, *Nurture the connection.* Indeed, parenting educator and author Pam Leo's brilliant distillation of the complexities of attachment research, *Connection Parenting*, tracks perfectly with the growth-versus-protection dynamic so central to parenting for peace. Writes Leo, "The model of parenting most of us grew up with was authoritarian parenting, which is based on fear. Some of us may have grown up with permissive parenting, which is also based on fear. Authoritarian parenting is based on the child's fear of losing the parent's love. Permissive parenting is based on the parent's fear of losing the child's love. Connection parenting is based on love instead of fear." And indeed, the growth-versus-protection dynamic can be framed in love-versus-fear terms. Leo's all-purpose guidance for parents who are overwhelmed with parenting advice from all corners (in-laws, experts, media) is to ask themselves, "If I use this technique, system or approach, will it result in a stronger connection or a weakened connection with my child?"[70]

Awareness Fosters Attunement

It can be immensely helpful to understand a few concepts about your child's social and cognitive development as he begins moving out at the end of the fourth trimester. For instance, if you realize that the most seemingly obvious reality is not always reality for a child at this age, it's easier to avoid slipping into the emphatic-*No*-every-nine-minutes pattern that is so common, and so not fun for anyone. A fascinating aspect of Piaget's classic studies is his assertion of the child's gradual development through infancy of *object permanence*—the ability to recognize that an object can still exist even if it cannot be perceived by the senses (the baby cannot see, touch or hear it). For example, a four-month-old will typically not look for an object after a cloth is put on top of it, even if she sees you cover it up.

By somewhere around the nine-month moving out stage, the baby will indeed look for an object after you hide it while she watches, but she may make the fascinating *AB error*: If she's allowed to find the toy in one place a few times and it is then hidden elsewhere, while the child watches you hide it, the child may very well *still search in the first location*. Once she finds the object at the new location, if the toy is again hidden at the original location (while she watches), the infant may now err by reaching back to the location that was most recently correct. Experts posit various explanations, including the infant's inability to yet integrate knowledge and action; constraints of memory (I doubt this); and the brain's current inability to inhibit what was earlier a successful response. I happen to find it enchanting that with all of our sophisticated diagnostic, research and testing expertise, we still don't have a handle on some aspects of the human mystery. This is part of the allure of parenting—discovering each day the wonders of how your unique child is growing and changing in her rapport with the world!

While the infant in his first year is working on this sophisticated endeavor of object permanence, he is also acquiring the first in a series of psychosocial developmental milestones as articulated by developmental psychologist Erik Erikson. Erikson cast the lifelong developmental arc as a series of psychosocial crises (lessons that must be learned) between the individual and society—a child's first society being parents and those in the home. The crisis of the first year (infancy) is *trust versus mistrust*—optimally leading to the baby's internalized experience of trust, that his caregivers reliably, consistently, and responsively meet his needs for food, comfort and relationship.[71] The successful resolution of each crisis (in which, as Erikson said, both polarities must be understood and accepted as both required and useful) results in the emergence of what he called a life-stage virtue. When a child has experienced a trust-building infancy, the lifelong virtues that emerge are *hope* and *drive*. And what more urgent virtues could there be for a generation inheriting tomorrow's world?

Another concept that I have found tremendously helpful in my practice with parents comes from the innovative Circle of Security program, an elegant approach to strengthening parents' ability to observe and foster their own capacity for nourishing connection.[72] It makes clear how the process of attachment is a basic, rhythmic pattern of connection-separation-reconnection that babies and children cycle through, over and over again: close, attuned, nourishing contact—the "secure base"—fills her up (both physically, in the case of nursing or eating, and social-emotionally, through engaged relationship), followed by a period of time during which she relies upon her own inner resources and fledgling experiments with autonomy, after which she needs to return to connectedness—the "safe haven"—for protection, comfort, cherishing and help managing feelings. In an infant the autonomous segment of the cycle may be just a short period of quiet-alert time when she simply takes in the world around her, processing it all, and fleetingly manages her own state regulation until that task is once more taken up by the adult caregiver when they are together again and linked up, social brain to social brain.

This cycle becomes more vividly noticeable once the child is a toddler, when he has the ability to quite literally walk away from Mama—to explore and then return when he needs to refuel. I had a big *ah-hah* moment when hearing one of the creators of this model introducing it to a conference audience, as he explained that depending on parents' own childhood experiences, they will usually find one or the other of these basic movements more challenging—either the moving out phase or the returning phase. I confess that when my son was little I was so undone by the relational demands of mothering—having grown up without secure early connections—that I delighted in his moving *out* (relief!) but sometimes anguished over his coming *back* (why must he need me so *much*?). One of my clients, Tina, had a more classically smothering type of experience with her own mother, which became her natural tendency to repeat (until we began gently working on it): Tina struggled with those moments when her son left her to explore, and she tended to hover anxiously, filled with relief when he would lift his arms to again be in her embrace.

For Tina it was the "venturing out" movement on the Circle of Security that pushed her old buttons, and for me it was the "returning" movement that did so. Identifying where on the circle you may feel discomfort is an excellent inroad to self-inquiry regarding the nature of your own early connectedness. It was only many years later that I realized one of the reasons for my distress over Ian's repeated returns to me was that I was unconsciously engaged in an inner process that was making us both miserable, and yet I didn't know it. I have since come to see, in my practice with parents, that this is a very common dynamic, yet rarely mentioned in parenting books: projecting your own unprocessed childhood experience and feelings onto your child, and then responding to *that* rather than to your actual child's experience and feelings in real time.

The authors of the extraordinary book *Parenting from the Inside Out: How A Deeper Self-Understanding Can Help You Raise Children Who Thrive* trace the contours of this and other parenting pitfalls related to our unfinished business from childhood. They also point out the good news that healing is possible, if we're willing to face "what at times may seem like unbearable feelings" as well as our "vulnerabilities that don't become apparent until we raise or work with children."[73]

Ian's birth and infancy had reawakened long-buried feelings in me from my own complicated infancy—grief, terror, rage. When Ian was around eight months old I spoke of my motherhood struggles with a therapist, who explained to me, "You never grieved for your childhood, and that is what's now coming up." The irony was laughable—several years and thousands of dollars worth of therapy had failed to do what my baby boy was doing effortlessly, without charge. Ian was eroding my defenses, stretching open my unhealed wounds, the losses of what I'd never received from my own mother—connection, security, predictability, attention. These were the things that Ian was calling on me to provide him, and in trying to meet his demands I was scraping an empty, aching well. Well, as those feelings bubbled up they threatened to undo the precarious construction that was me at that point, so I offloaded them onto Ian: I saw *him* as a bottomless, impossible-to-fill receptacle of attention, and then feared him for that. No wonder I felt anxiety every time he returned to me: not only did I have nothing to give, I saw it as a doomed task, since I'd obviously never be able to give him enough!

This tendency to unconsciously substitute our own history for our child's present reality is something to watch for, since it is very common and can insidiously undermine the effectiveness of even the most diligent, devoted parent.

Telling Our Birth Stories

Ancient warriors (as recently as World War II) returning from battle shared their stories of horror and heroics with their fellow warriors and eventually with their communities. In the past, birthing women also did this. Storytelling, dancing, music, poetry and chanting were all used to depict and relive the raw, powerful, transformative experience. The recounting of her personal story helps a new mother integrate the intensity of her birth experience into everyday life and into her own consciousness. It also introduces her experiences into the community, where the next generation of young women can develop a healthy understanding of pregnancy, labor pain, birth and motherhood. We have abandoned these kinds of postpartum rituals; in our culture, virtually all authentic expressions about the noble endeavor of childbirth are deformed into standard-issue sitcom punch lines.

Western civilization is notoriously cavalier about childbirth; as long as it results in a healthy baby, the birthing experience itself (from the mother's perspective) is seen as insignificant, a means to an end, nothing to dwell upon ("Oh, come on honey, Bill and Doris don't need to see the video..."). Any detours from a woman's childbirth expectations become largely irrelevant once a good outcome has been achieved. But new research suggests that we shouldn't be so quick to sweep birth bygones under the rug: negative emotions linked to childbirth may be pushed back by conscious cognitive processing ("Oh, it wasn't so bad, and look how beautiful she is!") and framed into a "wordless and unelaborated realm of experience" that can get in the way of the mother-baby relationship.[74]

And vibrant connection is the shining polestar of Generation Peace, the central, essential foundation for a person's lifelong development as an agent of empathy, innovation and sustainability. "How we connect with others," writes Goleman, "has unimagined significance."[75]

In one brilliant little study, women were simply supported in taking just fifteen minutes to write or speak aloud a narrative account of their child's birth—including all of their associated emotions and worries, without denying, prettying up or justifying them. Engaging in that short exercise greatly reduced these new mothers' symptoms of stress-induced avoidance, including a sense of "estrangement from others" and high levels of nervous system arousal, which lead to irritability, hypercontrol, and anxiety for forthcoming negative events. The reduced rate of these symptoms—often precursors to postpartum depression—remained consistent at a follow-up after two months.[76]

The Birth of a Mother

The Ticopia people of the Solomon Islands announce birth differently than most: rather than saying, "A baby has been born!" they proclaim, "A mother has given birth!"[77] A subtle but important distinction. When a baby is born, a mother is born; even if she already has children, each birth experience unfolds new facets of her, having to do with feeling powerful, capable, supported—or helpless, incompetent, insignificant. These primal feelings will weave their way through her ongoing life and her relationships—with her children, her partner, herself. Indeed, a mother's experience of giving birth leaves its indelible imprint, a faint yet distinct watermark on her soul.

Research shows that three primary aspects shape a woman's perception of her birth as positive or negative (and notice the interesting absence of anything about pain or hard work!): 1) her perception of control, 2) how supportive she finds the environment, and 3) her prior vulnerabilities.[78] The last chapter addressed the fact that the first two elements can be experienced across a broad spectrum, depending on where, how and with whom the woman is birthing. But the third element—a woman's history of vulnerabilities, such as loss, grief, depression, and the very story of her *own* birth and childhood—is rarely given the attention it needs so that a smooth way can be paved for a peaceful, enriching postpartum season. All too often, this time of life for mother and for baby is marked by a lack of ease, confidence, and joy.

When Joylessness Takes Over

Postpartum depression* is one of those terms like *love*—it trips off our tongues, we assume we know what it means, we do know that it is important and serious, but it remains quite abstract. What does it really look like (and *feel* like)? A web search can quickly turn up a laundry list of symptoms: extreme fatigue, disinterest in her baby, sleeplessness, sadness, tearfulness, anxiety, hopelessness, feelings of worthlessness and guilt, irritability, appetite change, poor concentration. But these are general, depersonalized descriptions that, in their generic broadness, risk failing to capture the precise texture of real women's actual

---

* I'm using the common term *postpartum depression* (abbreviated PPD) as shorthand to refer to something more accurately called *maternal depressive symptoms*, which suggests more fluidity to the timeframe and to the experience. The fact that these symptoms so often develop with new motherhood has misdirected us to assume that the powerful hormonal fluctuations are the cause, rather than the myriad, momentous psychosocial-spiritual growing pains that happen upon new parenthood. It should be noted that adoptive mothers also suffer from depressive symptoms, as do new fathers! So for thorough accuracy, we would call them *parental depressive symptoms*.

lived experience. Real women then slip through the diagnostic cracks and are left to struggle on their own.

Postpartum depression can almost always be detected by a single, simple screening question: *Is the mother feeling joy?* If she is suffering from any form of postpartum depression, the answer may be a straightforward "No." But more likely it will be, "Well, I know I'm *supposed* to feel joy...and sometimes...*occasionally*...there are brief *hints* of joy...kind of..." In Brooke Shields' self-portrait of postpartum depression, *Down Came the Rain*, she articulates in a raw and immediate way the terrifying, alienating, embarrassing, confusing—and most of all, countercultural—feelings and impulses that come with postpartum depression.

> I feel like a fraud. People keep saying, *Aren't you just thrilled to be a mother? You must be so in love! What a blessing.* All I can do is smile and say, "It's crazy."
>
> The thought of being the only person to care for her terrified me. She seemed pure and honest and raw, and it unsettled me. Her helplessness terrified me.
>
> These other moms didn't appear to want to be anywhere else, and seemed at peace. Motherhood agreed with all of them. What in the hell is wrong with me?? Why can't I be happy??
>
> It is as if I am trapped behind a thick glass wall. I feel like I'm moving further and further away from everybody. I'm so alone in how I feel.[79]

Many new mothers experience what I call Chronic Covert Postpartum Depression (CCPD). They suffer behind a façade of frantic perfectionism that effectively obscures the very possibility that there might be anything wrong. So information about or consideration of postpartum depression doesn't even make it onto their radar screens. Many years before research indeed turned up perfectionism as a risk factor for postpartum depression,[80] I wrote an about my struggles with perfecting new motherhood; it was clear that even ten years out I still wasn't recognizing those struggles as CCPD. I described my

> vague but persistent fears of incompetence, an intangible but relentless drive running deep inside me to always be trying to do it better, or at least do it right. Do *what* right, I couldn't define. I just knew that I

rarely felt a respite from this steady pressure that seemed to define my life after becoming a mother. And it seemed that I was angry, silently resentful, most of the time.

When there were no specific tasks to accomplish, like diapering or feeding or driving us somewhere, I felt deep discomfort at simply *being* with my baby. I had learned from my RIE parent/infant class that babies and children thrive on this "wants-nothing time," that it's as nourishing to their psyches as food is to their bodies. But as soon as I would sit down on the family room carpet with my baby, to just be there while he explored and played, the resistance would rise up and I would quell it by suddenly thinking, *Oh, I've got to jump up right now and call about those slipcovers,* or *Maybe I should plan tomorrow's dinner,* or *I'd better go wipe the water spots off that table.* The refuge of life's droning busywork.

We had planned for Ian to sleep in a cradle in our room during the early weeks, but on our first night home his snuffling baby noises kept me so on edge, his closeness so chafed at me, that he was alone in his own room beginning the following night. Then I could feel tense and guilty from safely down the hall.

My first years of mothering were thus: my need to escape Ian's crushing dependency on me, and the guilt, the anger, and the ever-present gnashing conflict of my two deepest impulses—to attach, and to pull away (not necessarily in that order). When Ian was about four months old I said to my husband, "I feel like he's sucking all the me out of me." But actually he was sucking the real me, terrified and enraged, out of hiding.[81]

And there it is, right there—a clue, a key, one way into the labyrinth of this sneaky, joy-stealing affliction: *I was hiding.* When we spend a lot of time with a child of a particular age, our own unresolved feelings from that age tend to surface. When a mother has a baby in her arms, the baby she once was is there too, fully present in her. Accordingly, a central postpartum focus is "the art of meeting yourself again." Is the mother prepared for this?[82]

We focus so much upon *childbirth* preparation and so little on preparing for what comes after! Has a new mother prepared to face again whatever might have been true for her in her own early days of life? And perhaps to meet her own long-banished feelings of longing, grief, or rage over her own babyhood experiences of separation or other difficulties in rapport with her mother? Or, will she tend to slip into the hiding place of postpartum depression? By contrast, a mother whose own birth and postpartum relationship with her mother was joyous, uncomplicated, and uninterrupted—or who has taken the time and care beforehand to navigate the memories and old feelings of more difficult experiences—is far less likely to suffer from postpartum depression.

Contrary to the most common conventional wisdom, there is little evidence that hormonal fluctuations *cause* postpartum depression;[83] rather, in classic chicken-and-egg fashion, they reflect, amplify and extend it. Our typical misperceptions about this naturally arise from the same medical-mechanistic viewpoint applied to labor and birth, which reduces postpartum depression to a primarily hormone-triggered malfunction of the body-machine. This leads to the common scenario of everyone walking on eggshells around the fragile and somewhat broken new mother, until her endocrine system rights itself and she can pull herself together. This poverty-stricken perspective on postpartum depression offers precious little hope for understanding, prevention, or healing.

An Organic Perspective on Postpartum Depression

To recap, the latest science of attachment and brain development reveals that it is in the context of the mother's gaze that the infant discovers who he is, and what the world is like, and fundamental aspects of brain circuitry wire up to match those impressions. It is this essential process that lies at the heart of parenting for peace. One of the first things we do when we're depressed is to avoid the gaze of others, including a baby's. A baby who cannot find his mother—and thus himself—within her gaze, is drastically handicapped in the complex developmental task of putting together a self. When a mother is unprepared to be seen, the child suffers deeply. And of course, so does the mother.

We are greatly handicapped around this issue by the way we handle birth, when biological realities clash with our accepted cultural norms—which aren't normal at all when we recognize that we are mammals! Recall cultural anthropologist Robbie Davis-Floyd's observation that a woman giving birth shares a similar psychophysiological profile with those involved in rite-of-passage rituals. By virtue of the cascades of oxytocin, prolactin and natural opiates that flow during an unmedicated labor, she is open to birthing not only her child, but entirely new layers and levels of herself. Neuroscientist Paul MacLean suggests that the birth of a child activates and opens multiple intelligences in the mother, previously untapped.[84] But when these profound openings and yearnings arise, and there is no one present to help mirror and support the mother through this awakening, and no cultural models to support the evolution they mandate, what we have labeled postpartum depression settles upon the mother's soul like a shroud, hormones and soul engaged in a recursive downward spiral.

The obstetrical establishment insists that postpartum depression comes out of the blue, with nothing in the mother's past to account for it. But the connection between PPD and disempowering, dispiriting birth experiences with postpartum separation of mothers and newborns, is supported by the fact that at The Farm Midwifery Center in Tennessee—run by famed midwife Ina May Gaskin—the rate of postpartum depression is virtually nonexistent (0.03 percent).[85] This contrasts with anywhere between 5 and 20 percent in the general population.

It is important to note that in the course of Harry Harlow's research with the socially inept motherless mother monkeys, they found that if allowed to simply spend time with their infants, the pitiful mothers got better at mothering with each successive litter. I was a motherless mother all those years ago, reeling like a rhesus in the headlights soon after my son was born. And what I needed was someone to know my story of separation, recognize my risk factors, and support my growth *beyond* my own pain and fear, by lovingly urging me to not give in to that deep impulse—a memory, really—to pull away. I most needed what felt most deeply unfamiliar: *the healing intimacy of connection*—to be physically and energetically with my son, with someone else nearby for support and reassurance. Our attachment would have gotten off to a much smoother start, and it is always easier to weave a foundation at the beginning.

Connection and Conscience: The Foundations of Peace

Whenever a heinous, violent act is committed, there is talk of a lack of conscience in the perpetrator. The question of what builds a conscience has long engrossed philosophers, psychologists, and even Disney imagineers (who decided Pinocchio's conscience looks a little like a cockroach, carries a watch fob and goes by the name of Jiminy Cricket). James Prescott's massive, cross-cultural study of the root causes of violence, together with the body of bonding and attachment research, point clearly to the fact that conscience is seeded in the nurturing, pleasurable physical and emotional connection of a baby and his mother. It's inescapable mammalian biology: in their poetic bestseller *A General Theory of Love*, the authors—three psychiatrists—explain that mammals who grow up in the absence of the coordinating influence of limbic regulation are "jagged and incomplete."[86] Central to this incompleteness is the missing foundation for the development of the entire suite of peacemaker capacities—including the basis of what we would call "conscience."

Childhood trauma expert Bruce Perry simplifies the layered neuropsychological process linking bonding, attachment and conscience to this simple calculus: *People = Pleasure*. When bonding and attachment unfold as nature intends, the connection between a mother and her baby remains unbroken after birth; she reliably tends to her baby's cries and coos in an engaged, responsive way, and delights in his delight, and he comes to associate her with all that is good. *Mama = Pleasure*. This association lays the foundation for the child, over the course of the critical first three years, to internalize myriad more complex associations as a foundation for a healthy self ("I'm effective in the world," "I can trust others to be there for me," "I make people happy," and so on), and also for his brain to eventually hardwire the broader association, *People = Pleasure*. It is this *People = Pleasure* association that underlies civilized behavior.[87]

But here's what seems to be the rub: before *people* can equal pleasure, there must be *one person* (usually the mother) whose consistent loving, sensitive care becomes associated, over the course of the first nine months or so, with the reducing of distress and the experience of pleasure. This is a critical first step and prerequisite for the child later extrapolating positive associations and empathy to others. Trying to skip this step is one big way in which we've thrown hefty monkey wrenches into Nature's elegant design: we let ourselves be lulled into the industrialist notion that we could substitute and rotate humans and get an equally good result. In many ways we've applied a factory model to childrearing: we thought that as long as a person had the right skills, he or she was interchangeable with a baby's mother.

And in our defense, the mechanisms by which any particular mother could be so *non*interchangeable have been unfathomable to us until the recent advent of brain imaging technology, and the field of attachment neurobiology that has made such informative use of that technology. We now know that there are dozens, maybe hundreds, of neurophysiological dimensions according to which a baby's mother is unique and utterly irreplaceable to him—at least if we want him to flourish in growth mode and develop to his optimal potential. As Perry and coauthor Maia Szalavitz writes in *Born for Love*:

> "Just anyone" with hands, food, and clean diapers won't do....This intensely tight bond rarely extends to more than one person—and will only extend even partially to others if those folks have been with the baby pretty much every day....Secondary caregivers like Dad or Grandma or a big sister might do for a while, but Mama is who they really want. Fathers often feel rejected by the strong preference that babies show for their mothers at [eight to nine months of] age and feel as though they've failed when they can't soothe them. But this is just a normal stage in the development of attachment, which gradually grows to accommodate more people as the child's brain becomes ready for this complexity.[88]

Indeed, the complexity and scope of a child's relationships is designed to sequentially expand the *Mama* = *Pleasure* association into a more intricate repertoire including ever more people, step by step. A child who is securely attached to his parents is deeply motivated to behave in harmony with them, which cultivates more pleasure all around; this becomes a positive feedback loop within the child that gradually expands outward to include the wider world in the category of "those who matter to me."

And that is conscience.

If we try to rush a child into this complexity by depriving her of what Perry and Szalavitz term the "intensive, particularized adult attention and affection" provided through a one-on-one attachment relationship, and instead subject her to an overly large or inconsistent rotation of caregivers as an infant, we cultivate a stunted social intelligence. Rather than the roots of conscience, what we see is the machinations of raw survival wit. An extreme example of this is seen in many children adopted out of overseas orphanages, and the indiscriminate friendliness they exhibit toward complete strangers. This is a pseudo-friendliness rooted not in authentic human connection but in the self-protective drive of *What can you do for me?* I believe that there are shades of this "What's in it for me?" motivation lurking in the relationships of far more of us than we'd like to admit—especially those who missed out on the fullness of that particularized Mama-is-pleasure experience as an infant. For Generation Peace to gain traction toward changing the world in a healing direction, people must not be a means to an end. For Generation Peace, people must be pleasure.

Yikes—Are We Up to This Calling?

No wonder we haven't yet gotten this parenting thing right as a human race. It's a tall order, requiring what sometimes feels like self-sacrifice on the part of those particularized primary caregivers—usually mothers—for those first few years. No wonder we're still spinning our wheels over the issues of domestic oppression, autonomy, choice and economic empowerment about which brave feminists raised our consciousness generations ago. I feel deep gratitude to them for generating a culture in which I had the freedom to choose whether I would stay home with our son and daughter or return to my work in television production and turn their care over to others. But in the mode of the many deep paradoxes that mark the evolutionary mandate of parenting for peace, I also feel unspeakably grateful that I chose (for reasons that at the time were incomprehensible to me) to devote myself to the transformational calling of fulltime mothering.

Let's remember that the first stirrings of the feminist movement grew out of the ideal of bringing value to women—to their voice, their needs and their contribution, which at that time was primarily made domestically as mothers and homemakers. Perhaps now that others have fought hard for us to have a choice in the matter, we can choose with more freedom and tranquility to dedicate a few years of our life to the most influential position we may ever apply for.

This ideal of parenting for a generation of peacemakers is so demanding, so sophisticated, and demands such a level of maturity, we are culturally only now barely up to the task. It took us all those eons of time to develop the balance of intellectual knowledge and heart, plus the technological machinery to free many hours in each day,* so that perhaps now is the first moment in our history when this is even possible! What do we think the industrial and technological

---

* With a car I can go to three places in a half-hour that once would have taken three hours each; rather than spending an entire day washing clothes in the river (and how would I dry them if it's raining?), I spend an hour; with a telephone I save a day or more of traveling it would have taken me to go see the person. The list of course goes on—email rather than the post office; running water rather than long, heavy walks to the well; with electricity, life and activity can continue past six in the evening; I can even go buy groceries at night!

revolutions liberated us for? Might it be that a key purpose of having our time
and our excellent minds freed up through all that brilliant technology, was so
that we can, for the first time, *have* the luxury of time we need to quicken this
next evolutionary leap? This is indeed the first time large swaths of the human
family have the time with which to reflect on our inner lives, to come to really
know who and how we are, and how we can become our very best—and then
to offer our best to our children, these future citizens who will inherit the
world at a most pivotal time in its history.

Time pressures aside, I also suspect that many of us, with all of our issues,
harbor fears that we aren't equal to the momentous role of shepherds to these
newly minted beings with limitless potential. We lack this or that virtue, we're
clumsy with intimacy, we're *imperfect.* We can barely wield a screwdriver and
we're being asked to build a space station. Take heart: our shaping force on
our children, which is huge indeed, need not be constrained by our own limitations and challenges, but is rather open to the wider horizons of the ideals
toward which we dedicate our energies.

Sorting through the din of modern life to simply figure out what your ideals
are requires time. Making the internal and external shifts that begin to align
your living to those ideals requires time. And being with children at the pace
and the fullness they require for optimal growth-over-protection development
definitely requires time.

Our ingenious innovations of the twentieth century gave us the gift of time.

Let us use that time to offer the twenty-first century the gift of a new kind
of innovation: a generation built for peace.

──────── PRINCIPLES TO PRACTICE ────────

Presence – And here we see the application of this principle in one of its truest
forms: just *be.*

- Because of its simplicity, its powerful protective effect in assuaging postpartum stress symptoms, and its positive impact on attachment, I would feel remiss if I didn't suggest that you take part in the brilliant birth narrative
  intervention I described earlier—especially because its ultimate outcome is
  to enhance presence. I heartily encourage you to get some paper—or a voice
  recorder—and do this exercise within a few days of your child's birth. Here
  are the exact instructions from the researchers: "In about 10-15 minutes
  please write about the thoughts and feelings you had when experiencing child-

birth. Please describe also feelings and thoughts that you would not disclose to others. You may want to include in your account other people, such as hospital professionals or important people in your present, past or future life. Everything you write will be kept strictly confidential."[89] When you're done, you can later decide whether you want to share it with anyone—or maybe do some kind of honoring or releasing ritual with the paper, such as burning it or framing it, or perhaps just adding it to a box of keepsakes for your child.

- A brilliant practitioner in the attachment field, Connie Lillas emphasizes that one of the most important things for *all* of human development is that right now, in these early days and weeks, the mother and baby have a falling-in-love experience. It may feel immediate or it may be a gently gathering process over time. You may feel it's the most natural thing or you may struggle—as I did and as so many women do, navigating this tender new territory of intimacy.[90] Even if you're not yet feeling deeply connected, continue to be close, have lots of skin-to-skin contact, nurse on demand, and do all of the caring things for your baby—this is your presence practice and his or her deepest need. The more you can fall into each others' eyes and atmosphere, the more kernels for future strength are planted—certainly in your baby, but also in you. A kind of template for meeting later challenges is formed in these days, a programming designed by Nature with utmost purpose: *Something essential and unrepeatable is under way!*

- Gabor Maté in his extraordinary book *Scattered: How Attention Deficit Disorder Originates and What You Can Do About It*, traces the connection between being present and *attending*, which he proposes is a fundamental, active form of loving. He points out that most parents don't need to learn to love their children in a feeling sense, "but we can all use practice in how to be actively loving toward them in day-to-day experience."[91] To *attend* to a child is to be present for them, attuned and responsive to their emotional cues. It is through the weeks, months and years of these attuned, responsive relational encounters that your child's brain's self-regulating system wires up—wiring up, remember, to mirror *your* relational and self-regulation style! Maté suggests that a child displaying the kinds of impaired self-regulating abilities central to ADD has indeed suffered a *deficit of attention* when it was needed—in the early years.

- If you have other children, invite them into this magic, out-of-space-and-time circle. Laugh and sing with them, envelope them in the love-drunk haze of new life. This, of course, goes for your partner as well.

- Taking a page out of Megan's book, do your best to have some well-considered support people and plans in place before the baby arrives; then just let yourself completely lean into them and let go of logistics, figuring things out, or fretting. No looking into the future, even by a few hours, as much as possible. Be here now.

- Partners, you may need to be present to feelings arising in you, having to do with being left out or left behind. As your baby's mother is making a narrative of her birth experience, you might find it helpful to make your own narrative of your impressions of how things have changed for you. Don't worry about doing anything to fix or change the situation; merely saying "hello" to it in this way is very helpful.

- Just as the baby she herself once was is reawakened when the new mother holds the baby in her arms, so too are your early experiences awakened when you spend time with your baby—or when *she* spends time with your baby and not with you. Again, simply turning your conscious awareness to this process is often enough to let it dissipate and move through. Jack Travis has written eloquently about this issue, under the ominous yet epidemically relevant title, "Why Men Leave."[92]

- Indeed, nothing prepares us for the joy—and often the challenge—of being so totally accepted, wanted and needed by this tiny creature. Not only can it fill us with unsurpassed delight, it can also bring up all of our imprinted resistances to the idea of "I am loved, wanted, and accepted." That can be terrifying, but allowing ourselves to acknowledge and be present with our feelings goes a long way toward moving them through.

- You will hear the incessant siren call to separate from your baby in many ways and on many levels. Well-meaning friends or family will insist that it is imperative for the new mother and her partner to take some time and space for themselves. But you've seen it countless times, our deepest instincts and intuitive inclinations to remain *with* our babies, parodied on sitcoms and in cartoons: over the most romantic candlelight and crystal at the restaurant… you end up talking about the baby. As much as you try to get into that mood of freedom and romance, nothing feels right—and this goes on for six or nine months. Nature has its own design, which urges you to *enjoy the baby!* Lots of messages will urge you otherwise, but surrender and give in to your preoccupation with the baby, knowing it is the path of peace and joy. It's easier to deemphasize our own peripheral needs—like a for a restaurant dinner or a night out with the girls—for a little longer, knowing that this temporary sacrifice is a sound investment that will pay rich dividends later on.

- Once the cocoon weeks have passed, rather than thinking in terms of "getting back to normal," as childbirth educator Tamara Donn points out, it is far more helpful and self-supportive to instead think of "going forward to a new normal." Be gentle with yourself, your partner, your baby. Let Life reveal the pathways forward through the magic of emergent novelty; the more presence you can bring to each moment, the more each moment can unfold with fullness and ease into the next moment…and on and on.

Awareness – Remember how we must strive to turn off the higher brain centers during labor, to help the process unfold with ease? If you can keep riding that impulse for the early days and even weeks of the postpartum period, it also helps the process of this foggy, sleepless time unfold with ease. In other words, turn *down* the awareness dial!

- Especially if you're a woman who's used to doing a lot and who may feel distressingly sedentary, it can help to realize that when you've recently given birth, you're burning somewhere in the neighborhood of a thousand calories per day, between milk production and all of the internal changes going on!
- Be aware that babies who have suffered any kind of distressing, intense experience need to discharge the energy that has overwhelmed their nervous system. They do this in physical ways that can be concerning to parents who don't understand what's up. This can include inconsolable crying (or the other extreme, virtually no crying at all), extreme startle responses, arching or stiffening at being held, spacing out or sleeping all the time, and severe colic or other kinds of illness. These are organic ways in which a baby's nervous system seeks to self-correct—one of many examples of the self-healing impulse with which Nature has imbued us. Common overwhelming experiences of varying intensities include cord-around-the-neck oxygen deprivation during labor or forceps or vacuum delivery; rough or invasive handling after birth, including airway aspiration; separation from mother due to adoption or NICU care; painful newborn medical procedures such as intubation, blood tests, administration of eye drops or injections; circumcision without anesthesia (or even with anesthesia, which itself can be traumatic—followed by a painful healing period).
  - By simply holding a mindful awareness of any such hurts, losses, or separations, you support and engage with Nature's self-healing impulse. This is an act of love that weaves a powerful foundation for your baby's trust in you: *My parents are capable of seeing me in all of my truth, no matter how*

inconvenient or difficult. And remember that this is the psychosocial stage in which he or she is indeed learning either trust or mistrust.

• One helpful aspect of awareness throughout your child's life is to know when developmental milestones typically occur, while also respecting the individuality of his or her unique timetable. Recalling Rudolf Steiner's model of development in which your child's gradual incarnation unfolds in roughly seven-year stages—aligning with his three major waves of brain development—you can think in terms of important aspects of your baby still in gestation.

  - One of the first of many milestones coincides with the end of the forty-day cocoon period, at around six weeks. Attuned parents will notice a change in the baby: Like Noah after the forty days, she is "ready to open a window on the world."[93] She's becoming more alert, more aware and responsive to the surrounding environment. Her journey toward relatedness is beginning. She is now ready to enter more into family life, needing somewhat less protection from the ordinary household noises, sounds of active older children, visitors, etc. Occasional gentle radio music is now acceptable. But television is still best avoided; the high quality of the sense impressions coming to the baby are fundamental to her newly wiring brain circuitry, making this one of the sensitive windows neuroscientists talk about.

  - One fascinating dimension of your baby's development to watch for is how he moves through the many stages of motor development in the first year. An imaginative observation of his body gestures through the first twelve months suggests that individual development recapitulates stages of the human evolutionary process. For the first six weeks, we see a plant-like consciousness. He is like a geranium, which has no awareness of its geranium-ness. The new infant benefits from being allowed to live fully within this "asleep" state of consciousness, yet many of our current cultural practices are designed to stimulate the baby from the very beginning, denying him this experience of a gentle landing into embodied awareness. Next is the "fish" stage (two-four months): she wriggles, often swishes her legs about and makes swimming motions with her arms. This calls for the opportunity to move the limbs and wriggle about when awake. Some babies at around five months make the "bird" gesture, with the arms becoming wings kicked up in the air as if in flight. This gesture speaks of the need for free movement, to allow for the increased mobility. (Many babies don't enact this bird—and instead move directly from the fish to the reptile. There are wide variations in the timetable and the specifics of these gestures.) Somewhere around eight months is the age of the "reptile" gestures: lying on the ground, reared up on his forearms, he's very sensitive to the slightest sound, swinging his head around to any slight noise. The legs—unlike the curled-in fashion of the fish stage—are now fully extended, resembling a lizard's tail. Next comes the "mammal" (quadruped) gesture: up on all fours. The freedom to crawl lays an important inner foundation, as it can metamorphose into a sense of soul freedom. And finally, she pulls herself up to the "human" gesture—which asks for an opportunity to explore, investigate, and learn about the world.

- The issue of vaccinations is a crucial one for you to develop your awareness about, beginning with the understanding that this is far from neutral. Shots are not to be simply accepted automatically. Homework is required. Some experts consider today's large slate of shots too much too soon for an immature immune system. Far from a black and white issue—to vaccinate or not, all or nothing—it is a complex health issue that calls for your thoughtfulness and discernment in partnership with a trusted healthcare practitioner.

Rhythm – The metronome setting the beat for your life these days is this tiny new human, with her ebbing and flowing alertness, delight, distress, waking and sleeping. Pooping and feeding. He is your calendar and clock—you're flowing with milk time now. Resistance is futile; but surrendering to these potent rhythms can bring unexpected joy.

- Take advantage of when the baby sleeps: nap, or maybe read, but try not to embark on endless phone calls! No projects to mount, no birth announcements to send, no emails to answer. (Well, maybe one or two, but only if it relaxes and delights you.)
- Each baby comes with a language, and this "molasses time" is the time to learn that language, to memorize him. And to learn your own new inner language as his mother. Nursing on demand is one way to richly do this—while noticing the ebbing and flowing rhythms of your milk to meet the changing needs of your baby.
- Even if at the beginning it's difficult to let go and freefall into the gauzy newness, do give it a try, to just let Life be with you. Be in a cocoon. There are very few parenting books that reassure the mother that she is *it*. Even the

most loving of mothers-in-law will insist to the new parents on day two or three that "you need to get out and have some time for yourself," which is well-meaning but not what is truly needed according to Life's timetable.

- Remind yourself of the capriciousness of time, and how what now feels like an eternity will one day feel like the faintest blink of an eye. (You might reread the Epilogue during your forty days!) It's not confinement, as if it were a prison. It's like being in the womb of Life again. Look what the lowly roots of a carrot plant do in the dark over time: they *become* the carrot itself. There is something mysterious here, about the power of beginnings.
- And enjoy sleep when you can!

Example – If you've not yet experienced caring for a baby, it may be wise to have someone present with you, modeling calm, confident newborn care. Via the wonder of mirror neurons, you will catch her confidence!

- The world of nature is filled with inspiring models for the mode you're striving to be in now—tranquil stillness that is nonetheless teeming with vibrant life. It may be gazing at a tree outside your window, reflecting on the tranquility with which it expresses its tree-ness or watching a bird sitting motionless on its nest for hours.
- One of the best sources of helpful human examples is a local La Leche League meeting, where you'll meet other mothers at all stages of their nursing experiences.
- Moms, let it be through your example (and not your lecturing) that you teach your partner the "right" way to diaper, carry, and hold the baby—and a few months from now, feed, play with, and entertain her. Dads bring a whole different and beautifully important set of qualities to baby interactions, and we gals have a nasty tendency to curb and quash that and instead get them to do it our way. Try and refrain from our womanly propensity for bossiness. Let his fatherly confidence flourish.
- A good deal of the Step Five chapter is about the latest science of attachment—the power of relationship to shape many aspects of your baby's brain potential in lifelong ways. As the process of interpersonal neurobiology works its unfathomable magic over these critical coming months and years, your example is everything! One of the most helpful guiding questions to ask yourself throughout your life with your child, beginning now, is "What lesson is

embedded in this encounter?" Your very demeanor—loving, attuned, tender, accepting, or otherwise—is a model for your baby in the most direct, physiological way: the circuitry of his social brain is wiring up to mirror yours!

Nurturance – The forty-day honeymoon period is a wonderful opportunity to really take in and understand that everything about you is a source of nurture to your baby. These early weeks and months give you the chance to cultivate a sensitivity for just how potent you are for your child.

- The look on your face, the quality of your touch, the volume and tone of your voice: let these all be conscious channels for your love—strands weaving an essential form of nourishment for your baby: the connectedness we call attachment.
- Now's the time to use those pastel silks to drape over her cradle or Moses basket, soften the edges of this new physical world and nurture the process of her brain's sensory integration system wiring up. By contrast, please, no trips to the mall…or anywhere else that represents a full-scale assault on fresh new senses.
- Avoid waking up your baby, particularly if it is just to feed him. It makes him cranky, and that interferes with digestion.
- Keep the atmosphere nice and warm, both emotionally and physically. Babies don't regulate their temperature well, so it's good to keep two or even three light layers over their torsos where their little organs are at work and growing. Also, take care to keep your own body warm—especially your feet!
- While, of course, there will be times when others are present while you're nursing and your attention is engaged elsewhere, do dedicate some nursing sessions to being completely there just for your baby.
- Be sure to drink plenty of water to help maintain your milk supply. Also, now is not the time to cut back on calories; your baby is sucking them out of you in a big way! Good nutrition, including enough protein, EFAs, and essential nutrients particular to this postpartum rebuilding phase, is key. Amanda Rose's book *Rebuild from Depression* is a great guide. (Don't let the title scare you off.)
- Touch is a potent sensory channel for both of you, and baby massage can be a lovely way to nurture your baby. As with most processes related to children, it's important to exercise discernment when choosing any instructional guides,

and *BabyBabyOhBaby: Bonding with your Brilliant and Beautiful Baby Through Infant Massage* is a DVD I can confidently recommend. Even more important, though, is to attune to your baby's cues; while most of them will enjoy it, there will be some who simply don't care for that version of love! (And keep checking in; one friend's baby didn't want anything to do with massage as an infant, but once she turned one—continuing now that she's twenty-two—she began loving massage!) The same goes for the sensory aspects of swaddling; many babies like such reassuring containment after so recently emerging from the enveloping womb to the wide-open world. But some won't, and you need to follow your baby's lead when making this surprisingly controversial choice.[94]

- Make no mistake—the early weeks are intense, and you may feel overtouched, underbathed, sleep-deprived and sucked dry. Take care to have some nurturing in place for yourself; even the smallest pleasures, if they are dear to you, can renew in untold measure without disturbing the cocooned atmosphere. A visit from a treasured friend; a wonderful book or enchanting Netflix movie; a bath with gorgeous salts; a home-visit massage—whatever makes you go *Mmmmm*.

- If you, like Megan at the beginning of this chapter, have concerns regarding your inclination toward depression, an important aspect of nurturance for your baby is that you tend closely to your own emotional balance. There are many helpful modalities for this, including a lot of skin-to-skin contact with your baby; feeling connected to others who are confident around new babies and mothers; homeopathic and Bach Flower remedies; energy psychology modalities such as EFT; acupuncture; various anthroposophic treatments for replenishing the tremendous amount of etheric energy expended during pregnancy and birth (oil dispersion baths, heat wraps, and lots of warmth in general); journaling; and having lots of help.

- Once the early weeks have passed and the forty days are over, and life finds its new normality, one of the most challenging aspects of fulltime parenting is the common experience of isolation and loneliness. You might make it a priority to find ways to share time and connection with other new parents. Even though she didn't think it was for her, Megan joined MOMS Club Int'l and found it to be wonderfully nurturing. La Leche League is another source of camaraderie.

  - One of my all-time favorite *Mothering* magazine articles is called "Find Your Tribe"—detailing the innovative arrangement two moms devised whereby they shared their days with their similarly aged babies and toddlers all together, alternating between each other's homes. Both husbands would even convene after work at the appointed home for a communal dinner. See mothering.com/parenting/feed-your-soul-while-feeding-your-kids.

- Croon, murmur, hum, sing and talk to your baby. My rule of thumb on this may seem odd but here it is: talk as much as you wish to your baby, until he starts understanding the explicit meaning of your words. That is when you had best dial back the stream of words and let your actions do most of the talking. One of the biggest adjustments I make with clients coming to see me for a spectrum of reasons, is, *say less and have it mean more.* But during this first year your voice is a river of love for your baby! My other guideline for parental chat, however, does apply beginning even now: let whatever you say spring from your knowing, your dreaming, your ideals—and not your insecurity ("Oh, sweetie-pie, why are you not sleeping?" "I'm not sure if your poops are looking the way they should..."). Keep those little conversations inside your own head; the self-discipline of doing so is also potent nourishment for her!

  - If you are supporting your baby in discharging the nervous-system over-arousal caused by earlier distressing events, your words are a balm that can greatly facilitate this process—an invaluable form of nurture: *You were expecting to stay connected to me but you were taken away, and that was scary, I know...You had lots of strange hands all over you, and you were missing me...They put that hard thing into your nose, I know, and that hurt, and I'm so sorry that happened...I'm not the mom you expected—my heartbeat isn't the one you know, nor my smell or my voice—and I know that must be so confusing and sad and painful, but I'm here for you forever, even if you're sad, or mad, and I want you to know that you're perfectly right and I love you, even if right now you can't quite let me in....* Rae, the adoptive mother of six-month-old Lana from Russia, emailed me that she had recently read an article about attachment, so the next time Lana awoke at 4 a.m. whimpering yet pushing Rae away and acting very uncuddly, Rae "gave Lana a bottle and spoke softly to her about how hard it must have been for her to see that her caretakers could be changed so quickly, without warning, when we took her from her babyhome in Russia. How maybe she was thinking it could happen again and that mommy would not be here with

her, but that this would never happen, and she did not have to be afraid—
that she could relax into mommy's care, that mommy would now always
be here with her. She finished her bottle, and for the first time in weeks,
she put her head on my shoulder and her arm around my neck, and sang
softly. We rocked for awhile, and then I took her into my bed like we used
to when she first came to us. It was wonderful. Whatever babies understand or don't understand, something changed in her behavior."

- The hero's journey of parenting for peace often entails swimming against the
  tide of the status quo, including the baby gadgetry and equipment one
  chooses to use. Rather than having the freedom to move about, infants are
  often strapped into bouncers, swings, snugglies, strollers, or car seats. While
  some of these may have their place when used mindfully and minimally (and
  of course, car seats *always* when in a car!), we want to watch our cultural tendency toward constraining our babies. I particularly discourage the use of a
  walker, which props the child into an upright position without her having to
  use her own muscles and to exercise her own will, and deprives her of activity
  that promotes healthy posture and body alignment. Recent research finds
  that they actually thwart the development they are ostensibly made to encourage.[95] The biggest surprise for most parents is walkers' negative impact
  on mental development.[96]
- While on the topic of negative impact on mental development, I want to re-
  iterate the fact that screened media has no place in the life of an infant. Only
  6 percent of parents surveyed were aware of the American Pediatric Association's recommendation that children under the age of two shouldn't watch
  any television, while 29 percent believe "educational" videos are very important for the intellectual development of their babies.[97] This is not so. Interaction with you, or with the three dimensions of her real, hands-on (and yes,
  usually mouth-on) world, is what builds her a most bustling brain-full of new
  dendrites, synapses, and pathways!

Trust – When we've been blasted off the planet and then landed "forever on
some *other* planet we hadn't packed or prepared for," as one blogger put it,[98]
what could be more important than trust? Trust that you'll find your way,
learn the terrain, uncover the secrets to survival in this new world, and the
pathways beyond survival—to thriving and even delight!

- The innumerable bioregulatory strands woven between you and your baby, physiologically and neurologically, represent a bankable source of trust—Nature's own baby monitor. Each time you wake just before your baby wakes hungry—and you will—it builds trust in this fundamental connection. Each time you get a sense that she needs her diaper changed, that he needs some silence, that she's becoming overtired, your trust becomes more vast.

  - Thanks to this meticulous attunement with which you're hardwired to so intimately know your baby from the inside out, you can trust in the safety of co-sleeping, as long as you are not altering your own neurophysiology with alcohol or drugs.

- Take the opportunity of these early months to cultivate a calm knowing that your baby's unique timetable of development is just right for her. You'll have the chance to practice and strengthen this tranquil assurance as you begin meeting with other moms and other babies, and the conversation inevitably turns to milestones and "Is he rolling over yet?" and "I don't know if I should be worried she doesn't have a tooth yet…" and the like. Trust that your baby is right on time.

- By contrast, don't easily trust the wacko things that our culture takes for granted are great for kids. If you need an example of what we unquestioningly embrace out of pure ignorance and assumption, take a look at the Baby Einstein phenomenon: in the absence of any shred of evidence that these videos are of value—and indeed, contrary to the APA's express guideline that children younger than two not watch television *at all*—Julie Aigner-Clark's little enterprise went from $1 million to $10 million in earnings over just two years, before she sold the brand to Disney. The kerfuffle over a 2007 University of Washington study finding that such videos actually *delayed* language development made nary a dent in the public's breathless love affair with such classics as "Baby Shakespeare" and "Baby Monet Discovers the Seasons." When Aigner-Clark went to court to try to obtain the raw data from the study, she emailed reporters, "I'm proud of what I made. Welcome to the twenty-first century. Most people have televisions in their houses, and most babies are exposed to it. And most people would agree that a child is better off listening to Beethoven while watching images of a puppet than seeing any reality show that I can think of." Those are the two choices? This is the brain trust whose (frankly bizarre, surreal) video collection was valued at $400 million two years ago, with no signs of pausing or rewinding. Trust your inner knowing and common sense, not the zeitgeist.

Simplicity – This is the watchword for the precious first forty days, going hand in hand with presence. In general, the simpler we can be, the easier it is to be present—to our baby, and to the important shifts taking place in the tectonic plates of our own identity. Complication, on the other hand, invites splintered attention, untended experience, and a dilution of joy potential.

- Remember that co-sleeping is a simplifying factor that can benefit everyone if it works for you. (And if you think it doesn't work for you, you might consider giving it a try before deciding for sure.)
- Our cultural tendency to clutter up a baby's room runs counter to this principle, which is so nurturing on so many levels. Sensory overstimulation insults the process of brain circuitry that seeks to wire up for optimal sensory integration. Mobiles in particular don't respect the natural focus-then-refocus aspect of an infant's attention; rather, mobiles—suspended as they are directly above a baby—somewhat forcibly assert themselves into a baby's focal process, grabbing her attention and making it difficult for her to turn away. (In that way they're like training wheels for television.) A few beautiful pieces of art on the walls, a bit of color, translucent curtains that let in light (babies love windows!)—enough to make it a pleasant space for you and not overwhelming for him—is simply right.
- Our R.I.E. teacher introduced us to the gift of simplicity for choosing our babies' toys by giving us a few criteria with which to select playthings that would foster rather than thwart their motor skills, imagination, and healthy will (the sense of "I *can*"). Few of the objects in the R.I.E. baby spaces were actually toys, but rather, items chosen to richly meet these criteria. First, it doesn't *do* something of its own accord or even at the push of a button; the jack-in-the-box is the ultimate nonrespectful toy in that the action of the child (turning the crank) creates a startling, even scary, result not at all cognitively related to his action. Second, the optimal toy does not have just one dedicated use or action, but through imagination it can be or do many things. One of the most versatile playthings for the youngest baby is a square of colorful fabric that is stiff enough to be "tee-peed" on the floor near the baby who—on her back where she has the freest, fullest range of motion of her head, spine, arms and legs—can easily (first accidentally) grasp it and manip-

ulate it. One of the most popular playthings among the babies was a flexible plastic basket filled with those metal disks from the tops of frozen juice concentrate!

- This principle shares an intimacy with the first one, presence: we can see presence as an inner simplification. In this spirit, poet Andrea Potos sees the call to mindful motherhood as an invitation to "unclench your life." Do less, buy less—*just be,* more. Depending upon your own experience of babyhood, and whether someone was able to "just *be*" with you, this might be an incomprehensible concept, maybe even a little bit terrifying. It was for me. But babies and children are our Zen masters, inviting us daily to our own renewal—and with it, their most vibrant flourishing as peacemakers.

Resources

La Leche League: www.llli.org, and their wonderful book *The Womanly Art of Breastfeeding.*

Breastfeeding USA (BFUSA), breastfeedingusa.org.

MOBI Motherhood International - Mothers Overcoming Breastfeeding Issues: www.mobimotherhood.org/MM/default.aspx.

Mothering online: www.mothering.com (including a "Finding Your Tribe" forum, at www.mothering.com/community/forum/list/7).

Resources for Infant Educarers: www.rie.org.

Step Six

The Enchanted Years— Toddlers through Kindergarten: Playing, Puttering and Peace

If a child has been able in his play to give up his whole loving being to the world around him, he will be able, in the serious tasks of later life, to devote himself with confidence and power to the service of the world.

RUDOLF STEINER

The Rubber Hits the Road

Your child is on the move, and parenting has taken on a different pace, more physical than ever now that you're also on the move—after him! In this past year you have accomplished a rainbow of transformations: the baby proofing you've done around your house in some ways is a metaphor for the many inner adjustments and remodeling that have taken place within your psyche—simplifying the landscape, deciding what's precious. For some, this has included reprioritizing your financial values—choosing to live less grandly, with fewer luxuries, in order that one of you can stay home with your child.

Regardless of whether you have returned to work or opted for full-time parenting, you have navigated a minefield of difficult, sometimes painful, choices. It is disheartening that a country with our technological and military prowess has made so little progress, in the forty years since the advent of the feminist movement, in attenuating the agony involved in the at-home v. working dilemma. The U.S. lags behind many other Western countries in prioritizing innovative social policy measures that support the needs of parents to work, as well as the needs of children for their parents (and parents for their children!). Our versions of parental leave and workplace innovations such as flex-time and job sharing have a long way to go to bridge the disconnect between the needs of our families and the demands of our employment.

It is also dispiriting that a country founded on diversity tolerance cannot seem to dig out of its entrenched polarization of stay-at-home motherhood and working motherhood. One need not have a psychology degree to realize that one strand of this eternal tug-of-war is woven from the divergent feelings and experiences of these two classes (and make no mistake—they are indeed social classes): the working mother wrestles with brands of guilt and stress the at-home mother is largely spared, while the mother at home often suffers isolation, a dearth of adult stimulation, and a sense that her work is not valid or valued according to our cultural clout-o-meter.

Burton White, director of Harvard's Preschool Project and author of the classic *The First Three Years of Life*, has held to his highly unpopular position about day care for over thirty years. "Controversy notwithstanding, I remain totally convinced that, to get off to the best start in life, babies need to spend a great deal of their waking time during the first three years of life with older people who are deeply in love with them. Although this ideal circumstance does not always prevail in families, it is much more often found there than in any substitute-care arrangement."[1]

While, of course, there are mothers for whom working is a given and not a choice, research reveals something that came as a surprise to me, and yet not: a significant portion of women choose full-time work over caring for their children not because of economic pressures, but rather, writes Mary Eberstadt, "because they prefer to arrange their lives that way,"[2] and that the higher up the socioeconomic ladder one goes, the *more* likely are mothers with young children to leave home:

> Faced with the endemic uncertainties and boundless chores of domestic life, many adults, male and female, end up preferring what Hochschild calls the "managed cheer" of work. Modern office life, she argues, not only competes with the home as "haven in a heartless world," in the phrase popularized by Christopher Lasch; for many women (and men), it partially or fully *supplants* the hearth, offering simpler emotional involvements, more solvable tasks, and often a more companionable and appreciative class of people than those waiting at home.[3]

If you indeed choose to return to work, or have no choice but to do so, keep in mind the central implication of attachment neurobiology: your child's social brain is going to wire up to echo that of the person with whom she spends the bulk of her time, so let that guide you in choosing substitute care. White's extensive research led him to recommend that the best kind of substitute care is individual care in your own home, followed by individual care in the home of the caregiver. Next is family daycare, followed by nonprofit center-based care (such as at a church, temple, or other such organization). At the bottom of the list is for-profit center-based care. Keep in mind White's overarching guideline for the person with whom your young child spends the bulk of his day: someone "deeply in love with" him.

In her wonderful manual *You Are Your Child's First Teacher,* Rahima Baldwin Dancy acknowledges, "To expect a thirty-seven-year-old PhD candidate, or a woman who has had an exciting career, to be fulfilled spending her days in an apartment with a two-year-old is idyllic but hard to find in reality."[4] It is my hope that the insights in this book help you recognize not only the supreme importance of your ongoing presence in your child's daily life, but also some interesting facets of what can, admittedly, be the tedious job of day-in-day-out parenting. And, you can rest assured that following attuned conception, radiant pregnancy, and empowered birth, parenting is far easier than conventional reports warn. You are teed up for some really joyous adventures—and yes, continued avenues of challenging discovery and growth.

Full-time mothering can bump us up against our own most tender, unresolved material—memories we carry within us of how we were received and mothered—and I believe that along with a love of our careers, there is often an element of avoidance: we don't want to go there. But these very memories, our stories, contain the power to heal us and in turn, heal the world. The current consciousness revolution unfolds within each of us, and with exquisite intensity when we become parents. If we can bear it, mother-child communion reveals to us ourselves.

And sometimes it's hard to watch—all that imperfection so vividly spotlighted. But as Nancy Jewel Poer reminds us, it is not our perfection but our *striving* that teaches our children. And if we have been able to continually reshift our worldview to one of wholism and sustainability, our entire parenting landscape is transformed: ongoing striving and growth is the whole point, not merely a pesky obstacle. If we can see our children's development in layers and dimensions that include physical, emotional, cognitive, and spiritual, we begin, writes Dancy, "to perceive the whole child and how he or she unfolds." Then things make eminently more sense and our choices "will begin to have coherence. No longer wanting a cookbook of 'how to's,' we will trust our own decisions, based on our understanding of the developing child and observation of the resultant flowering of our children."[5]

You Are Your Child's First Teacher

In an understandable desire to help assure our children's success, we try to give them a head start by beginning earlier and earlier to teach them the alphabet, numbers, maybe a little prealgebra. (I'm just kidding—I think! I'm keeping a close eye on that *Yo Gabba Gabba* robot for surreptitious math tutoring.) Intellectual work at this age actually undermines the young child's development by diverting energy from critical organ growth, and enlisting areas of the brain that are not yet meant to be "on line." The latest science of brain development supports what Waldorf education founder Rudolf Steiner taught almost one hundred years ago: early academics does not strengthen the young child's development, but instead undermines it! And it is in the social-emotional realm—his peacemaker potential—that we most seriously derail a child's development by pressing him into cerebral, rational pursuits during these early years.

How a Young Child Really Learns

Since the sensory-motor areas are the most active parts of her brain in the early years, the young child—up until around the age of seven—relates to the world primarily through her *senses* and her *body.* Her primary modes of perception, therefore, are through sensing (seeing, hearing, tasting, smelling and touching—indeed, lots of touching!) and doing, through the most active mode of learning, which is *imitation.* Understanding this basic fact about their child should help parents with two very important issues:

- knowing that for a child to *touch* something, or to *do* with her body, is similar to an adult *thinking* about that same thing
- recognizing that activities which engage these two aspects—sensing and doing—are the richest, healthiest, and most effective learning environments for the young child.

It also raises a third issue: the adults in a young child's life have a responsibility to create an environment—including themselves, their speech and actions—that is worthy of his *unquestioning imitation.*

What is the learning activity that most powerfully engages the child's two primary modes of taking in and processing her world? And that quickens her imitation-driving learning? Play! Play is the all-important world of the child until around seven—or should be. But in our hyperaccelerated culture we've lost an understanding and appreciation for just how critically important play is in the healthy development of our children. We tend to see it as a waste of time. A toy cannot simply be a toy—it has to be educational. Play cannot be for its own sake, it needs to be organized, improved upon, and packaged as enrichment.

When a child engages in open-ended play (that is, *un*organized, *un*-"improved upon," and *un*packaged), he engages the all-important *senses* and he cultivates perhaps the most important peacemaking capacity of all, *imagination.* As he imagines the wooden crate as his pirate ship, he *sees* the tall mast, *hears* the crashing waves, *feels* the salt sea spray. As he climbs in and hoists the sail (Mom's favorite guest towel), his body and brain are engaged in a stunningly intricate series of sensory-motor interactions and important "prelogical mental frolic." In an hour of such play, he is stimulating robust growth of important new neural connections. This play-centric activity not only cultivates his greatest peacemaker potential by fostering creative imagination, social intelligence and a healthy will, but also serves as an important foundation for later academics.

A recent study compared four- and five-year-olds enrolled in a play-based school to those in a more typical preschool ("typical" meaning it emphasizes academics). The students in the play-based school scored better on cognitive flexibility, self-control, and working memory—all aspects of the executive function mastered by the prefrontal lobes—which have been consistently linked to academic achievement. (The results were so compelling that the study was ended early so that all of the children could be moved into the play-based curriculum!)[6] Child psychologist David Elkind has devoted his professional life at Tufts University to studying the costs of hurrying children. On a visit to Stanford University, he noticed that bright young architecture students had to play with erector sets in class, because they hadn't had enough hands-on play as children. As a result, the sophisticated computer drafting technologies weren't serving them because these play-deprived young adults didn't have a real-world, three-dimensional frame of reference for the two-dimensional images on the screen.[7]

The same problem arises when we introduce abstract intellectual concepts to young children—like the alphabet. Letters are symbols, and the areas of the brain that process and make sense of symbols are not yet available in an integral way in the young child. Children live in the realm of the concrete world of the brain's right hemisphere—what they can sense (see, hear, feel, taste, smell, etc.). Symbolic thinking is governed by the brain's left hemisphere, so if introduced too early it is "learned" in a rote, mechanical way. It has little depth of meaning for a child, and leads to a more superficial interaction with words, ideas, and concepts. As Elkind points out, "The language of things must precede the language of words, or else the words don't mean anything." Not the best way to begin a child's lifelong learning, and certainly not conducive to the flexibly innovative, layered thinking capacities needed to forge peace, innovation, and prosperous sustainability.

Decades of learning research has consistently turned up the same result—that the strongest predictor of school achievement is the frequency with which parents read to and share stories with their child during the preschool years, not the early age at which the child masters reading. Because the most important element of early reading skills is *comprehension*, which is developed through the child's imaginative, whole-brain engagement in stories, not through rote, superficial flashcard learning of letters and phonics.[8] It is mostly English-speaking countries that have become intent on starting children on reading while they're still in this naturally dreamy, prelogical stage of life; studies of international data don't suggest an advantage for earlier reading, and it may make stressful demands on a brain not yet properly wired for it.*

Then the child gets slapped with a label—ADD/ADHD, for example—with which he is saddled in perpetuity; shame, discouragement, and insecurity can then drain him of his innate affinities toward learning to read. Indeed, the professionals who work with children—occupational therapists, development specialists and neuropsychologists—see early academics as directly related to the growing incidence of attention and visual processing disorder diagnoses. Developmental pediatrician Susan Johnson says there are behavioral clues parents can look for to see if their child has developed the hemispheric integration signaling true reading readiness. One is the ability to easily (without intently concentrating on doing it right) do a cross-lateral skip, in which one arm swings forward with the opposite leg.[9]

Brand new longitudinal data—the first of its kind—has found that readers who start at age five and those who start at age seven show no differences in reading ability by age eleven.[10] Researcher Sebastian Suggate says that this finding "emphasizes to me the importance of early language and learning, while de-emphasizing the importance of early reading. In fact, language development is, in many cases, a better predictor of later reading than early reading is."[11] Having credibly disproved the widely presumed advantage of early reading, Suggate is now researching whether it might actually incur developmental costs.

Despite this new research and the virtual absence of data supporting the advantages of early reading, it is still cultural blasphemy to suggest that the hundreds-of-millions-of-dollar programs to teach reading skills to three-to-five year olds might possibly be missing the intended mark. We would do bet-

---

* I'm referring to coaxing, coaching, and flashcarding; in the unusual instance in which a child spontaneously begins reading on his own at, say, three or four or five, that is different. In that case it is important for parents not to seize on this exciting development and fast-track him into Hemingway and the local school's GATE program, but to continue fostering rich play, imagination, story time and a matter-of-fact enjoyment of his precocious ability.

ter by enriching the daily lives of at-risk youth with one or two reliably at-tuned, interested adults in whose orbit they could engage in meaningful hands-on activities, play, conversations and storytelling. I believe that Head Start's success is largely a result of the epiphenomenon of this kind of relational enhancement in the lives of at-risk youth—a circumstance that naturally co-occurred with its stated objective of "teaching."

Elkind makes the point that true reading readiness emerges only once a child has attained the neurocognitive milestone of syllogistic reasoning ("All men are mortal; Socrates is a man; thus Socrates is mortal"), which dawns during the *concrete operational* stage of cognitive development. This "con-op leap" happens around age seven, and is a *biologically based* milestone, just like the shedding of baby teeth or the onset of puberty. How many parents fret if their son hasn't managed to lose his first tooth as soon as his friend did, or if their daughter is thirteen and "still just has not been able to get her period"? We wisely recognize that biology has its own internal timeline, but where *neuro*biology is concerned, well, that's a different animal. We get anxious. We want to get in there and…tinker and tweak…optimize…accelerate…give them a head start.

One reason for the widespread presumption that early reading predicts higher academic achievement is also a knotty problem parents face as they contemplate schooling choices: early reading is simply assumed within, and central to, our conventional educational system. As homeschooling mother Beth Clarkson articulates it, this precludes any latitude for the naturally idio-syncratic developmental timelines of children. She suggests that beginning as early as kindergarten, "so much of the curriculum is designed assuming a cer-tain level of reading ability, if a child is behind in reading ability, they will fall behind in all other subjects. With homeschooled children, if a child is not reading, the parents simply help them learn in other ways and thus, they need not fall behind in other subjects."[12]

Clarkson astutely points out that research finding that students suffer long-term as a result of late reading is an indication of "the inability of the school system to adequately adjust to the individual needs of the children rather than an indication that it is supremely important for every child to be reading by a certain age."

Play researcher Kathy Hirsh-Pasek, author of *Einstein Never Used Flashcards*, sees our cultural devaluation of play—shoving it aside in favor of academics for preschoolers, the extinction of recess through the grades, the erosion of unstructured time in kids' lives—as a crisis whose consequences may take years to be recognized. If, as the new research suggests, our conventional preschools with their low-play, prematurely academic focus are turning out children who struggle with executive function, then "we may be raising a generation of kids with less self-control, shorter attention spans, and poorer memory skills."[13] Crisis, indeed—of the peacemaker kind.

How Parents Can Build Their Child's Brain

One very important area of the child's brain does need parents' active participation for optimal healthy development—the *orbitofrontal cortex,* or OFC. It isn't just the first year that is a critical window for OFC development, but the first *three* years, during which time its circuitry in the toddler's brain wires up in *direct response to the nature of his or her primary attachment relationships.* The watchword for these essential early years is relationship, relationship, relationship. Empathy, connection, presence are OFC nourishment; they reciprocally cultivate the capacities for empathy, connection and presence in the child.

Because of its essential functions, the OFC is what I call the "Human Being Success Center" of the brain. If you forget every other function carried out by the OFC, remember this one: self-regulation. The implications of a child's self-regulation brain circuitry are immense and enduring: it lays the foundation for the very sense of self—so much so that one of the godfathers of the field of attachment neurobiology titled his landmark textbook on the subject *Affect Regulation and the Origin of the Self.*[14] Bottom line is, optimally developed circuitry in the brain's OFC is paramount to personality development, peacemaker potential, and lifelong success.

According to Steiner, the life-giving forces that support the optimal unfolding of a child's innate intelligence are a phenomenon of human development, and these newest findings about the importance of developing a child's healthy orbitofrontal cortex are amazingly consistent with what Steiner taught a hundred years ago about how the mind develops. He referred to these inner organizing forces as the *will energies* of a child. A robustly healthy will—which correlates directly with robustly healthy OFC circuitry—is central to success in every dimension of a person's life, and certainly to their capacities for peace, pleasure and innovation.

Learning Peace by Living Peace: Nourishing a Child's Will

Child psychiatrist Bruce Perry points out that the young child's healthiest early brain development is nurtured by consistency and predictability in her daily life. I have a poem on my wall that says "children learn what they live"—and this is especially true in the early years at the basic, unconscious level of brain organization. When a child *lives* regulation, consistency and stability, the child's will energies are fostered, and his brain is wired to *be* regulated, consistent and stable. This is the foundation for peace in the home and in the world, for achievement in school, and success in life!

In the midst of our speedy, complicated world, how do we create an atmosphere of regulation, consistency and stability? How best can we nurture our children's capacities for peace, creativity, ingenuity? The answer is quite simple, actually, but not always easy: we do it by supporting their life-building will energies, which in turn foster optimal brain development. As with a rose, we ensure the unfolding of a beautiful mind and body when, during these first seven years, we enrich the child's soil—her home, her days, her parents—with the four elements most important to the young child: nourishing diet; physical and emotional warmth; consistent rhythms; and an atmosphere of reverence, awe and beauty.

Diet — It seems to go without saying that during these critical years when the child's body and brain are undergoing such intense, rapid growth, he needs a wholesome, nutritious diet—including plenty of protein, fresh vegetables and whole grains, ideally locally and organically grown—to provide the construction materials. But many parents don't realize which nutrient is *most* essential to the life-giving forces at work now: fat. Children need a variety of high quality fats and oils, from both animal and vegetable sources. Myelin, the protective sheath that covers communicating neurons and facilitates optimal functioning of the nervous system, is being created and laid down at a tremendous rate in the young child's brain. Myelin is composed of 30 percent protein and 70 percent fat. Indeed, optimal formation of the brain—the organ of utmost importance to a child's future success and peacemaker potential—relies on an abundance of essential fatty acids (EFAs). In today's excessively antifat diet culture, children are at risk for not getting enough. Care must be taken by vegetarians and meat-eaters alike to provide their young children quality sources of EFAs. With today's obesity epidemic among children, avoiding the wrong kinds of fats, especially trans fats, is of utmost importance—as well as making sure physical activity is part of your child's daily life.

Warmth — As mothers through the ages can attest, children rarely feel cold (and thus are not inclined to "Put on a sweater!"). This is because of their accelerated metabolic rate: so much new growth is going on inside of them—organs, bones, blood, brain cells—it's like a little furnace in there. A young child or infant may not even feel cold until she's on the verge of hypothermia. Like so many other mothers living in warm climates, I let my summer baby sport nothing but a diaper on many occasions, but I have since learned it would have been far healthier for him to have on a couple of thin layers of cotton or even lightweight wool, especially over the center of his body, where organs were developing. (This is why little vests are wonderful—they warm the center while leaving the playful arms free.) Advises developmental pediatrician Susan Johnson:

> If we don't provide them with the layers of cotton and wool to insulate their bodies, then they must use some of their potential "growth" energy to heat their bodies. This same energy would be better utilized in further developing their brain, heart, liver, lungs etc. In addition, being cold decreases our immunity. We are all more susceptible to the germs and viruses that are always around us when we are wet and cold. When our body has to expend extra energy to keep warm then less energy is available to "fight" off infections.[15]

So the question becomes, how do we get our children to wear jackets? Well, we can develop the habit of always having a child put on a hat and coat when they go outside during cool weather, and we can also tell the child that they will actually run faster and have much more energy to play if they wear a coat. If they don't wear a coat then their body has to expend a lot of energy just warming up, and they will have less energy to build muscles and to play.[16]

The warmth of a fever is also important for a child's healthy development; it's one of her immune system's key tools for the ongoing remodeling of her body throughout childhood. Fever is the body's wise way to get hot enough to digest and expel layers of what needs to go—so wise parents won't automatically reduce it with children's Tylenol or Advil. Once they determine—

with the help of a doctor, especially in a child younger than two years—that the child doesn't have a serious illness (e.g., strep throat, pneumonia, meningitis), it's important that they consider supporting the fever process in various ways, such as properly breathable yet insulating clothing and even such unexpected yet effective approaches as lemon wraps.[17]

As author Melissa Block points out, "Each fever and acute inflammation is like a labor pain. While it's hard to welcome and embrace the intense discomfort of a contraction, each one brings you closer to holding your baby in your arms. Each fever and inflammation is trying to bring to birth a new balance in your child, helping her to make a new step in her development."[18] Many parents notice that their child takes a big developmental leap directly following an acute illness.

Besides physical warmth, the young child needs to be surrounded by emotional warmth. This may seem obvious, but it's actually not such a given: if you were the proverbial fly on the wall looking in on how people are living in today's sped-up, must-go-faster world, you'd find that many homes of even the youngest children echo with the chill of cool, expedient efficiency. We've become a hyperpractical, results-focused culture too often too busy to slow down to child time, which is inherently more molasses-paced. To kneel down to our child's level to listen to her story, to put our arms around our son and look at that bug he just caught, doesn't often jibe with our lockstep schedule.

One of the biggest obstacles to joy and tranquility in the home of young children is adult agendas of what must get done. As everyone who has ever raced with the clock knows—whether it's in the workplace, out in the world doing errands, or at home—one of the first casualties of time pressure is simple *kindness*, in our demeanor and speech. It's bad enough when this happens with our peers and fellow adults, but in the life of a child the evaporation of kindness is incalculably risky: it erodes the bedrock of all development and also, remember, they are watching, imprinting, and will soon be imitating it all. *Social Intelligence* author Daniel Goleman highlights genetic research demonstrating that "small, caring acts of parenthood can matter in lasting ways—and that relationships have a hand in guiding the brain's continuing redesign."[19]

I vividly remember that one of the most blissful weeks I ever spent with my two children when they were very young—six and three—was when their dad was out of the country on business and I had cleared my schedule, resigned to getting nothing done…except remaining sane! Once my own agenda was dropped, I was able to be present for my kids in a way that my habitual, hyperefficient approach usually didn't allow for. To this day, almost twenty years later, I remember the extended game of Pirate Ship we played together... the feeling of Eve's breath in my face...the sound of Ian's giddy laughter...the intimate connection we shared and the sense of infinite expansiveness in those moments. That taught me the value of being flexible regarding my own thoughts of what I needed to accomplish on any given day.

If parents were to consider *every* day with young children as such an extenuating circumstance—and just as temporary—as I considered that unusual week when my husband was away, they might lean more naturally into modes that nourish their children's healthy will (and bring themselves more tranquility). And when you think about it from a big-picture perspective, these early years truly *are* extenuating and temporary—a relatively fleeting, unspeakably precious window of time in which to accomplish perhaps the most important work you'll ever do—weave a core of peace and joy within your child(ren).

A rarely considered facet of our tendency toward overpermissiveness is part of where we've veered off course in our collective approach to parenting: a sense that we must instill the lesson early on in our children that they can do it themselves. Whether it's prompted by anxiety that they'll remain helpless forever, or our uniquely American value of rugged individualism, all this nudging and cajoling we do so that our kids get on with the business of growing up doesn't serve anyone. It was a huge *ah-hah* when I learned that the best way to foster true independence in a child is to allow her to be *dependent* for as long as she needs to be. The parenting strategy by which parents either distractedly leave children largely to their own devices or consciously choose not to indulge their "childish" needs in an attempt to cultivate self-sufficiency, actually backfires and results in what therapists call *unmet dependency needs*. These get expressed in all kinds of unconstructive, self-defeating behaviors later in life, part of a constellation labeled narcissism.[20]

The common perception of a narcissist as someone who is overly confident and in love with themselves is a *mis*perception: the narcissist* masks the fact that he (usually unconsciously) feels deeply insecure and unworthy, and does

---

* I dislike this pejorative term for someone struggling with a developmental imbalance that results in a certain kind of vulnerability; while I understand that narcissism can result in behavior that is hurtful to themselves or others, it would be like labeling someone with diabetes a *diabeticist*!

all the wrong things and looks in all the wrong places to find the mirroring—the adoration reflected back to him in his mother's "eyes of delight"—that he missed when he *should* have received it in copious amounts. Meaning, in his first three to five years. And thus the irony: many parents' well-meaning attempts to raise a person who *isn't* self-centered and narcissistic can actually result in exactly that!

Aside from the missing experience of being significant and cherished, the chronic experience of insecurity and fear experienced by a child who doesn't feel allowed to be "needy" or "weak" or "a baby" leads her to construct an inner emotional fortress and an outer brave face: *I don't need anyone.* This insular, protection-rather-than-growth orientation toward the world—which becomes part of her neural circuitry—is the antithesis of the constellation of personality traits that mark a person of peace and enlightened, innovative action. Most importantly, it snuffs out empathy.

Carolyn Zahn-Wexler, a psychologist specializing in the development of empathy, antisocial behavior, and depression, writes, "In adverse environments (such as a chaotic family life, child maltreatment, parental mental illness) children may become frightened, threatened, or angry and lash out or turn away from others in distress. In steeling themselves against their own pain, they may also become inured to the pain of those around them, which can adversely affect later social relationships, and the ability to discover peaceful solutions to conflicts."[21] Indeed, children aged three to four who display fearless behavior show less empathy and more aggression toward their peers.[22] They are also "emotionally shallow" and have a hard time identifying (i.e., relating to) facial expressions of fear.

Also of particular interest to the central growth-versus-protection theme of parenting for peace, the preschoolers were studied according to the "approach and withdrawal dimension" of their neurological functioning—the tendency to approach new stimuli (to gain information and acquire new skills) and withdraw from unfamiliar stimuli (to avoid danger). Ideally a child strikes a balance of exploration and caution—i.e., a healthy integration of growth *and* protection impulses. Fearless children fall at the caution-free end of the spectrum, which the researcher says involves neurological and genetic predisposition—but predisposition is not predestination: a child who is closely nurtured in the attuned way described in these pages is unlikely to have his or her normal fear response as dampened as was found in the children in this study.[23]

The researcher suggests, "As a society, we must discern the optimal stimulation that can be provided in the child's natural surroundings, in order to awaken those emotions that are necessary for the development of empathy toward another and for refraining from aggressive behavior."

This means enveloping the child in the emotional warmth he needs—which includes mirroring, kindness and the security of being supported and nurtured with all of his individual needs, fears and dependence. And then as if by magic, usually imperceptibly but sometimes overnight, he will organically outgrow the childish expressions of those needs, fears and dependencies—not because he had to repress or deny them, but because he will have internalized the healthy capacities for regulating them within his own being. (Once again, the magic of *projection of function outside until the capacity is built inside*.)

We Americans feel the need to begin training our children from the very beginning that "the world does not revolve around you." But the fact is, the world (the little world of home and family) *should* rightly revolve, to a great degree, around the young child's needs (not necessarily *wants*—an important distinction). This is the age when she is internalizing the experience that she has an impact on her world, that her needs matter, that the world and the people in it are responsive and she can thus feel confident rather than on guard. These are fundamental templates through which all her future experiences and relationships will be filtered. It is not possible to "spoil" a child of this age with too much love, attention or cuddling!

This does not mean we become doormats, doormen, servants, or sacrificial offerings to the unbridled whims and wants of our children. Which brings us to the next of the four basic elements needed by the young child.

Rhythm — "As biologists have learned in the past decade," writes author Jennifer Ackerman, "time permeates the flesh of all living things—and for one powerful reason: We evolved on a rotating planet."[24] She observes the many ways in which we carry inside us a model of the cosmos. It is thus no wonder that we find rhythmicity so nourishing. The young child most especially thrives on rhythmic routine, consistency and predictability. It weaves a sense of security into the fiber of his very cells as they are busy building brain and organ tissue. Rhythm should permeate the child's daily, weekly and even seasonal life. Meals and bedtimes are consistent and regular. Activities at home as well as outings take on the predictability of ritual, which the child can count on and keep a sort of internal beat to: *today we wash the sheets, then we go to the market, now we go to the post office, now I turn the dial on the box, now I am bored at the bank.*

We have become so frightened today of subjecting our children to—dare I even utter the word?—*boredom,* that we pack their lives full of extraneous, exciting, new adventures that will stimulate their imaginations. Ironically, it is sameness and routine, the steady rhythm internalized by the child and embodied in well-mapped brain circuitry, that frees him to engage his imagination, creativity and, later, intellect.

Will energies are embedded in the body, experienced in the body, and are most nourished by the experience of *doing.* The child who is developing a healthy will helps fold the laundry, stirs the soup, sweeps the floor. She stacks blocks and bangs pots. She putters, she plays, she dabbles, she peeks at her mom from behind the door, all in the course of a day that has a comforting, secure structure and rhythm, which helps her brain hardwire for regulation and stability. It is through the doing of these simple activities that the child's will forces take shape and are strengthened. The regular recurrence of the daily rhythm in which one element flows smoothly into the next is calming, and offers children a sense of security through which their forces of will, expressed particularly in their play, can be nourished and their imagination take shape. Such rhythm used to occur naturally when work was homebased in preindustrial America; today it requires dedicated effort and ingenuity to meet these developmental needs of the young human, needs that have not changed to keep pace with the technological revolution.

Common antirhythmic activities that adults take for granted but which can overtax the child's life-building will energies are visiting new places in tourist mode; time spent in the car; participation in competitive sports; crowded places like supermarkets, sporting events, or malls; literature meant for older children (e.g., *Harry Potter*); and rock and roll, jazz and other music meant for adults. All of these influences—like the rock music that when played in a greenhouse causes plants to wither—will weaken and dissipate a child's life forces. (We'll discuss TV in its own section a bit later.) The very pace at which we tend to live is itself a taxing influence on the child's development.

Reconciling these two somewhat incompatible realities is a big part of the peaceful parenting challenge. Sitting in a parent's lap while he or she is riveted to a computer screen is antithetical to the needs of the child for activities done by hand—routinely, repetitively, and in joy. The child needs to see real work

---

A Peaceful Parenting Conundrum

Technology has careened forward and changed our world dramatically, even in just the past fifty years.	*Human beings haven't much changed— in how we're built or how we function— in thousands of years!*

---

modeled by his parents. Here is where the conundrum really shows itself clearly: so much of what we adults consider meaningful activity happens in the abstract, virtual world of computers, screens, social networking technologies and the like. You will rarely hear me romanticizing the past (as in "We've got to return to the old ways of…" or "…back when things were simpler… "), because we have never lived in an era with less brutality, more freedom, or greater opportunity as we do now. There are, however, certain aspects of earlier, less-sophisticated life that you would do well to embrace for these few years when your children are young, for the simple reason that it will best help you harness and leverage Nature's innate plan for their most vibrant flourishing.

The child's need for a worthy example brings us to a central feature of this need for rhythm—the solid bass line of that rhythm: the parent as a calm, loving authority figure who is grounded in his or her life, which is not balanced on the child as its fulcrum. So many power struggles and discipline issues begin to arise in toddlerhood, and as Jean Liedloff explains, it is often because in their devotion to being good parents who respect and honor their children, parents have "gone overboard in the other direction" in which they center their attention and activities on the child, rather than engaging in "adult activities that the children can watch, follow, imitate, and assist in as is their natural tendency."

> In other words, because a toddler wants to learn what his people do, he expects to be able to center his attention on an adult who is centered on her own business. An adult who stops whatever she is doing and tries to ascertain what her child wants her to do is short-circuiting this expectation. Just as significantly, she appears to the tot not to know how to behave, to be lacking in confidence and, even more alarmingly, looking for guidance from him, a two or three year old

who is relying on her to be calm, competent, and sure of herself. A toddler's fairly predictable reaction to parental uncertainty is to push his parents even further off-balance, testing for a place where they will stand firm and thus allay his anxiety about who is in charge.[25]

I would invite you to see if you can incorporate a sense of life oriented around some basic, hands-on activities that your child can watch, then imitate and help with. And to also cultivate an inner, abiding confidence in your authority; unlike in so many of today's families, in which parents seem to have developed an aversive allergy to their children's unhappiness or upset, your child needs to know that you will not be shaken by her crying, whining, or protests.

The Challenge: Cultivating Calm, Loving Authority

We all know the feeling of being in a situation—a new class, a new job, a new city—in which we're not quite sure what's what. Where do we go, what do we do, who do we talk to? In those cases, it's always a relief when someone on the scene confidently and reliably knows the score and kindly lends us authoritative guidance. It helps us relax and experience the new situation more fully, rather than being in the on-alert state that tends to come over us when we're unsure of things. For the toddler and young child, all of life is a new situation!

An important function of both the predictable routine and a dependable authority figure is that they provide a secure form that allows children to live in "dream consciousness," a hallmark of the first seven years. The slower brainwaves of the young child do in fact resemble that of a dreaming adult.[26] Children need to be able to unselfconsciously and wholeheartedly participate in the day's experiences without worrying about what comes next or what they need to be ready for. But these days it seems that even very young kids are savvy and alert and in-the-know about everything that is going on in the household.

It is best if we don't awaken the young child from her "dream"; therefore, we shouldn't offer a stream of choices or involve her in democratic family policymaking, and we should definitely not *overexplain*. In my practice, and in observing families out in the world, I've come to see this as an epidemic—young children having too many choices and too much say in what takes place in the family. Now I myself will admit to once believing that having many choices in the course of the day (*Which pants would you like to wear, the blue ones or the brown ones? Do you want bananas or blueberries on your cereal, and do you want oatmeal or corn flakes? Yellow bowl or red?*) imparted a sense of empowerment in the young child, helped him feel a bit more involved in his own daily destiny, and built self-esteem. As with so many of our parenting missteps, giving a child this opportunity for autonomy errs not in its noble intention or even in its content, but in its timeframe: these are choices and freedoms that are not yet age-appropriate. My term to describe the myriad ways in which we perceive or treat young children as older children or even grownups is *adultifying.*

When we offer endless choices to the child, or engage in extended explanations, justifications or negotiations, or phrase our language in equivocal terms ("How about getting your PJs on?") we undermine our standing with him. If you were to listen in on many a parent's conversations with their young one, it wouldn't take long to hear what is in my opinion a most damaging (when used with a question mark) four-letter word for a child: *Okay.* As in, "It's time to get ready for bed now, okay?" And then there's the friendly, four-word discipline-disaster-in-the-making, "Do you want to..." As in "Do you want to get your sweater so we can go to school?" Talking to a young child in this way essentially enlists him as a co-decision-maker, with a level of influence and responsibility that makes him extremely anxious—though he doesn't know why. This anxiety and insecurity ("Mom doesn't really know what should happen now...") reorients his biochemistry and neurophysiology toward protection rather than growth. Also, the young child learns first and foremost through imitation, so if you negotiate and debate with her, she will soon get better at it than you!

This is a vicious cycle: the more the child perceives that you are looking to her to participate in important decisions (and to a young child even the basics seem very important), the less trust she'll have in you, the more insecure she will feel, and the more controlling (i.e., difficult) she will become. Before long, she won't do anything without opening and closing arguments, along with exhibits A, B and C. And it shouldn't be regarded as cute when a child repeatedly corrects a parent; it is the basis for his loss of respect and turning away from the parent later on.

Another effect of having too many choices and discussion is a prematurely awakened sense of her own self (self-consciousness) and a premature focus on what she likes and doesn't like. (So here we have another irony: we all want our children to grow up generous, considerate of others, and not so material-istic, but all this mental activity focused on preferences tends to foster quite the opposite! We parents can also serve as models in this area; let's not make an issue of everything we feel and want. When parents show restraint—in eat-ing, in buying, even in speaking—and demonstrate *joy in what we already have*, this is a great lesson for the child.)

The sad thing is, children naturally want to please the adults to whom they feel connected, and the child who has become controlling and demanding due to this kind of insidious insecurity desperately (though unconsciously) *does not want to act like that.* She fervently wants you, her parent, to be the calm, loving authoritative figure she can look up to, rely upon, and joyfully follow! Indeed, the word *discipline* is related to the word *disciple,* a "joyful fol-lower." If you can stand centered as the calm, loving authority figure, your child will relax and take joy in following you; discipline will not be nearly the issue it is for most families. But what I find so often in my practice is that par-ents bump up against tremendous inner resistance and insecurity in trying to step into that place of calm authority. This is when *their* own templates from when they were young children kick in and suddenly they're being driven un-consciously by such guiding convictions as "I'm not worthy of being listened to," and "I have no impact upon my world." Thus, they feel little confidence in their own ability to lead, and fall back on cultural parenting conventions based on coercion, manipulation, placating, shaming, etc.—none of which allows for optimal growth mode in their children.[27]

Over-explaining almost always covers up a lack of truth or conviction in the exchange. We need to always check the reason why we want to say some-thing to a child: Is it based on our wisdom or our anxiety? Does it come from a place of real knowing, or a place of fear? If it comes from a place of real knowing and complete conviction within you that it is correct, the child will usually behave in harmony with it. (A good example is that children almost never fuss over putting on seat belts, largely because within the mind of the parent there is 100 percent conviction: seat belts are an utter nonnegotiable and the child picks up on this conviction.) If it's coming from worry or inse-curity, we best refrain from speaking. Yes, we're still feeling the fear, but it is your self-discipline in *containing the feeling* the child picks up on.

One of the newer findings from attachment neurobiology is that *what we say* is far less important than *who we are*, and this is one of the reasons: the way in which we manage the ebb and flow of our own feelings and impulses, our mastery of the currents of our inner lives, is what makes the greatest impression on the child, rather than the content of the currents themselves. This is good news: again, it is not our perfection but our striving that influences our children!

The most precious commodity we have in our ongoing relationships with our children is *trust*. The young child's trust is staggeringly complete: he will reach for the hand of his mother to cross the street and not even look to see if a car is coming. This is the level of trust that later we are meant to have for God; indeed, parents are the young child's first model of a higher power. Trust, however, erodes little by little when we engage in standard parenting techniques that are not rooted in our authenticity. This insidious evaporation of trust underlies many of the conflicts and power struggles between parents and children as they get older.

I have found it remarkably helpful—sometimes downright transformative—for a parent to envision, in great detail, herself in a typical discipline situation with her child that doesn't tend to go well, and then to revise the scene—see herself responding as the calm, loving, and self-assured mother she would choose to be. Ditto father. We know from sports psychology how powerful such visualizing can be, as well as following the basic tenet of "Fake it till you can make it." Think of a parenting figure you admire, even a character from a book or movie, and adopt him or her as your own role model to emulate and help you elevate yourself to the level of confidence, inner poise and perspicacity (a great word with no good synonym) that your child dearly hopes to find in you.

Reverence, Awe, and Beauty – Another fundamental need of the young child is an atmosphere in harmony with his natural impulse to celebrate beauty and feel reverence and awe about almost everything. But what does our culture do in this techno-materialist age? We foist upon even the youngest child a flat world of facts and commentary. At a time when the child most needs wonder and reverence, we explain away all sense of the miraculous with our cold, adult intellect, with the good intention of helping prepare them for the real world. ("Daddy, look at that bright star!" "Oh yes, Esmerelda—do you know that a star is just a very dense concentration of gases—just air!—that burns very, very hot...thousands of light-years away..."). Mystery eradicated, poof!

Sheltering your child's natural sense of wonder—and indeed, cultivating your own if it has atrophied over the years—is a gift of lasting wellbeing. That sense of "Wow—water out of the tap! or "Wow—text sent over phone lines through squeaky little noises!" is a route to vast inner horizons. When we lose that, we need ever more stimulation—more shopping, more drama, more drugs and alcohol, more thrillers (which feeds the collective propensity toward societal violence), more sexual excess, and so on—to fill the void of disenchantment.

We dress babies in black T-shirts with hiply ironic slogans that make us adults laugh—at the expense of respect for "the kingdom of childhood" as Steiner called it. Kim John Payne suggests that we're living in an "undeclared war on childhood," in which sarcasm and cynicism—poison to the young child's soul—are primary forms of entertainment and humor, especially in so-called children's entertainment![28] So speaking of that, we can put it off no longer, the issue of TV—a hugely important topic for parents and children.

Staring into the Void

There are several excellent books entirely devoted to the thorny issue of children and television (and screens of all kinds), and, so I'm going to "nuggetize"—from the standpoint of its known effects specifically relevant to a child's developmental orientation toward optimal growth rather than defensive protection. I venture into this knowing full well that television addiction—I *mean* it, addiction!—is not only culturally sanctioned but encouraged and cultivated. Hi, my name is Marcy, and I'm a tube-aholic. I'm not proud of it, but I am. And chances are, you are too. Unless you're that rare specimen (like people who don't care for chocolate—*what?!*) for whom TV is a take-it-or-leave-it proposition, the whole television situation will likely present an ongoing challenge you'll negotiate throughout the childhood and teen years. I know it did for our family. If it's not a big thing for you, then consider yourself freed of a considerable parenting hurdle—for now. (Just wait till your sweet one starts going to sleepovers...)

In 1999, a year after *Teletubbies* landed on U.S. television screens from Britain, the normally reticent American Academy of Pediatrics issued a statement that said children under two should not watch television, and that no child of any age should have a television in his or her room. They added, "Maybe it should be phrased more positively, that children do best with the maximum free play, the maximum interaction and maximum face time with their parents."

These early years feature some of the most vigorous brain growth your child will undergo, particularly in the orbitofrontal cortex—the command center of capacities for intellectual flexibility, innovation and peace that we want to encourage. The maturing of the young brain is experience-dependent, meaning that the wiring of enduring neural circuitry happens in direct response to what the child encounters in his or her daily life. Put another way, how a child uses her brain during these early years determines to a great extent how her brain—particularly her *social* brain, but also her intellectual capacities—will develop and function lifelong. The scientific research is unequivocal: the healthiest psychosocial development of the young brain is achieved through close and near-constant human relationship, hands-on interaction with the world through imaginative play, and connection with nature.

Sitting in front of a television runs counter to all of those brain-nurturing pursuits, and is in fact a highly unnatural activity for a young child: sitting motionless for thirty, sixty, ninety minutes at a time, watching the flicker of electronic signals play across a backlit screen was never part of Nature's plan for the unfolding of social or cognitive intelligence. Rather than nurturing rich neural connections in the social brain through human interactions, and building structures of knowledge through imagination-igniting engagement with three-dimensional elements of the real world, the child watching TV passively receives preformed images, slogans, goals and values while his unique human powers of consideration, comparison, and imagination go to sleep. (Very often a child—or for that matter, an adult—is unable to tell you in much detail at all about what he just watched for thirty minutes, because a lot of the content slips in beneath the radar of conscious processing. Advertisers have been leveraging that fact for decades.)[29] This is starkly evident from looking at scans comparing the suppression of higher brain wave activity during television viewing as compared to drawing or other pursuits.

When presenting a talk to an audience, Joseph Chilton Pearce gets particularly animated when scribbling out a rough schematic on the overhead projector of what happens in the higher centers (neocortex) of a child's brain when she listens to a story about a dog: a blitzkrieg of synaptic connections lights up as the words stimulate her neural structures to create images, then more connections to connect images as the story unfolds. New interconnections between separate neural fields in the child's brain are woven with each new story. During this process the child seems almost catatonic, but it's drastically different than the classic flickering-blue-glow catatonia conjured by TV: the child engaged in a story is deploying all the energy of all her online brain centers. Her creative brain is *hard at work*, in contrast to the inertness of the creative brain centers watching television.

At least a decade before research conclusively showed that babies don't learn language from screens but from people,[30] Waldorf teacher Carol Toole raised a concern with electronic playmates for children—ironically, years before the massive proliferation of screen-based learn–to-read programs for even the youngest of children. She points out how such devices undermine the central need of children to learn in the context of relationship and imitation.

> The budding orator needs to hear speech that bears the undivided attention, enthusiasm, and interest of the speaker. Studies reveal that language experienced via television or other electronic media does little to increase a child's vocabulary. Such disembodied speech does not nourish the child in his learning to speak. Even the speech of real and present people, when it is curt and clipped and seeks only to convey information, does not truly nourish.[31]

Most of the solid research on television's effect on children has centered on physical health and behavior, and such consequences as obesity, increased aggression, desensitization to violence, gender stereotyping, warping of reality perception, increased materialist drive and susceptibility to commercialism. While these together with television's known negative impact upon a child's cognitive and intellectual skills[32] are bound to be of concern to parents, and obviously have implications for our discussion, I want to zero in on effects that strike at the brain's developing capacities for peace, joy and innovation. How might television undermine a blossoming generation of peacemakers? How might TV viewing redirect a child's developmental orientation toward defensive protection rather than fully elaborated growth?

The cuts, pans and zooms that happen every few seconds on a television show elicit our brain's instinctive reactivity to novelty, movement, and sudden changes in vision or sound. This *orienting response* is part of our mammalian heritage, designed to help us survive predators and other lurking threats. The television age marked the beginning of a vast neuropsychological experiment whose subjects are innumerable and who are us—from every race, country, culture, and socioeconomic group. What happens to people when for the first time in human experience they spend hours at a time having their orienting response subliminally triggered every few seconds?

At the level of the brain's automatic systems, the countless incidents of novelty programmed into a TV show—specifically engineered to keep the viewer's attention from veering away from the tube[33]—are double-edged swords that swipe Zorro-style at neural pathways so quickly as to be imperceptible. The lower brain centers are snapped to attention for possible danger (with the attendant neurochemicals to prepare the body for fight, flight or freeze) and then are immediately relieved of the threat as the brain calculates at light-speed that there's in fact no danger. This triggers the dopamine system, the brain's pleasure center, which evolved to reward us with a heady sense of euphoria when we escape harm or engage in other activities that promote survival of the individual and thus the species (think eating, drinking, sex).

The result is a brain that is alert, but not focused. Placated but not engaged. One effect of this alert-relief dialectic inside the brain is that television viewing has a numbing action, with a reaction in the body sometimes like that of a tranquilizer. Also, the repetitive dosing of the dopamine receptors can dampen the receptors in the brain's pleasure center, making joy harder to come by through simple, human, nontechnological means. When regarded this way— the actual *process* of television and not so much the *content*—it's not hard to understand the growing body of research linking television with such neural regulatory problems as depression and attention deficit disorders.[34]

I have long suspected that many cases of ADD or ADHD are actually children in the grips of chronic, inarticulable anxiety, such as happens in the wake of trauma or possibly after sitting through dozens of novelty events on TV. The child cannot focus on any one thing for a length of time because she has to continually reorient in search of the threatening stimuli; it's just that the stimuli aren't out there in the world, but rather, internalized imprints on the brain, irritable neural pathways that are hypersensitive due to being continually triggered. And indeed, brand new research demonstrates that the more fast-paced the programming (e.g., *SpongeBob* as opposed to *Mr. Rogers*), the more impairment was seen in the executive function of children's brains while performing tasks following viewing. This includes such critical aspects as self-regulation, attention and problem solving.[35]

Numbing Them Down

We see in brain scans that the level of gamma waves—the highest frequency brainwave, associated with perception and higher brain activity, which is present when we're actively focused in on something—drops to almost a flatline during TV viewing. Is this what we want to train the young child's brain to do? I understand the common complaint from frustrated parents that sometimes television is the only time an active child will sit still and pay attention; the problem is, the child isn't really *paying* attention but rather having his attention *involuntarily stolen*!

And all the while, the child's own nascent powers of voluntary, conscious attention—the capacity to *attend* and be present, a central feature of the Generation Peace profile—languish and atrophy. Remember, the way a child uses his brain largely dictates how his brain develops. The brain regions meant to be engaged and bustling with activity at this age for optimally healthy psychosocial development essentially go to sleep when a child watches TV—establishing what Jane Healy in her book *Endangered Minds* refers to as the kinds of "habits of mind" that put them at a disadvantage at school.[36] Do we want to routinely flatline the higher brain centers responsible for perception, engagement and attention?

Does this mean that an occasional episode of *Sesame Street* will undermine a child's trajectory toward unfolding into a person of peaceful innovation? Of course not—especially if she shares in that episode with one of her close adults. But because of that pesky trick it plays on the pleasure center of the brain, television is a slippery seductress: one episode a week so easily and insidiously becomes two, then a few, and then a daily dose, and so on. Power struggles ensue. It's not a path I recommend starting down; it's like tossing a handful of landmines onto your own road ahead.

I realize that *Sesame Street* is a sacrosanct institution, but even with a show that features engaging characters, socially conscious story lines and attention-grabbing formats, we have to constantly ask ourselves, Is this hitting the sweet spot of what I want to nurture *at this time* in my child's life? (If pressed, I'd rather children who are older than the two-to-five-year-old target audience view *Sesame Street*; seven or eight is when letters, numbers and stories of social mores become more developmentally appropriate.)

Aside from the neuroerosive aspects of television, another troubling issue with children's programming (as well as children's literature) is that the message and values conveyed become unguardedly accepted as valid and true. This has implications across a range of dimensions, from tot consumerism to the veiled depiction of aggression and violence. And there is also the issue of the young child's need for reverence and beauty. Research tells us quite precisely what physical properties in a creature we innately find compelling and attractive, having to do with the proportions and symmetry of eyes, nose, and mouth, as related to the size of the head. The fact that all of this is such meaningful data for us humans brings a concern regarding a reverence for beauty in form and expression. Everything from *Rugrats* to *Simpsons* to *Sesame Street* to *Yo Gabba Gabba* features gross distortions of human anatomy, calling it funny, cool, or, most insidious of all, cute. Many of the caricature traits are designed to tap into our hardwired receptivity to the baby of any species, often featuring large eyes, large foreheads, and almost no nose. These are then distorted through a mélange of other features—like that card puzzle game in which you put one person's eyes with another's chin, etc.

And there's often a high-pitched voice. The hallmark of our human species is our articulated speech, an aspect that places us at the pinnacle of the animal kingdom, but television insists on regaling children with voices that are unmelodious and whiny. As any actor knows, when we want to convey superficiality, awkwardness or even mental disability, we speak with a nasal voice. It is universal, our human perception about this vocal "less-than"; children know at a deep level they're being talked to as second-class citizens—citizens whose brand loyalty can be wooed as early as age two. Meanwhile, their humanity is subtly demoted by the grotesquely formed yet amusing characters, and wisdom is trivialized when it is announced by a big bird with eyes that cross. (And that *voice!*) When raising peacemakers, do we really want to subliminally train them in the devaluation of wisdom and humanity? (And as one dad astutely points out, the wisdom conveyed by a big bird in half an hour of "educational television" could be taught in three minutes by a parent, leaving twenty-seven minutes to go outside and jump in puddles.)

So what's a mom or dad to do, at the end of a trying day, when everyone's tired—when all they want is a few free minutes to prepare dinner without juggling junior at the same time? Before resorting to the electronic babysitter, try:

- a sink of soapy water and unbreakable items for him to wash
- a floor-sized puzzle
- bubbles
- a basketful of a few treasured items she enjoys that only appear at this time of day
- ditto a sand tray
- ditto a pot of clay or play dough and cookie cutters
- a clothesline with kitchen towels clipped to it to make a peek-a-boo fort

- a solo game of Twister he plays with your rousing encouragement
- giving her a heavy piece of moistened art paper with two harmoniously matching colors of gouache and a thick paint brush and letting her go to town

Ever a pragmatist, and wanting to keep an eye on what works while still supporting a child's inner connectedness and imagination, I sometimes suggest parents in my practice consider introducing their young children to the joys of audio stories and music. If you begin early with the notion that these are a special treat, you will have a win-win resource for your family: audio stories (such as the treasures my kids used to listen to from Rabbit Ears Radio) or a child's favorite CD of songs can hold a child rapt for the twenty or thirty minutes of solitude you might crave, while still engaging her active imagination as she sings or dances along, or envisions the scenes in the tales—maybe even drawing or acting them out with her dolls or wooden figures. These are also a boon for long car trips.

Wondering about the DVD screens currently embedded in the backs of car seats? Here's the thing: car rides come with many naturally occurring sensory stimuli as standard equipment (everything passing by outside the windows, not to mention the conversation inside). If we distract and essentially hypnotize a child away from possible *boredom* (the dirtiest word in our current parenting culture) by plugging her into video entertainment, we deprive her of a regularly occurring, ideal opportunity to practice the important developmental task of learning to soothe and regulate her own fluctuating internal states of attention, interest, distress, etc.—and to engage in the kind of open-ended thought stream of nothing-in-particular (mind*less*ness) neuroscientists now recognize is as important to the health of our social brains as is mind*ful*ness.[37] *This could not be more essential to her growing Gen Peace capacities!*

Next best after audio recordings, if you're really desperate to occupy your child with programming, is to lay in a small supply of those rare videos that feature gentle visual formatting, unsophisticated production values, and no rapid cuts or special effects. When our son was young we had a video that was simply a twenty-minute walk around a farm, with no editing and only the natural sounds of the environment—quite a novelty for a city boy. He also enjoyed an occasional episode of *Mr. Rogers' Neighborhood*, and we all loved the two volumes of *Mother Goose Treasury of Sing-Along Nursery Rhymes*. (The latter was born in 1987, just like our Ian—and it held extra appeal for him since "Mother Goose" was actually a friend of ours!)

Just keep in mind not only the slippery pleasure center slope of any kind of video entertainment, but that the more we offer children appealing prefab scenarios, even the most seemingly benign or enchanting, we *un*invite their own unique creativity that might have sparked a brand new little crop of peace-buds within. Many Waldorf early education teachers can recognize "media children" in their classrooms by observing the nature of their play, which is more chaotic and mechanical, in imitation of what they have seen on television. The flexibility of their play is impaired, as they tend to get stuck replaying a story line over and over, or become obsessed with one particular character from a show.

In their book *Magical Parent, Magical Child,* Michael Mendizza and Joseph Chilton Pearce point out that the kinds of qualities essential to an innovative peacemaker—curiosity, playfulness, willingness to experiment, flexibility, humor, receptiveness to new ideas, eagerness to learn—all rely upon imagination. Just as chips and candy are junk food for the child's developing body, so are television and computer images junk food for her developing imagination. Stories, conversation, and meaningful hands-on activities feature descriptive words, symbols, and metaphors that the authors say "act as nutrients. They challenge and feed the developing brain, growing and expanding the capacity for imagination." Their primary criticism of screened media, especially for the young child, "has to do with the way these technologies create counterfeit images for processes the developing brain is designed to create itself." The implications could not be more sobering when we're envisioning a peacemaker generation:

> The creative play of these images results in the discovery of new patterns and possibilities that we then use to change our environment. The inner affects the outer, which affects the inner in an unending reciprocal, creative dynamic. Fail to develop imagination and this expansive creative cycle ends. We literally can't imagine new forms and possibilities. We are stuck in a reflexive, mechanical, cause-and-effect world over which we have little control. Hope, the passionate vision of a new alternative, a better future, has no meaning whatsoever without imagination.[38]

Television and media in general tends to fall into the "adultifying" category: not only does its very process undermine healthy development in anything beyond the smallest doses, but its content tends to be inappropriate for young children—even so-called children's programming. And the effects feed back into the most fundamental substrates of a child's blossoming personality. I'll leave this topic for the moment with one last fascinating word on the adultifying effects of media, stated eloquently by the late social critic Neil Postman:

> To a certain extent curiosity comes naturally to the young, but its development depends upon a growing awareness of the power of well-ordered questions to expose secrets. The world of the known and the not yet known is bridged by wonderment. But wonderment happens largely in a situation where the child's world is separate from the adult world, where children must seek entry, through their questions, into the adult world. As media merge the two worlds, as the tension created by secrets to be unraveled is diminished, the calculus of wonderment changes. Curiosity is replaced by cynicism or, even worse, arrogance. We are left with children who rely not on authoritative adults but on news from nowhere. We are left with children who are given answers to questions they never asked. We are left, in short, without children.[39]

TMTS (Too Much Too Soon)

Television and other media—as well as media-saturated technologies like computers and cell phones—are just some of many ways in which our culture seems hell-bent on saddling children's lives with adult things. (I'm reminded of an old Six Flags commercial in which a father and his young daughter sit side by side on their front steps, both frantically noodling away on their individual PalmPilots trying to schedule some time together. It would be amusing if it weren't so sadly realistic.) I believe that we do it out of genuinely good intentions—to prepare our children for all of the things they will face in the world. But if we keep in mind how differently a child's brain and psyche work from those of an adult, and the purposes for those differences, it's clear that the "helpful information" we adults offer young children is often counterproductive to our goals of raising responsible, informed adults.

Here's an example: in our efforts to instill in children a sustainable sense of money, we begin at the earliest ages to make sure they know that "money doesn't grow on trees," and the like. Requests for toys or treats at the store are often answered with "We can't afford that," and so on. But it is central to remember that during these early years generalized *lifelong templates* are being shaped for who the child is, how the world works, and what his or her relationship to that world will be. Until the age of five, the child needs to see, experience, believe and know that *Life is abundance.* So we don't teach or demonstrate the lack of money or anything else.

This doesn't mean you buy everything she wants; on the contrary, giving a child everything she wants, or letting her do everything she wishes, is a perfect recipe for a cruel human being later on. Instead you respond in a way that is consistent with abundance at every level—including abundance of respect for her request, and abundance of inner tranquility: "Yes, it's a beautiful doll,"—find something about it you can admire with the child, as a way of having connection with her at her level of wanting—"but we're not going to buy her today." The power of saying "No" with complete tranquility is the key.

It's important to never demean what a child wants ("Oh, that's a silly thing, and you already have one like it"), or the wanting itself ("You want everything you see!"); to do so is to bleed off some of the essential will forces that are developing and that will later contribute to her abilities to carry out her noble goals and visions. And if she cries you can empathize: "Yes, I know that you are suffering with this 'no,' my love." Hopefully in this particular moment she has the resources of having eaten recently, has had enough water to drink, enough sleep the night before, a pleasant breakfast time—and also, you are not in a stressed or resentful place as her parent. You get the idea: nothing happens in a vacuum.

Even in homes where media and other popular culture is curbed, one way children often suffer from TMTS is through being inadvertently overexposed to adult life in general. Having worked with children suffering post-traumatic stress disorder (PTSD) in southeast Asian refugee camps and such war-torn areas as northern Ireland and Israel, Kim John Payne was struck by the similarities between those young PTSD patients and the students he was treating years later in his private counseling practice near London. Nervous, easily startled, controlling in their behaviors, attention-challenged, troubled by novelty or transitions, explosive in their outbursts of anger—these children from a relatively affluent, stable Western country were displaying symptoms of PTSD, Payne finally admitted to himself despite all counterintuitive reasoning. He came to realize that underlying these children's similar suffering, despite their extremely different living circumstances, ran a common, caustic thread: "…for both groups the sanctity of childhood had been breached. Adult life was flooding in unchecked. Privy to their parents' fears, drives, ambitions, and the very fast pace of their lives, the children were busy trying to construct their own boundaries, their own level of safety in behaviors that ultimately weren't helpful."[40]

Parents need to buffer their children, not from the normal vagaries of childhood—the daily frustrations inherent in being a child, the disappointments with parental restrictions, the spats with friends, the famous skinned knees, all of which are essential for their budding resilience—but from the vagaries of *adulthood*, one of which is simply a flood of too much information: CNN, NPR, World News Tonight, *Modern Family*, family politics, political intrigue, intriguing reality shows, community gossip, environmental crises and the like. (I still vividly remember a conversation between my mother and stepfather about whether, in the course of their daily lives, they were frightened of the Mafia!) And it isn't just about the quality of information (such as "too adult," although that is often an issue), it is about the sheer quantity of sensory input with which children, like everyone, are bombarded by virtue of living in this information-revolution era. They feel the world is "coming at them," which shifts them into protection mode.

This is one of the many good reasons for an early bedtime for your child: to preserve enough adult-only time during which you can engage in data-rich discussions to your mind's content!

Discipline, or Being a Leader of Joyful Followers

This is the age when discipline first becomes an issue and often brings discord, but when you understand and embody a few key principles you'll parent more effectively and joyfully. As we begin to discuss discipline, it's helpful to have a long view of the territory. Payne points out how our culture along the way has gotten the timeline of our discipline styles utterly flipped 'round: we give way too much autonomy and too many choices to the young child, and then tighten the reins with too much limitation and scrutiny during adolescence! He sees the discipline focus of the first seven years as "the will, and creative compliance," during which children are trained to accept limits and adult direction, and to comply with rules.[41] It's within the sturdy form traced by the child's boundaries that his or her healthy will forces can fully expand.

First and most central, the young child learns primarily through imitation, taking our cues about everything, and becoming our most exquisite mirrors— so always ask yourself, *Am I worthy of my child's unquestioning imitation?* If you can answer *Yes*, then you have resolved 95 percent of your discipline issues before they even materialize. All true discipline is ultimately *self*-discipline, and the more mastery we develop of our own inner being, the more harmonious family life will be. Writes psychologist Gordon Neufeld, "Our ability to manage a child effectively is very much an outcome of our capacity to manage ourselves."[42]

Indeed, when you marshal your inner resources in striving to be the calm, loving, authority figure your children will take joy in following, peace emerges in your home and in the very fiber of your children. But ah, this so much easier said than done! A toddler who is practicing his newly discovered autonomy by defying you can push your buttons of powerlessness like nothing else—buttons that were installed when you were his age, possibly when you weren't listened to or respected in the way you're devoted to doing with your child. I still vividly remember the one and only time I swatted our son's behind: he was six or seven and was stubbornly, defiantly ignoring me right to my face. Something primitive inside me uncoiled and I whacked him. I regretted it immediately and ever since, not just for the obvious reason of having been violent with him, but also for the modicum of his respect I lost in that unbridled moment.

We lose the admiration of our children when we "lose it." It's a mammalian thing: all animal behaviorists know that our ability to have authority over— and thus the ability to train—a dog or a horse is severely eroded if the animal sees or feels us get angry. Credible leaders don't lose their composure, it's as simple as that. Of course, children aren't dogs, but we can learn so much from understanding the mammalian similarities! When it's necessary to reprimand your child, strive to not do it with a raised voice or the look of disgust or cruelty in your eyes. Aside from the corrosive effects of shaming, the child will lose trust in you over time, and will look toward others as models. "He doesn't respect me" will be your (accurate) complaint later, especially at an age when he most needs to be able to learn from his parents, such as during his teen years.

And while we don't speak of training a child, it is in fact what we need to be doing with a young one. This flies in the face of many so-called progressive, child-centered approaches that are based on the notion that the child left to his or her own devices will blossom perfectly well without the impingement of our adult meddling. If we do not guide and direct, we abdicate our sacred responsibility as a parent. Prenatal specialist Laura Uplinger, also a mother and a lifelong researcher of esoteric principles, clarifies this little-understood distinction between the perfection of a child's *essence* and the need to guide a child in the *expression* of that essence:

> We would be cruel to not provide guidance. For their empathy to flow, and for the fostering of their grandeur of soul, magnanimity, and intelligence that isn't oriented to destroying things, children need pedagogy. They need to be given a model. A garden is different from a forest because someone went there and did something. We're so afraid of managing life too much, but we never refer to the "woods of Eden" or "a prairie of paradise"; we refer to paradise as a garden. That is the image for parents as the true meaning of parenthood: respecting the child's essence while bringing your own experience to help the structure of the child blossom. (And you don't remain neutral—your own structure changes too!) This is the great invitation—to collaborate with Life in a great adventure.
>
> It's politically incorrect, but true: for the young child, there should be no freedom! Nature has sent children to parents precisely because they're not meant to be free, they're meant to be governed, to learn *how to become free one day.* Freedom is a very serious thing; it isn't a right, it is something you earn through self-mastery. The more you obey the natural and higher laws, the more you are free. An example is someone who has self-discipline regarding food or exercise: they are so much freer in these realms than those who are constantly abusing or struggling with their physical organism. We easily fall slave to our lower tendencies, so our apprenticeship toward freedom is a long one.[43]

My favorite nonviolent interpretation of the oft-mistaken-for-biblical discipline slogan "Spare the rod, spoil the child" is one in which the shepherd's rod is used not to hit but to guide errant sheep in the right direction when they stray off the path. Just as sheep aren't plotting to annoy the shepherd when they stray, the young child's brain simply isn't equipped to marshal the kind of complex planning and detailed motivational linkages that would enable her to systematically drive you crazy (much as it may sometimes seem like it). Children need guidance and instruction, not punishment. And it is often far more effective to simply use a gentle, redirecting arm around the shoulder of a young one heading toward trouble—while perhaps also singing a soothing little melody, like the Pied Piper—than to deploy a string of words to reason with or explain ("...for the umpteenth time!") the prohibition to the errant child.

As I've said, a central goal in parenting for peace is to cultivate an atmosphere in which our children are able to live as much as possible in growth-flourishing mode rather than protect-and-defend mode. It ensures the correct wiring of their social and cognitive brain circuitry, as well as their optimally healthy bodies. This doesn't mean insulating them from every possible stressor; preventing them from experiencing life's daily ups and downs would be counterproductive to the developing vitality of the critical self-regulating capacities of the orbitofrontal cortex. But heavens, just *being* a two-, four- or six-year-old is inherently steeped in near-constant frustration: each of the emotional, motor and cognitive skills that lies tantalizingly, maddeningly out of their reach at each stage is enough to give their nascent stress-management systems all the strengthening workouts they need. One of our huge jobs as parents is to have our children's backs (brains?) when their own emotion regulation isn't quite yet up to the task. Like the spotter who stands ready to help lift the massive barbell if the guy on the bench can't quite summon the strength from his weaker position, we help our child lift the load of his distressing emotions until his own neural regulatory system can manage the task on its own.

As we help our children regain balance after big and little upsets, we foster strength and flexibility in their all-important self-regulatory capacities, by helping stress biochemicals recede and pleasure chemicals flow. We also help them orient in a healthy way toward the universal and perennial experience of frustration. Together these are core features of the all-important quality of *resilience*—the ability to regain inner and outer balance following a stressful experience. Self-regulation is also centrally related to *self-control*, which researchers are seeing emerge as a fundamental determinant of a child's successful adult future—"so important that it may play an approximately equal role with other well-known influences on a person's life course, such as intelligence and social class."[44] A newly released study followed three thousand people from birth to age thirty-two and found that differences in self-control that begin to show up as early as age three reliably predict health, financial, familial and even criminal status decades later.

Asked what self-control looks like at that age, one of the researchers explains, "A three-year-old with good self-control can focus on a puzzle or game and stick with it until he solves it, take turns working on the puzzle nicely with another child, and get satisfaction from solving it, with a big smile." As for a child with poor self-control, he "might refuse to play with anything that required any effort of him, might leave the puzzle in the middle to run around the room, might lose his temper and throw the puzzle at the other child, and might end up in tears, instead of feeling satisfied."[45]

If a child is consistently left to his own devices when he's overly frustrated, he doesn't develop the inner self-regulatory capacities he would were he to have the assistance of a connected adult; his brain will be hardwired with the tendency to respond to future frustrations in one of two basic modes—lashing out, or rolling over and going internally numb. (There tends to be a sex differentiation to these responses, with males more often responding with the *outward* aggression, and females with the *inward* aggression.) But when frustrated children have the benefit of parental support, presence and modeling, not only do they develop essential self-regulation, but their brains also hardwire a more healthy reflexive response to frustration, which is to *act*—to try and change the frustrating situation. So here again we see how closely self-regulation is tied to the formation of healthy will energies and how all of it is key for raising Generation Peace.

It's of foremost importance to strive to keep your own self-possession when the pressure's on, like grabbing for your dangling oxygen mask on a depressurized airliner so that you can assist your child. New research suggests that just as the fetal brain adapts to the world as interpreted by mom's perceptions, the same kind of elemental shaping continues through childhood: parents' stress during the early years can leave an imprint on their children's genes—an imprint that lasts into adolescence and can affect how those genes are expressed later in life.[46]

What you might not realize is that pretty much every kind of conventional disciplinary measure elicits a cascade of hormones in the child's nervous system that curtails optimally healthy brain development. Even just the threat of such discipline—a spanking, a time-out, or even a disgusted look from her parent—can instantly shift a child's biochemistry into protection mode. Every time a child receives a punitive rebuke or scolding, it's like a small shock to her system. (I mean, imagine yourself, today, receiving sternly delivered negative feedback about something you did; it is the rare person who can hear that without feeling a tightening in the stomach or a flush in the cheeks—and we're adults, supposedly possessed of all our state-regulation neural software!)

A child's self-regulation capacities are in nascent form, wiring up to suit the experiences she is encountering; her natural response to these kinds of relational concussions, over years of repeated such incidents, is to erect protective inner barriers that become increasingly difficult for parents (or anyone) to broach. How many times have we heard the parental lament, "I just can't seem to get *through* to her!"? This is one key reason why. And if we lose the ability to get through to our children, we lose our special role as their most powerful booster rockets for becoming agents of positive change.

How to De-Peace Your Child: Spanking, Shaming and Isolating

Spanking – In our modern, supposedly civilized society, hitting as a means of teaching is still shockingly prevalent, despite numerous studies proving its destructiveness.[47] Any perceived effectiveness of swatting, slapping or spanking is nothing more than short-term compliance rooted in a child's fear of the parent. (This is a hallmark of the *authoritarian* style of parenting—in which children's unquestioning obedience is the goal—rather than *authoritative* parenting for peace—marked by the parents' decisive yet respectful leadership role and an ever deepening bond of loving trust between them and their children.) Rather than internalizing any moral message or noble value by being spanked, a child grows resentful and avoidant of the parent. This, together with the inner contortions of denial and dissociation from the distressing negative feelings that a child must perform, exact a steep, enduring toll on their wellbeing. Spanked toddlers are less likely to listen, are less compliant and have more poorly developed motor skills; spanked adolescents are more likely to suffer depression, alcohol addiction and suicidal thoughts. Children who are hit are more likely as adults to hit their partners and their own children—and so it goes, the transgenerational-go-round of violence, which ripples outward from family to community to society. In *Parenting for a Peaceful World*, Robin Grille writes:

> The school bully or juvenile delinquent is an emotionally injured individual trying to compensate for an inner feeling of powerlessness. The same is true for those who grow up to become autocrats, dictators and bullies in business....Bullies are not a fact of life but an artifact of history.[48]

Grille raises the compelling idea that there is likely a connection between the U.S.'s legal sanction of corporal punishment in schools in twenty-one states (*and corporal punishment at home in all fifty states*), and some of the harsher aspects of U.S. domestic and foreign policies and social issues: we have the highest documented rate of incarceration worldwide and the highest homicide rate among affluent democracies, and are the only western democracy to retain the death penalty (despite its researched ineffectiveness at deterring crime); we are one of only five countries (together with Iran, Nigeria, Pakistan and Saudi Arabia) to retain the death penalty for juveniles; one of just two (with Somalia) that has declined to sign the U.N. Convention on the Rights of the Child.[49] The list goes on, but you get the idea. The scourges of violent social, institutional and public policy are grown from tender shoots in the home.

Shaming – Punishment need not be physical to exact a toll on a child's developing personality and the lifelong neural templates for how he will relate to himself, others, and the world. And indeed, a far more common form of violence routinely used in disciplining children is *shaming*. Shaming is more subtle than hitting, but in many ways, more insidiously damaging because the child cannot consciously point to the hurtful moment of impact. Rather, shamed children sustain an incremental erosion of their competent, loving, "good enough" selves with each verbal rebuke. Shame researcher Brené Brown, in her 2010 TEDTalk, aptly defines shame simply as the fear of disconnection: "There's something about me that if other people know it or see it, I won't be worthy of connection."[50]

Such exclamations as "Bad boy!" or "You're very naughty!" are clear examples of shaming, in which the message is a diminishment or accusatory diagnosis of the child. One problem with shame is that it's not always so obvious—and thus so readily available for reconsideration by parents seeking a more constructive mode of parenting. Experts through the years have counseled parents to focus on expressing displeasure with the behavior and not the person doing the behavior, but this can easily lead to shaming as well, as in, "Your whining and crying is not okay."

(And focusing on behaviors—and on extinguishing those we don't want— is a short-sighted, limited approach, like focusing on symptoms and medicating them away: it doesn't address the underlying cause. In fact, one of the ways adults shame children is to quiz them, "Why did you hit your sister / put syrup on the dog / lie to Mommy?" A child usually does not consciously know why she did something "naughty," so this puts her on the spot and adds another layer of shame related to the unmet expectation that she should be able to answer you.)

Shame is like the stealth bomber of emotional zingers: it can slip into almost any verbal exchange. It all depends on what's going on in the mind and heart of the person uttering the words. For example, "That's so silly" can be delivered during a loving, playful exchange in a tone that cultivates warmth and connection, or it can be landed as a shame-based dismissal of a child's earnest feelings, thoughts or actions. And this lacing of garden-variety words with something as corrosive as shame is a process that is virtually unconscious. Few parents— or should I say, few parents who'd be inclined to read this book—open their mouths with the conscious intention, "I'm going to shame my child now."

And it's practically universal in our culture; the vast majority of us have been shamed as children by parents, siblings, teachers, peers. For us to become aware and sensitive to shame is like a fish becoming aware of water. But we may be aware of shame's fallout, either in ourselves or in those close to us. Its immediate effect is to "unravel connection," says Brown. Then over time, shame becomes a part of us. Those who have internalized shame tend to specialize in—and often fluctuate between—one of two polarized patterns of expression: emotional muteness, paralysis and dissociation from their own feelings and needs; or bouts of hostility and rage, which is either expressed outward toward others or internalized as depression, self-destructive behaviors and even suicide. Shame corrupts social intelligence by inhibiting the development of empathy and the ability to take responsibility for oneself, leading to a habit of blaming.[51] The effects of shame begin in the earliest moments of a child's life; a comprehensive August 2010 *New York Times* article on depression in preschoolers zeroed in on the shame that parents (unintentionally and unwittingly) inflicted on their young children as a causal factor.[52]

With respect to parenting for a more peaceful, constructively interdependent society, Robin Grille points out that "So many of our most problematic social behaviors are compulsive covers for inner feelings of shame. To conceal our shame, we sneer at others, we criticize, we moralize, we judge, we patronize and we condescend....Finally, the shamed tend to anticipate feeling humiliated and disapproved of by others, and this can lead to hostility, even fury. Quite often, shame makes us want to punish others. When angry, shame-prone individuals are more likely to be malevolent, indirectly aggressive or self-destructive—their anger finds no appropriate expression."[53]

Isolation – So here you are one afternoon, at the end of your rope with an out-of-control three-year-old. You know you won't spank her, and you have become mindful of avoiding shame-based measures, so what's left? Is time out the answer? At risk of incurring the frustrated wrath of parents everywhere, my answer is no. While time out was conceived as a more humane alternative to spanking, it lands a blow to the brain and psyche rather than to the bottom. Right at the moment when the child is overwhelmed by a flood of emotions that she cannot manage, and she most needs the regulating presence (that is, close *physical* presence) of her attachment figure, she's banished to her room or her "naughty chair" or her "thinking rug" or her [fill in the blank with any of a list of prettied-up names people have devised for this particular form of exile].

What a tantruming child (or, more helpful to think of her instead as a *struggling* child) most needs is time *in*—that is, *in* secure, soothing arms, *in* the steadying, regulating sphere of your engaged presence. Time out is developmentally and neurobiologically counterproductive: it deprives a child of regulation just when she needs it most, throws her system into protection mode, and erodes her trust in and relationship with her parent. After all the fussing is over and order is restored, the memory trace etched in her social brain is, *When I'm having trouble, I'm on my own.* This is not the foundation we're striving to offer Generation Peace. We wish for them the suite of healthy social and relational capacities of resilience, which includes being comfortable reaching out for help when needed. Let's not extinguish that skill with our well-meaning attempts at positive discipline!

The foregoing three forms of "discipline"—punishment is not true discipline, thus the quotation marks—short-circuit Nature's plan for the unfolding of peace-loving intelligence. And they don't happen only in my-way-or-the-high-way authoritarian homes. Because of the unconscious, reflexive nature of how parenting often goes—in which we either reprise with our own children the way we were raised, or, in an effort to never do to them what they did to us, seize on predominant cultural parenting modes—these corrosive approaches also feature in homes where well-meaning parents regard themselves as progressive and enlightened. Indeed, in the course of a single generation, Time-Out has become the gold standard in discipline for savvy parents. And thus the cycle of (usually unintentional, often subtle) parenting violence continues. As Robin Grille points out:

> Child rearing has historically been so violent…that almost all of us are either battered children or descendants of battered children. It is no wonder that violence persists in so many forms, across all age groups, and that most of us are capable of slipping and treating our children violently on occasions, even if we strive against it.[54]

Fostering Growth While Keeping Peaceful Boundaries

As a sound alternative to all three of the above measures, consider using a time-out in the way it was originally conceived in sports: for a team (not just one struggling player) needing to take a pause to regroup, rethink its strategy, and return refreshed. Used in this us-as-a-team manner—"Let *us* take a time out"—it is a demonstration that while you're not happy with the way things are going or the choices he has just made, you are on his side in this challenging moment—and always. You can find your own name and style for this regrouping process; in psychologist Lawrence Cohen's family it's A Meeting on the Couch:

> Discipline is a chance to improve your connection with your children instead of forming another wall that separates you. The best way to make discipline more connecting is to think *We* have a problem instead of *My kid* is misbehaving.
>
> Sometimes just changing the scene and making reconnection a top priority can create a dramatic difference, and the tension is gone as soon as you get to the couch, so you might end up just goofing around and being silly together.[55]

Indeed. In his wonderful book *Playful Parenting*, Cohen offers a roadmap for parents wanting to enrich their family life with more play—and that is a worthy goal for all of us. Parenting for peace is all about providing the most fertile ground possible for the blossoming of our children's social and cognitive intelligence, and among the animal kingdom—in which we are supposedly the crowning achievement—it is a fact that the more intelligent the animal, the more it continues to play throughout adulthood. There are rich layers of meaning to even the most casual play, Cohen points out, and not only is it the primary way children sift through, practice and integrate the massive amounts of new incoming data they encounter in the course of a day of life, it is also their way of processing hurts and frustrations. "Play is where children show us the inner feelings and experiences that they can't or won't talk about."

But somewhere along the way to adulthood the vast majority of us forgot how to play. Life became serious business—and parenting along with it. And especially for those of us who had less security in our childhood, who may have never really felt safe to enter that imaginary frolic zone,[56] when invited by our children to play, we're like deer in the headlights. For some, every detail of parenting is a grave matter; the stakes feel intangibly yet dangerously high (*It's got to go right this time*). Our own uneasiness seeds uneasiness in our children and this itself can evoke challenging behavior. The sad irony in this negative feedback loop is that these are the parents whose buttons are particularly sensitive, their own childhood "stuff" so ready, like a dry tinder box, to be set off by the sparks of a child's unwanted behaviors. The beauty of Cohen's approach is that it offers a playful way out of that contracting spiral that is helpful and healing to everyone: "As long as we are grown up enough to handle things like keeping them safe and getting dinner on the table, our children want and need us to loosen up."[57]

If I'd had the gift of this perspective back there in that painful moment with my son, I might have used one of Cohen's many playful ideas to free us both out of that tight spot—such as *pretending* to be angry. "Okay, so let's play the game of 'Mommy pretends to be really angry at Ian': (making an exaggerate lion face) I'm *soooooooooo* angry at Ian…I may have to steal his shoe!" At which point Ian would have felt drawn in by my silliness, rather than pushed away by my own lack of inner regulation, and of course, by my physically violent act. The fact is, parenting can actually be a whole lot more fun and lighthearted than we typically realize, once we get over our culturally imprinted worry that if we use humor to diffuse and redirect a disciplinary jam, we're somehow failing our parental role by not taking it seriously enough… or rewarding or reinforcing "misbehavior" by not bringing the hammer down…or slipping down that slippery slope of being their friend rather than their parent. The fact is, the more confident, credible and authoritative a leader truly is, the lighter the touch he or she needs to use to be effective and admired.

"Misbehavior" is a trap of a concept in the first place—a term only appropriate for situations in which someone truly understands the alternatives and consciously chooses to engage in bad behavior. But for the young child, this is simply not the case. The young child is a scientist figuring out the world, gathering data and conducting experiments. Her behaviors that don't please us are more helpfully considered as "mistakes" rather than misbehavior. Do we punish people for mistakes? Not if we want improvement, excellence and growth!

And even the most suspiciously flagrant "mistake" of a child reflects an *unmet need*. Figuring out what that need is, rather than focusing on the inexperienced way the child expressed the need, or ineffective strategy he used to meet his need, is central to parenting success and peace in the home. Lawrence Cohen boils these needs into two basic categories—the need for connection, or the need to feel effective and successful—and gives myriad examples of how play can a) help us figure out a child's underlying needs; and b) unfold solutions to meeting the child's needs. And most importantly, play provides a bridge through which parent and child can reconnect after any of the many disconnections we experience in the course of the day. And as we've seen, connection is the heart of parenting for peace.

So for example, "stealing" a piece of your jewelry or some other precious item—yes, even your money—can be a child's way to get close to you, to keep you with her. Hitting or teasing another child is also sometimes a young, inexperienced human's misguided strategy to connect. And yet that same behavior—hitting, or even biting—will be used by another child (or the same child in a different circumstance) as an attempted strategy for meeting an entirely different need, such as the need to feel less fearful, embarrassed, isolated, or envious.

Waldorf kindergarten teacher Barbara Patterson[58] shares some wonderfully unexpected, lovely and effective healing approaches to such things as hitting and biting—which can evoke strong feelings, and sometimes, reactive, unmindful reactions in parents. Having some creative responses at the ready can help us maintain the calm, loving authority children so need from us.

Healing actions for unacceptable behavior:

- *Hitting*: Wrap the child's hands in a comforting scarf and sit next to him: "When your hands are warm and strong, they don't hit." (Same for kicking.)
- *Biting*: Give the child a large piece of apple or carrot, and have her sit next to you to eat it: "We bite the carrot, not our friends."
- *Violent play*: Real work is the cure for violent play: digging holes or moving stones in the garden, carrying wood, stacking bricks.
- *Defiance*: Between ages two and four, children can be very stubborn, and it's best to simply overlook some of their negative reactions (remember, they're always imitating!). Just go with the child and begin doing with him what you want him to do, without anger or lots of explaining. Don't waiver or allow him to wriggle out of it. For example, rather than butting heads about him picking up his toys, just begin rhythmically picking up a toy or two and putting them into the bin. Like with a yawn, he will hardly be able to keep himself from joining in. Then you can thank him for doing it!
- *Tattling and other upsets with socializing*: Chronic problems in this area suggest difficulties or weakness in the child's developing social brain or will energies. Involve her in your work to let her feel the adult's creative strength focused upon a particular activity. Washing dishes is a wonderful healing action here, as is baking. Sometimes merely listening to children's upset or tears will ease up the problem enough so that they can respond to a suggestion as simple as, "Just go start over."

These all feature an important theme in constructive discipline: it is always more effective to focus on what the child *may* do, rather than issuing a "You may *not*…" prohibition. This approach also reduces the risk of putting the child into a disconnected neurobiological protection state. And in fact, Patterson suggests that the very word *may* can have seemingly magical properties, as in, "You may put the forks on the table now": it presents no question for the child to either answer or ignore, and it implies the notion of *privilege* to be doing what the adult is suggesting. And indeed, a child enjoying a secure, connected relationship with her parents *does* find it a privilege and a joy to behave in harmony with their wishes. In this way, robust attachment is like the power steering of parenting!

In his compelling book on key dynamics in attachment, *Hold On To Your Child*, Gordon Neufeld cautions that this "power assisted" aspect of the parent-child relationship requires "careful nurturance and trust":

It is a violation of the relationship not to believe in the child's desire [to behave well] when it actually exists, for example to accuse the child of harboring ill intentions when we disapprove of her behavior. Such accusations can easily trigger defenses in the child, harm the relationship, and make her feel like being bad....It's a vicious circle. External motivators for behavior such as reward and punishments may destroy the precious internal motivation to be good, making leverage by such artificial means necessary by default. As an investment in easy parenting, trusting in a child's desire to be good for us is one of the best.[59]

Keeping this sacred trust in mind, along with the foregoing principles regarding the importance of your example, of relationship and play, of clear messages and limited choices, and of healthy rhythms, remember that the single most pivotal ingredient in harmonious, joyful parenting is *you*—your confidence, conviction, and trust in yourself and in your child.

What's All This Hoopla About Praise?

While on the subject of trust between you and your child, let us tackle the topic of praise. Somewhere along the way it became generally assumed that praise builds self-esteem, leading to the daily parental litany of "Nice job!" and "Great throw!" and "Gorgeous painting!" and on and on, ad nauseum. When our second child was a toddler, our R.I.E. teacher gently suggested that we parents reconsider our attitudes toward praise. She presented the counterintuitive (and definitely countercultural) notion that praise—especially the kind that is routinely doled out to kids as standard practice these days—can insidiously erode a child's intrinsic motivation, pleasure, and self-satisfaction in a given task or activity.

Indeed, praise deflects a child's focus away from her inner will to create, play and do, outward to our response to *what* she creates, plays and does. In his book *Punished by Rewards* Alfie Kohn points out that praise "sustains a dependence on our evaluations, our decisions about what is good and bad, rather than helping them begin to form their own judgments. It leads them to measure their worth in terms of what will lead us to smile and offer the positive words they crave."[60] Their natural intrinsic motivation, delight, and sense of just-rightness wear away, and they become dependent on the illusory glow of pseudo-self-esteem coming from outside in. One of the most helpful things I ever heard Dr. Laura say on her radio show was that self-esteem is about whether you impress *yourself* through how you act. Or as the saying goes, "Self-esteem is an inside job."

We now have a generation of young adults whose addiction to the constant flow of external rewards and positive feedback has become an issue for employers. There are even companies who specialize in providing flashy workplace demonstrations of praise and acknowledgement for employees whose motivation and morale flags without such external bolstering. This is not a dependence that we want for Generation Peace; rather, we want them to feel an abiding sense of rightness, worthiness and "enoughness" from deep within.

One morning Sarah's three-year-old daughter Emma called to her—"Come look, Mama!" When Sarah rounded the corner to the family room, there was Emma's new puzzle, all put together. Rather than the standard, "Great job!" or "I'm so proud of you!" Sarah said, "Emma, you finished that puzzle all by yourself!" She simply reflected what was true, with no judgment attached. Her gratifying reward was Emma's own assessment: "I *smart!*" Self-esteem doesn't come any more vivid than that, or any more authentic. It was Emma's, given by herself to herself, via an appraisal she made of her own accomplishment. She truly owned the doing of that puzzle, and the pride that came with it.

As Kohn points out, "...*the most notable aspect of a positive judgment is not that it is positive but that it is a judgment. Just as every carrot contains a stick, so every verbal reward contains within it the seed of a verbal punishment...*"[61] Praise is just one side of a two-sided coin, whose other face is criticism. Sometimes well-meaning parents sidestep the double-edged nature of praise by sticking to words of reflection, encouragement, and acknowledgment—"I notice you set the table by yourself," "You've climbed up really high on the jungle gym," and the like. But author Naomi Aldort points out the pitfalls here as well, especially when our goal is to raise self-directed, secure individuals with whom we share a strong bond of trust: "Sensitive and smart, [our children] perceive that we have an agenda, that we are manipulating them toward some preferred or 'improved' end result....Gradually, a shift occurs....No longer do they trust in their actions, and no longer do they trust us, for we are not really on their side."[62]

Regarding a parent's offering encouragement or demonstrating loving support by commenting on what a child is doing, Aldort says, "Even when we intervene with casual commentary on our children's imaginative play, doubts sneak in. What children are experiencing inwardly at these times is often so remote from our 'educated' guesses that bewilderment soon turns to self-denial and self-doubt." As I reflected on what seemed like a radical notion of Aldort's back when my own children were small, and continued to observe interactions between other parents and their children, I came to wonder why we feel this need, this near-compulsion, to constantly comment. *Why do we have to say anything at all?* Aldort thoughtfully suggests that one cause of our verbal meddling involves our own histories: what we don't trust in ourselves, what we weren't *supported* in trusting in ourselves, as children—our natural impulse toward self-directed, un*adult*erated learning explorations—we have a hard time supporting in our own children.

Another factor in our commentary compulsion is that nowhere in our society is something allowed to simply *be*, without blurbs, hype, or headlines—and never has this been truer than in today's iTwitterFaceLinkedInPod culture. Along with sheltering our young children from screened media itself, we do them an important service and honor to spare them the self-referencing, aggrandizing, "look at me" sensibilities that saturate these technologies, and our very society. Parents may worry that their children will be left behind if not allowed to participate in this high-tech web of supposed connectivity, but a decade of Waldorf school graduates (in which computers are excused from the curricula in both lower and middle school) suggests that this concern is unfounded: teens quickly pick up computer technoskills as if born to it. Indeed, the current generation takes to these technologies with a natural ease and affinity; let us give them the gift of unfolding their own imaginative and will capacities before letting them loose into the realm of the digital, which when introduced too early curtails that development. (It bears noting that the chief technology officer of e-Bay, as well as employees of tech giants Google, Apple, Yahoo and Hewlett-Packard send their children to a Waldorf school.)[63]

The Cost of a "Head Start"

Our current culture's lifestyle tends to undermine a child's will energies, draining rather than building them up. We ask them to think, reason and "get smart" at ever younger ages, much to the detriment of their healthy development. The child's life forces (remember—like the life forces at work in a plant to unfold the blossom) are needed for the complex activity of building up the physical body until around age seven. (A milestone event signaling the completion of this phase is the emergence of the first permanent teeth.) When we engage the young child in academics and other intellectual pursuits—in which the jobs of memory and structured thinking consume tremendous amounts of physiological energy—the life forces are diverted from their main tasks, and the healthy development of the body and brain can be compromised in life-long ways.[64] We can use the metaphor of electric power to understand the importance of protecting and nurturing the young child's will energies: our children are born with a vast supply of latent wattage—all their intelligence, their passions, personality, *everything*—but without a grid or infrastructure through which this power can be effectively utilized. Supporting their life forces (the development of their etheric body) during early childhood is how we foster this infrastructure, so that when the latent power begins to course—during the seven-to-fourteen stage—there is a strong, flexible and integral deployment system for it.

Academics and other pseudo-mature pursuits—including organized, competitive sports—may indeed produce a child who is very bright and capable, and who may very well enjoy the work, but who later—by middle- or high-school age—can burn out, become depressed, cynical, or disengaged, because there is little inner foundation to support this intellect. It's like having tons of wattage without a strong grid to deploy it—dangerous. Supporting the healthy development of a child's will during early childhood is an investment in her future; it builds a sound infrastructure that will contain and conduct her future interests, passions, and intellectual pursuits.

Our current ignorance of this developmental need is surely a significant contributing factor to the multiple crises facing our children. Developmental and learning disorders, along with behavioral problems, are epidemic. Depressive disorders are appearing earlier in life than in past decades; indeed, The National Institute of Mental Health has over the last generation documented substantial increases in the use of myriad psychotropic medications, including antidepressants, in *preschool-aged children!*[65]

Many of our middle- and high-school children have become jaded; they do not seem to find in school, in learning, or in life, anything about which to be excited, enthused, or inspired. Their will forces, whose development ideally should have been supported in early childhood, instead often languish, latent yet unrealized, sapped by the adultifying activities with which parents packed their young lives. Without these will forces, which are transformed in later childhood and young adulthood into *interest in the world,* our youth fall prey to cynicism, ennui, and yes—ironically—*boredom.* Along with the Generation Peace qualities I mention often, there is one hugely important quality I haven't yet mentioned: *curiosity*. A person can have the kindest heart, but if she has no interest in the world around her, she isn't going to be a vital agent of innovative change, is she? All parents hope that their children will be interesting people as they grow up, but of much more importance is that members of a peacemaker generation be *interested* people. When young children have the opportunity for a kind of constructive boredom—i.e., calm, predictable, home-based rhythms—then as teenagers they can scarcely understand the notion of boredom, for their interest in the world is so robust!

Family physician Philip Incao suggests that the ever growing numbers of youth suffering from "Is that all there is?" ennui, myriad psychosocial and learning disorders, stress, anxiety, depression and even suicidal thoughts,[66] are telling us that they aren't finding what they need when they come into this world and into their families. Warns Incao, "They are the canaries in the coal mine."

Protecting the Bud, Envisioning the Blossom

Your child is not a blank slate or empty vessel who needs to be filled up with copious amounts of excellent information. Your child comes to you with a nascent intellect that is consolidating energy and waiting to unfold in good time, like a flower in the bud. You would never pry open a rosebud to somehow optimize or improve upon it! Instead, you would make sure it has the best soil and nourishing fertilizer to support its optimal unfolding.

So it is with our children. But *we* are the soil in which our children grow. For those precious and critical early years, we are their earth, their sun and their water. If we are willing to embrace that daunting and magnificent responsibility, then the potential for their lifelong wellbeing is virtually unlimited, as are the prospects for their unfolding as socially adept agents of peace, innovation and planetary evolution.

PRINCIPLES TO PRACTICE

Presence – Our children's healthy development calls on us to pursue our own development, and presence practice is one of the richest, most versatile ways to do this. In any moment we can align and attune ourselves more deeply to what we're engaged in: gestures can become prayers, thoughts can become meditations, comments can become blessings. It may come naturally to you, or it may feel foreign and awkward, no matter: striving toward the gathered moment is the heart of presence practice—to become more present to yourself, to Life—to the onion, the computer, the bathtub, the car—and to your child.

- Throughout these steps I have encouraged you to engage in some kind of meditative or contemplative practice, including mindfulness, which can be seen as bringing presence to the daily movements of life. This helps you to answer this important question in the affirmative: *Do I, as the parent, have mastery over something as fundamental as the movement of my own thoughts?* Your level of parental self-possession is perceived by your child, and when the answer is Yes, this in turn fosters a respect for you that is deep and implicit, and which rarely wavers.

- One presence practice that can be very helpful is a daily review just as you're about to go to sleep. Simply play in your mind the day's events—the good, the bad and the ugly. The critically important aspect to this exercise is that you do so *without any judgment*: make this as objective a viewing as possible, like a movie of someone else's life. If you insist on having any feelings about it, let them simply be gratitude for most of the scenes, and for those that didn't go as well as you'd wish, simple compassion—as you would feel when watching a stranger who is struggling. This is one of those mysterious, seemingly simple practices that when done regularly can bring more ease to life and effect astonishing transformations within. The next morning some events might stand out in your mind, calling for action; notice how you benefit from the clarity this practice can bring—how you are enabled from within to address tough situations.

- At this step when discipline issues first arise in earnest, it's good to remember what I pointed out in Step One: whatever you put your attention on, you get more of. When we're upset, we're choosing to be present to that which we *don't* want. When we get annoyed or angry with our children the same thing happens—we're being present to everything we don't want, rather than standing in that loving, authoritative center and focusing on what we *do* want (and calmly expect) from our child. Becky Bailey writes in *Easy to Love, Hard to Discipline*, "Learning to focus your attention on the outcomes that you desire will bring you enormous power. It is probably the most important technique you can learn for living peacefully with children (and with other adults), and for finding joy in life."[67]

- Related to this is the understanding that our unconscious doesn't process *negation*; it doesn't really hear the "don't" when you admonish, "Don't put your muddy shoes on the kitchen table." (So he'll also hear just "… touch the priceless crystal lamp!" or "…cross the street alone.") A good rule of thumb, then, is to try and say what she *may* do rather than what she shouldn't do: "Sweetheart, put your muddy shoes on the mat by the door."

• One of the best times to share moments of connected presence with your children is just before they go to sleep. The bedtime story—and quiet conversation before or afterward—is perhaps the most important time to shelter and cherish with your children, right up into their adolescent years. It is when they are often at their softest and most tender—when their hearts are open and they are most apt to share what is living inside them. For many parents, this is precious time in which they nightly continue to learn and be present to the truest essence of their child.

• Parent-child conflict often arises when the parent's reality collides with (and usually overrules) the child's reality. Kim John Payne offers a way of weaving the two realities into a harmonious shared presence that helps immensely with the practical kinds of struggles we can have with young children on a daily basis—especially volatile times such as the dinnertime example he gives. The classic evening scene plays out like this in untold millions of homes, in which the child is deeply engrossed in playing, then Mom calls to him, "Ten minutes till dinner!"…then "Five minutes till dinner!"…and so on until the countdown is over and she says, mildly (or more than mildly) annoyed, "Spencer, dinner's ready now, hurry up and go wash your hands," but he does not change gears whatsoever, is still deeply engaged in building his Lego castle, and a struggle ensues. Payne calls his alternative approach "My World, Your World, Our World,"[68] and it can work magic at these kinds of touchy transition times, in which agendas tend to collide and struggles arise: "Mom goes to the child who is engrossed in playing, sits next to him for just a few moments, just simply present. The child turns his attention to her—he cannot help but do so, he's wired for it!—and that's when she says 'Dinner's going to be ready in a few minutes—I'd better go back and grate the cheese just like you like it.' They each return to their worlds, and then she comes back another time or two in this way, so that there is an *intersection* of her world and his world. They don't collide, but become 'our world.'" And things happen with much more ease and harmony in "our world"! (There are, of course, as many variations on this as there are parents, children, and imaginations; I seem to remember when Ian was deeply engrossed in his trains I might show up and say that the train's engineer has requested that he come have dinner in the dining car of another train—"over here, toward the dining room table!")

- Bath time is one of those daily events that can take on the character of a tedious chore, or the opportunity for a smorgasbord of playful, intimate time to be present with your child. The deciding factor is simply your own consciousness. There is something freeing about the very element of the water you're sharing as you bathe your child—let your imagination fly with every wish you have for her, giving thanks for the health and beauty of her physical being. It's a wonderful time, as you're soaping and rinsing, to demonstrate reverent, joyful celebration of her body and your blessings on what she might do with it: "May your strong legs walk you across this marvelous planet"… "May your creative hands shape beautiful ways of joy"…"May this beautiful face bring smiles to many others…" And when shampooing it is helpful to engage a most elaborate imaginary scene on the ceiling for her to gaze at while you rinse: the gazillion stars in the night sky, or the colorful fish in the ocean's underwater universe…? We can also greet and bless the water itself—the true elixir of life. Barely of speaking age, one little girl clearly had developed an appreciative rapport with the living water, when as it drained away at the end of her bath, she exclaimed "Bye bye, water!" Yes, the bath's warm, watery atmosphere invites delicious whimsy—particularly helpful for the parent who may not be naturally whimsical. Let your child draw you into her world of wonder as you share this time together.
  - The warmth and wetness of bath time suggests a return to the womb, and it is indeed between about the ages of 2½ and 3½ when children have been known to relate prebirth or birth memories. At this age you might occasionally ask, "Do you remember the time before you were born?" or "What was it like for you when you were in Mommy's tummy?" You might get a delightful surprise one evening!

Awareness – One helpful aspect of awareness for this step is to understand a few key developmental turning points during this stage of your child's life. It can help enliven your job as a parent to watch for and delight in these milestones.

- Last step I described the baby's gradually developing cognitive awareness of *object permanence*; somewhere between eighteen and twenty-four months this complex shift completes, freeing the child from the limitations of the concrete information brought in by his senses. This is epic: he can now construct a mental representation of the world and locate objects after a series of visible displacements that include hidden conceptual transitions (e.g., the potato moved from the box under the cloth.) He can *imagine* where an item might be even when he cannot see, hear, or touch it.

- The second of Erik Erikson's psychosocial stages begins around eighteen months and lasts through roughly age three, as the child gains more control over her body and its movements. (This is the time of toilet training as well as myriad experiments by this wee scientist in her exciting environment.) Erikson suggested that this is the stage at which the child internalizes a fundamental sense of either *autonomy* or *shame and doubt*. The child begins to experience a sense of independence, and this impulse may first emerge as her demand, "Me do it myself." It helps parents to know that even though it may not seem like it, the child is also beginning to develop some self-control in her environment (including the basic self-control involved in toileting). Her budding autonomy can be supported with loving, authoritative boundaries and the opportunity to make mistakes without retribution. The life virtues gained through the positive resolution of this psychosocial crisis are *self-control*, *courage*, and *will*.

- Following his cognitive achievement of object permanence, the child embarks on what will be several years (from about two to about seven years of age) of what Piaget called the *preoperational stage*, in which not only can he hold a mental representation of objects, but now he can mentally manipulate them (as opposed to last stage's limitation to physical manipulation of objects). He can now perform such mental actions as imagination and symbolic encoding (which Gen Peace parents will do well *not* to exploit to introduce early academics). These are all the wellspring of his important endeavor of playing.

- From infancy through the child's third year she experiences a gradually dawning awareness of her own individuality separate from her mother and the rest of the world—first as a basic bodily reality and over time as a deeper existen-

---

* Each of the three seven-year phases of a child's life is marked by a significant developmental milestone in his or her awakening, maturing sense of self relative to the world, occurring roughly two years into the cycle—at age two, age nine and age sixteen.

tial reality. This process has some pivotal moments, such as when she turns two.* This time has earned the unfortunate nickname of the terrible twos because it can come as an unsettling surprise to parents when their "easy" child suddenly begins practicing her individuality by saying "No" in countless creative ways. It helps to have a big-picture sense of what's going on in order to maintain your equanimity and not get flummoxed by your child's sudden obstinacy. Watch for the fascinating self-referencing transition taking place in the language of the two-to-three year old, when "Baby do it" evolves into "Janie do it," and then, one magical day, "*I* do it." It is in the sacred ground of this new name "I" to which she has now awakened that the seeds for her future sense of self are planted and will flourish.

- The third stage of Erikson's psychosocial development runs from about ages three to five, during which the child internalizes a sense of either *initiative* or *guilt,* as he sees and imitates the adults in his world and takes the initiative to imagine, elaborate, and direct new scenarios through play. In this way he experiments with prototypical grownup experiences and asserts his budding power over his world. If he is supported with both encouragement and boundaries, he develops a sense of being capable of leading himself and others, and gains the life virtue of *purpose.* Guilt can come over the child by virtue of the huge, earth-shattering things she contemplates (and sometimes does) in the sheer exuberant enjoyment of her new motor and mental powers. His conflict is between "What I *can* do, and what I'm growing increasingly aware of what I may and may not do..." as he is slowly beginning to internalize a self-regulating "parent" part of himself. If his efforts at initiative are dismissed, shamed or thwarted, he can internalize lifelong guilt, self-doubt and a lack of initiative. Parents can foster initiative through offering the child the chance to find pleasurable accomplishment in wielding tools, cooking utensils, meaningful toys and objects—and even in caring for younger children.

- No matter how much awareness and presence practice you have engaged in, preparing for being with a young child, now you really *are* with a young child, and that can push lots of buttons! Continue to foster compassionate awareness of your own history of being parented, and let that awareness breathe space into the interactions you have with your own child—the space needed for peaceful intention to take root and flourish.

- Within the kind of Gen Peace disciplinary framework outlined in this book, whose intention is to foster a growth-over-protection posture in the child—and thus does not feature fear-based training of what to do and not do—it's important to realize that it's only around the fifth year that a truly organic, internalized sense of right and wrong awakens in the child. Until then, patient parents with their eyes on the big peace picture will realize that discipline necessarily involves loving repetition of right action—again and again, over and over, day in and day out—for the child to imitate.

- The fourth stage of Erikson's psychosocial development begins during this step—around age five—and resolves around age eleven: *industry v. inferiority*. During this stage the child's psychosocial milieu widens considerably to include peers and teachers, who join parents in influencing this outcome. It is a time of learning many new things, accomplishing new tasks, and cooperation with others, all of which can contribute to the child's deeply felt sense of industry. It marks the origin of the work ethic, wherein the child incorporates a sense of what society values. She is ready to learn avidly, and to become bigger in the sense of sharing obligation and performance during this period of development. He is eager to make things cooperatively, to combine with other children for the purpose of constructing and planning, and is open to guidance from teachers and to emulate ideal prototypes. Positive regard and encouragement by peers foster industry (and by contrast, the lack of it can seed a lasting sense of inferiority); parents, teachers, and other adults who offer worthwhile tasks and meaningful challenges will also help foster a sense of industry—and the life virtues of *competence* and *method*. It's important to note, in this era of early academics, that the assignment of tasks that are beyond the child's ability will tend to produce a sense of failure and inferiority.

Rhythm – This is a parent's best friend. Rhythm is one of the greatest needs of the young child, but also a fundamental human principle, often forgotten in our supercharged, 24/7 world. (FYI, the first thing Super Nanny does is put every family on a schedule, and just that improves the situation tremendously!) Young children thrive on and crave rhythmicity to their days, their weeks, even the seasons: "This is when we eat, this is when we nap, this is when we have play time. Tuesdays we go to the park, Wednesdays we go to the Farmer's Market, Sunday we visit Grandma, and summer is beach time!" Seems monotonous to us as adults, because we're essentially different creatures inside our skulls. The limbic or "feeling brain" structures developing in these early years are critical to the formation of all later brain-based capacities. Rhythm's external consistency and predictability allow the growing child to gradually internalize regulation and stability, which we now know are *the* foundation for all human success, including intelligence, relationships, and joy.

- The three-year-old son of one of my clients recently said, "The leaves are turning red—my birthday is coming!" Ecologist Sandra Steingraber writes, "When one is not yet old enough to read the calendar or the clock's face, when the difference between 'next month' and 'tomorrow' still seems a little fuzzy, it is comforting to know that the year's longest day comes when the strawberries appear, that one's birthday falls during apple-picking time, that the geese fly away when the pumpkins are ripe..."[69] Even when one *is* old enough, these knowings bring a deep level of connectedness, which itself is a warp thread of peace and joy. Pulsing through all of these natural rhythms is *etheric* energy—the life-giving force that animates all elements of the natural world. Only minerals have solely a physical body; everything else, including plants, and of course, animals, has an etheric body. It is the etheric body of your child that is still in gestation during this seven-year period, and rhythm is a primary form of nourishment. As Thomas Poplawski notes about the etheric, "Its rhythms are like those of the moon and the tides and, if supported by external rhythms, will hum along quietly and smoothly."[70]
- The two most fundamental rhythmic aspects for your child's daily life are mealtimes and bedtime; they should fall at the same times each day as consistently and smoothly as possible. The child's dinner should be early—5:30 or 6:00—to allow for an appropriately early bedtime. This may mean that the adults in the household have dinner together later...or Mom eats with the child earlier and has a wee snack as her partner dines later...or any of numerous other arrangements that respect the child's rhythmicity needs.
- The two key aspects of bedtime are: 1) it should be early—during the seven o'clock hour so that she is asleep by eight at the latest—because it is healthiest for her and also it allows you and your partner time every evening that is yours alone, which brings joy into the family; and 2) it should be organized around the understanding that the child's last impressions are taken into the night life of her psyche, and will have implications for her growth. (Children do their growing at nighttime, like plants!) This should guide your choices for the entire bedtime ritual—the stories, the singing, the coziness—so that it ushers them with delight, peace, and tranquility into their mysterious night of dreaming and dancing with the angels.
- Consider your child's naptime sacrosanct, as it really is an elixir for him. I recall how my friends mercilessly teased me about my obsessive "rigidity" in

holding to Ian's nap schedule ("No, I can't do a park date at noon"); not too many years later those same friends were commiserating about their kids' regulation and sleep issues, saying how wise I'd been to establish and so fiercely preserve his sleep rhythms. Sleep is the royal cradle of growth; protect it and Life will thank you.

- Perhaps the most precious gift you can give yourself and your children throughout these early years is *time*: one of the handiest, all-purpose tips that makes virtually everything easier is *Slowwww dowwwwnnnn*. Remember the langorous pace of "milk time" after your baby was born? Well, here's the thing about the "new normal" that follows: a child's pace is naturally poky. Kim John Payne points out, "We're confronted with the often simple requests of these small beings (whom we love immeasurably), and yet their pleas seem to be coming form a galaxy far away, from the planet 'slow.'"[71] Attuning when possible to your child's unhurried rhythms makes everyone's life sweeter. As I like to say—and this pretty much applies to all aspects of life—"slow down, pleasure up." Allow twice as long as you think it should take to do anything— a trip to the grocery store, a visit to the playground at the park, a stop at the library. Put this formula on your fridge: *Perceived Time Requirement x 2 = Sanity, Joy & Peace!*

- Support the internal rhythms of your child's self-regulatory system, which needs to be worked and practiced to fully develop. This calls for some interludes of *(gasp!)* boredom, which are essential for the fully articulated wiring of the brain circuitry that mediates her own inner capacities to manage and balance her emotional states—stress, boredom, pleasure, and a basic sense of being connected to Life. This serves as a significant protective factor against high-risk behaviors not too many years from now, which are ways of attempting to manage such emotions from the outside in. Regular intervals of not much to do are also a boon for her flourishing imagination.

- By contrast, one enlivening activity that's wonderful to include in your rhythm is a weekly gathering at the home of one of the mom friends you've met by now—at the park, or a La Leche League meeting, or way back at your prenatal yoga class. As you rotate homes each week you all mutually enrich your child's and your own experience through, say, the mom who is a wonderful baker...and this other mom who is a master at sculpting beeswax... and this one who knits.

- Take a cue from Waldorf kindergartens, where each day goes with the cooking of a particular dish. (I still vividly remember the teacher reassuring the other children as my daughter and her friend were picked up as usual before lunch on Wednesday, "Yes, Eve and Julia leave early on soup day." This *is* how children mark time!) You need not be rigid about it, and you can even consider it liberating: you don't have to wonder what side dish you'll serve! ("We have pasta on this day, sweet potatoes on that day.") It may seem boring, but trust that there is still the five-year-old inside you that will take comfort in it. You can elaborate this to include such child-friendly activities as sweeping floors, folding laundry, and weeding in the garden. ("Monday is broom day"... "Thursday is dirt day..." and so on.)

- The kitchen is especially fertile ground for peaceable episodes with our young children, as it features such basic, hands-on activities that result in near-magic alchemy. Having a day when you cook—bread, cookies, soup—maybe not once a week (daunting for many of us!), but on a regular basis, maybe every other week, is like a bank deposit for your child's will energies. There is rhythmicity to so much of the process—chopping, stirring, kneading—and we can enhance it with singing or chanting ("This is the way we bake our bread, bake our bread, bake our bread..."). Follow your child's affinities, for he will lead you to his favorites. There was a leek tart that became one of ours. And remember that it is the process and not the product that is the whole point! The conversations that will unfold are like no others, such as when one of my clients added a bit of cognac to a chocolate cake she was making, and her son licked the mixing spoon, winced, and asked, "Mommy, are you sure this is for *humans?*"

- Any rhythm designed to support the etheric energies needs to include regular time outside in nature, particularly when they are very little, either walking alongside you or in a stroller. Walking in the rain is especially recommended (followed by drying off and warming up afterward)! Bare feet on the earth is rich; one particularly wise teacher told me that he makes it a point daily to walk across the grass and soil in his front yard for the morning paper in his bare feet, summer or winter, says it grounds him. (Granted, he lives in California!) Having a child by your side—looking out through her eyes of wonder—gives you permission to be especially exuberant in expressing delight in a world in which everything is magically alive. "Hello, leaves... hello, pebbles...hello, wind!" A central tenet of esoteric psychology is that once you acknowledge the life in everything, it awakens life (etheric energy) in you. Perhaps this is one reason behind the success of mindfulness for treating depression.[72]

- Back in Step Two I mentioned the concept of a nature table. Children delight in this tangible portrait of life's rhythms. During each season Nature offers treasures for her to discover while on your outdoor adventures. In spring you can find interesting seed pods…in summer wild grasses and flowers…and in autumn you can gather beautiful leaves—some for the table and perhaps some to glue into a journal, each leaf facing a page with a little description of where it was picked up, what was going on that day, etc. As children grow they can get quite elaborate in their depiction of the seasons on the nature table, complete with mirrors for frozen ponds in winter!

- Seasonal rhythm can also be nurtured through certain fairy tales. The symbols, numerical themes, and repetitive rhythms of classic fairy tales hold deep meaning for children. (A more thorough discussion of fairy tales—most appropriate for the school-aged child—follows in the next step.) Here are four season-specific tales that are wonderful for the younger child, four and up. During the fall months: *The Three Little Pigs*; during wintertime: *Mother Holle, The Shoemaker's Elves*; at the New Year: *Jack and the Beanstalk*; in the springtime: *Briar Rose*.

Example – Rudolf Steiner said that the young child is really an eye, taking in everything, registering everything, *without analysis*. They don't so much hear our words, but pick up everything else. And they imitate everything. So recall the master question: "Am I worthy of my child's unquestioning imitation?"

- One great Waldorf kindergarten teacher, Patty McNulty, taught me an important aspect of this principle for this age: mothers, find the queen in you, and fathers, the king. Seek out and cultivate your inner nobility, benevolence, and knowing authority. This can be a tall order if you grew up with words that undermined your sense of deserving respect. I have often engaged my counseling clients in guided imageries with surprising success in addressing this very important aspect of inner development: they call to mind a familiar discipline scene with their child and then vividly see and feel the experience of responding in this unfamiliar, "beneficent parent" mode to their child. A child needs to sense a dignity about her parents, and their attitude toward parenting (and thus, to her). Sometimes parental insecurities are expressed as silly humor that undermines this dignity. One father used to deliver his son to the kindergarten classroom by lifting him off his head and announcing in a goofy voice, "Here's my trained monkey!" Such a scenario doesn't fit this elevated atmosphere I'm speaking of. Of course you can—and should—be playful on a regular basis, but let it be from a place of deeply sensing and owning your own dignity and that of your child.

- Find what it is that you deeply know—that you know best—and bring that to your child. Let them see you deeply engaged in it, let them feel your passion for it. In age appropriate ways, involve them in it. It could be engine repair or the cultivation of orchids—whatever for you is a source of confidence, of 1,000 percent inner knowingness, which is a powerful form of peace to model. Best not to *talk* all about it—just do it, revel in how it feeds you, and allow your child to absorb everything in that deep rapport.

- Perhaps the truest, most potent teaching example for the child is for her parents to live a profound inner life, without putting it on obvious display (as in Jesus instructing us to "pray in a closet"). Rudolf Steiner said that the child learns most from who we are *when no one is looking*. I was always touched by the remarkable dedication and commitment Ms. McNulty devoted to her calling of working so intensely with young children. She didn't watch television, she took care to not even listen to much (if any) news of world events, even current events that seemed to be on everyone's minds and lips. When I asked her about this, she said, "The children feed on our consciousness." I found that profound, and so sensible. Young children do live mostly outside the realm of words—they pick up and sense what is far beyond the things we yammer at them. They pick up on the truth that lies beneath, behind and before our words. So yes, children feed on our consciousness, and once we can swallow that daunting reality, let us choose: *What do we want to be feeding them?*

- If we complain about chores—even just in the way we make the gesture of doing the chore—it will be emulated (perhaps not right away, but years from now). So, for example, take care that the books you read to your little one also interest you; if you are forcing yourself to read to your child (again, as a chore), you risk his imitation in the form of resisting the desire to read!

- A dimension of daily life that is potent in its regularity and its constant presence is that of eating. Through your example, instill the idea and the habit that we eat with consciousness in the name of friendship with our fifty trillion cells whose work and joy is to keep us alive. To bring presence and mindfulness to the simple act of eating is a lifelong gift to confer on your children. (One excellent—and quick—blessing before a meal or even a snack: "Here's to the health of all of our cells.")

- Sandra Steingraber shares dietician Laurine Brown's simple, child-friendly food groups, of which there are only three: "*go foods* (whole grains and complex starches for energy), *grow foods* (protein for building body parts), and *glow foods* (brightly colored fruits and vegetables, full of vitamins)."[73]

- One of the challenges many parents meet in setting boundaries, redirecting unacceptable behavior, and denying dire requests (another term for whining, usually as you run the gauntlet of a toy store or any supermarket checkout, for example) is confronting their own guilt, insecurity and fear of disappointing their children. (This is often related to them confusing their own childhood experience with their child's. I love John Breeding's bluntly sage invitation: "Make peace with disappointing your child or go crazy.") Along with that is the discomfort many of us have—it's cultural—regarding the value of emotional expression, when our children cry, scream or melt down. The example you set by surmounting your inner struggles to attain the self-possession to kindly but firmly say "No" despite a full court press is one of the greatest gifts you can give your children—for it won't be many years before you will want them to be able to do the very same thing: say "No" in the face of conflicting feelings, high emotions and intense peer pressure!

- Children learn unfortunate lessons of cynicism (a subtle violence) when their parents take pleasure in criticizing friends, acquaintances, politicians. Children take our cues about how to treat themselves, others and the environment—with compassionate care or mindless disregard. They absorb the inner and outer atmosphere we create. Consider Kim John Payne's suggestion to go on a "shame, blame and put-down diet." He further offers wise counsel: ask yourself "What need was not met in *me* that prompted that put-down?"[74] You might also take Eleanor Roosevelt's cue: "Great minds discuss ideas; average minds discuss events; small minds discuss people."

- Sing often—softly or right out loud: it helps leaven and brighten the atmosphere. Even just humming works wonders in the brain, bringing oxytocin into your bloodstream. The quality of every gesture we make percolates into the psyche of our child: the way we set the table, wash the dishes, make the bed, vacuum, or respond to a wrong number on the phone. In these situations, when we are flowing we give them the gift of a flowing attitude. The way we even *touch* objects matters; we can cultivate a precision in our gestures that is a tremendous gift to our kids. This self-mastery is perhaps the single most potent influence we have on our children.

Nurturance – This is the practical demonstration of love, the giving of ourselves to our child: how we cuddle them, feed them, speak to them, look at them. Everything is an opportunity for nurturance of our children, from how we choose their toys and books, their clothing, the colors for their rooms, what to feed them, even the attitude we hold while preparing their meals! And we must also take care to apply this principle throughout the household—to people, pets, fruits and vegetables, our cooking pots, and of course, to our partners and especially to ourselves.

- If there is one quality to most strive to express on a daily, even hourly, basis in our lives with young children, let it be the warmth of *kindness*. Kindness with them, as they struggle with the many frustrations that come with being little in a big world and wishing to do more than their capacities will yet let them. Kindness with ourselves, whose own tender places are so often laid open anew when we give ourselves over to the tumultuous adventure of parenting for peace. I was blessed to be friends with Laura Huxley, the late widow of Aldous Huxley, best known as the author of *Brave New World* but also a pioneering researcher who had studied various psychological, philosophical and spiritual systems aimed at furthering human potential. Laura often told the story that during a lecture near the end of his life, Aldous was asked what the most effective technique was for positively transforming a life. He answered, "It is a little embarrassing that after all my years of researching and experimenting, I would just say, 'Be a little kinder.'"

- Laura's nephew Piero Ferrucci devoted an entire book to illuminating, through the latest research in many different fields, that we are "designed to be kind"—and how imperative it is for us to make the conscious choice to *do so*! In *The Power of Kindness* he writes, "In this exciting but dangerous moment of human history, kindness is not a luxury, it is a necessity. Maybe if we treat each other, and our planet, a little better, we can survive, even thrive."[75]

- Hand in hand with kindness, at the pinnacle of parenting for peace, is empathy—the actively nurturing posture of feeling the experience of another, and caring deeply about it. Not only is empathy the golden ground from which loving responses spring, it is an essential capacity for Generation Peace. Your child is watching and downloading your styles of relating, and every time you respond with empathy to her…to your pet…to your UPS person… and so on, you foster within her greater depths of this fundamental peacemaker quality. Robin Grille, in the very first paragraph of his epic *Parenting for a Peaceful World*, writes that "the human brain and heart that are met primarily with empathy in the critical early years cannot and will not grow to choose a violent or selfish life."[76]

- Empathy—seeing and feeling the moment through your child's eyes—together with your calm, loving and authoritative mindset helps make discipline a source of nurturance, growth, and greater connectedness for your child, rather than shame and disconnection. One spiritually oriented mother's empathy for her daughter—a spiritual being having a newly physical experience, needing to learn so many basics—led her to issue the gentle, rather enchanting correction: "Darling, that's not how it's done here on Earth. Let me show you…" This harnessed another quality that is so helpful for disciplinary moments—humor! When we can have a sense of humor, to laugh *with* him at a mistake (not *at* him), it adds tremendous ease to what could otherwise be moments of struggle. This is a boon to parenting a toddler for peace, but will remain a helpful staple throughout the teen years.

- If you go to any park on any day in any city, you will see a child fall and start to cry and then you will see his mother swoop him up and begin to chant incessantly, "You're okay, you're okay, no blood, you're okay!" Meanwhile, the child wails. Only very occasionally will you see a mother who calmly reflects her child's true experience: "Yes, love, I saw that you tripped over that bucket and fell down. And that hurt, didn't it?" Or maybe, "That was pretty scary, huh?" She reflects *what is so*, not what she wishes were so. Her child's crying ebbs, and he is quickly ready to get back to his business of playing. He has been *heard*. This kind of nurturance fosters connection—between a parent and child, and between a child and his own inner knowing.

- In almost every choice you make for your child, there is the opportunity to nurture him with reverence, awe and beauty. Will the walls in his room be the common off-white, or will you choose instead a soft pastel hue that envelops him with warmth and beauty? Will you absent-mindedly crack the eggs for his breakfast and toss the shells in the garbage can, or thank the chicken that gave this perfectly formed, protein-rich slice of perfection? This is an invitation to leaven and enliven the days for you and your child. (Of course there will be some eggs cracked without a story or a blessing!) One helpful way to approach this is to imagine looking out at the world through your child's eyes, which brings the uplifting quality of *wonder* to the fore. The more we can live, as Joseph Chilton Pearce puts it, "in constant astonishment," the more we can attune to the aspect of our children that seeks reverence, awe and beauty.

- One of the simplest ways to increase a sense of reverence and awe is to put yourself on a zip-the-lip regime. Say less, let it mean more. There is an epidemic raging, which I call TITD (Talk It To Death) syndrome. I gave one example earlier in this step, but one only has to spend a little time with any American family to see TITD in action: "Why is there a rainbow on the wall?" "Well, Samantha, the sunlight is being split into seven different wavelengths by the refractive index of the crystal on my watch sitting there on the counter." Wonder and awe quotient abysmally low. David Elkind offers an illustration of how young children's questions are usually focused on the *purpose* (why) of things rather than an explanation (how): His preschool aged son asked him, "Daddy, why does the sun shine?" At first tempted to give him a scientific answer about the relationship of heat and light, he remembered this principle behind the young child's questions. He simply answered, "To keep us warm, and to make the grass and the flowers grow."[77] In this spirit, a more nurturing response to Samantha's question about the rainbow might have been, "To make our morning more beautiful with the special qualities that sunlight can have."

- Your young child (especially at four and five) will generate a seemingly unending stream of questions—one of the ways he is working on developing intellectual and social initiative. There is a delicate balance for the attuned parent to strike—between falling into the TITD trap on the one hand, or being dismissive or unresponsive to the child's earnest inquiries on the other. If we brush off, demean or ignore a child's questions he may associate curiosity with a feeling of guilt or shame, which is a catastrophe for the future peacemaker, in whom curiosity must remain a crackling blaze. To support and foster his robust sense of initiative and curiosity, strive to feel your way into the lifeworld of the young child, which wants to know in a way that preserves wonder and reverence for a still-magical world. There is time aplenty for the bottom-line, scientific knowledge of "reality."

- Here are two handy responses to have at the ready, which work in virtually any situation in which you're caught off-guard by your child's question (like one our son asked, "Do people grow *down* before they die?"). The first is, "I wonder..." This leaves the child's own imagination to all the possibilities that will come her way, and allows her to remain in the dream-space that is a child's right. I fear, however, that in our hyperintellectual culture many parents would feel remiss in giving a response like this, afraid of failing the child by not providing an "answer." Yes, "I wonder" can be considered an advanced maneuver that you can work toward saying with confidence and tranquility. The second is Elkind's suggestion to ask the question back to the child. "Well, why do *you* think a rainbow has appeared in our kitchen?" This will often elicit a stream of enchanting insights into your child's imaginative capacities—all of which should be met with the utmost interest and respect for her opinions on the matter, never "corrected." Remember, there will be time aplenty for "reality."

- The nurturing power of stories cannot be overstated. Stories told out of your own imagination or memory are the gold standard, but it is the rare parent gifted with this talent (I certainly wasn't). One way to begin to cultivate the knack for just telling a story is to relate some of your own adventures—those, of course, appropriate for the age. Stories of your travels, your own childhood, your activities while expecting him, are all great fodder. And children always love to hear about the day they were born. The point is to highlight the sensations, the beauty, the wonder, the feelings, rather than "just the facts, ma'am." Children love repetition and will ask for the same story over and over—and will often protest if you miss a crucial detail. Story time can become a soaring collaborative event as the child gets a bit older and adds her own fanciful embellishments.
- When choosing books for your child, it is helpful to have a few basic criteria with which to sift out the gems from the glut of so-called children's literature out there. To me the most basic is that there is beauty (as opposed to just cleverness) in the illustrations, especially in the depiction of the human form. So many illustrations portray people in caricatured, exaggerated and even grotesque ways, which has a subtly discouraging effect upon a child's psyche. Another is that it draws on wonder, imagination, and reverence for its subject, whereas countless books feature overly adult perspectives and tones such as irony or sarcasm. And remember to choose the books that *you* resonate with; your little one will be nurtured by the resonance you feel with the story and illustrations.
- It is important to keep the question before you, *What can I do to nurture myself?* These are demanding days. It has become cliché because it's so true: full-time parenting is the most difficult job. Have a favorite book or magazine to read on a subject you find fulfilling and nourishing. Have someone close at hand who is a friendly voice for you; a chat with him or her is nurturing time, even if it's brief—in person or via Skype or even the quaint old telephone. Friendship connections fire up the oxytocin system, they replenish you.
- Research demonstrates the power of giving to restore and refill our own psyche. There are some moments when we can make a space inside, a silence, and connect through our imagination with parents around the globe, wish-

ing them the best, dedicating to them an echo of the joys we have. When you open out a dimension of your days in this way, it can fill you with an expanded sense of appreciation for what you're living—a potent antidote for cabin fever.

- Time in nature is an absolutely essential form of nurture, for the young child and for us. Science has now even quantified some how's and why's of nature's important role in human wellbeing: natural settings engage our attention in subtle, relaxed ways—the rustling of leaves, patterns of clouds, colors of a sunset, birds taking flight, the gnarled shape of an old tree. Contrast this with the manmade world of a cityscape that demands the active attention of the person strolling city streets—Walk/Don't Walk lights; the pedestrian about to bump into you with her hot Starbucks; the ambulance passing, siren blaring; together with the bombardment of sensation of bus-bench ads, traffic, and the overall noise level. Constant exposure to such an environment is like running an engine at high RPMs without a break. Natural environments give our brains' "attention equipment" a chance to reset, refresh and renew. In fact, out of this research has even emerged something called ART—Attention Restoration Therapy! So as it often happens, science has now "proven" what philosophers have long known—in this case, Henry Thoreau: "We can never have enough of nature."

- Remember the nurturing power of warmth, and use your imagination to bring this quality into your child's home life in a variety of ways. Not only is it a fundamental need of the young child's unfolding will forces, it is needed all the more in today's world in which, writes Piero Ferrucci, "we are all in the midst of a 'global cooling.' Human relations are becoming colder."[78] Fire (candles included), teas, soups, yummy natural fiber layers of clothing, the tone of your voice, the colors on your walls—these are all opportunities for warming up the atmosphere. Bedtime is especially a time for warmth: a candle burning during the bedtime story can be very soothing.

- Family traditions warm the soul and reinforce a deep sense of connectedness. Creating a few meaningful traditions when your child is young pays untold dividends as they grow up and hit the teen years and still find great comfort and joy in them. Holidays offer particularly ripe opportunities for developing your own unique touches—some of which may not catch on while others will become sacrosanct within the family. One friend has the simplest, most elegant Christmas tradition, in which all of the gifts that Santa brings are wrapped in white paper, period. (How brilliant is *that?!*) In my own family I carried on a tradition begun by my own mother: on Christmas Eve when I went to my room to get ready for bed, there was always a gift of new PJs waiting on my pillow—as there now is for my son and daughter (even though they're 20 and 24!). Perhaps the most fervently adored tradition in our family became the Easter egg hunt, whereby my husband, John, did a maestro's job at hiding eggs (that had been dyed by the kids earlier in the week) in and around the house.

- One great idea is to choose one special, consistent event every year (or most years) and record it on video. (For us it was indeed the increasingly competitive world-class egg hunt.) I think it would be great to shoot the classic "measuring the kids on the closet doorway" event each year. Whatever event you choose, it makes for a great growing-up montage when your kid is eighteen!

• One of the key decisions you will be faced with is preschool: whether to send her, and if so, when to start and what kind. Parents today are offered far less choice than when my children were this age; managing to find a nonacademic preschool these days is kind of like Dorothy managing to get the witch's broom! The downward thrust of the former first-grade curriculum into kindergarten and now into preschool means that years four, five, and six (and sometimes even three and two) are spent on preacademics and kindergarten preparation. This is a catastrophe for every dimension of Generation Peace potential! David Elkind's *Miseducation: Preschoolers at Risk* is an absolute must-read, even if you skip his compelling analysis of why we're so hell-bent as a culture on hurrying our children, and his excellent explanation of children's developmental needs and abilities at these ages, and flip directly to the section on exactly what to look for in a healthy preschool for your child.[79] Keep in mind that early education has a more fundamental and enduring impact on the very shape of your child—his social intelligence, his capacities for peace, innovation and enjoyment of life—than does college. So if it's a question of finances, my motto is, spend it at the front end, and let the back end take care of itself.

- I have explained the importance of play for fostering the capacities of a peacemaker. One portrait of a *truly* developmentally appropriate (see below) preschool curriculum comes from Waldorf education: "In the nursery-kindergarten, children play at cooking, they dress up and become mothers and fathers, kings and queens; they sing, paint, and color. Through songs and poems they learn to enjoy language; they learn to play together, hear stories, see puppet shows, bake bread, make soup, model beeswax, and build houses out of boxes, sheets, and boards. To become fully engaged in such work is the child's best preparation for life. It builds powers of concentration, interest, and a lifelong love of learning."[80]

- Preschool administrators throw around the buzz-term *developmentally appropriate* somewhat loosely in my experience, sometimes using a child's interest in an activity as evidence of its developmental appropriateness, which isn't valid. Young children will often happily embrace colorful workbooks, spelling tests, and group drills (none of which are appropriate); for one thing, they are exquisitely receptive: they pick up on what *we* want them to do, and they are eager to please us. It doesn't mean that it's the right thing to do, any more than it would be right to let them have all the sweets or toys they *think* they'd like to have!

Trust – As the mother with a child in her womb trusts that his organs are forming correctly, that trust in the hidden inner process of your child's vibrant development continues into childhood. The days go on and on, each flowing into the next, and we don't readily see the transformations that are happening. You can trust that the forces of life are working in your child. Sometimes we need little boosts of inspiration to continue fanning the faintly glowing embers of our confidence in the notion that this too shall pass (whether it's colic or potty accidents or sleep droughts). Then we hear one of countless stories like that of a colleague whose child barely smiled until the age of seven, when he seemingly overnight came out of his cocoon. Trust that this mysterious, magical being called your child has his or her own timetable for the unfolding of everything.

As I write this it's impossible to overlook the epidemic rates of ADD, ADHD, sensory processing, autistic spectrum and other psychosocial disorders. Many of these would no long be considered epidemic but have become endemic: tragically common. While this book is not geared to the child with special needs, nor to a child with serious developmental delays, all of the principles nonetheless apply as enriching adjuncts alongside whatever specialized guidance you receive from your child's healthcare professionals.

- I know many women—myself included—who never thought they were mother material, who didn't think they had the capacity to surrender to "just being a mother." By trusting the mysterious streams of Life and your own inner capacities—your imagination, your insight, your savvy—you'll discover activities suited to your child *and* you, which will beautifully foster his sense of joy in being alive. And it is this, ultimately, that must flourish vibrantly in the peacemaker—the joy of being alive.

- Cultivate trust in your own affinities rather than in any preconceived ideas—from the culture, from your in-laws, even from me! You have embarked on this hero's journey that is an existentially solitary endeavor, and if bucking the status quo brings loneliness, let it also bring delightful exhilaration.

Simplicity – Recall that simplicity is a portal to joy, and joy lies at the very foundation of health, wellbeing and peace. Cultivating a sense of wonder and imagination fosters rich simplicity, because then everything becomes something amazing: wind through the trees is fairies dancing…a piece of wood becomes an alligator or a doll…a spoon becomes a great flag or a king's scepter. Then we don't need to constantly purchase things. (Laura Huxley once mused to me that the two overriding cultural messages with which we are bombarded are: 1) "Buy it"; and 2) "Throw it away.") When anything can become a toy, the child experiences such freedom! And a child—or parent—who can wonder and imagine is on a path toward unlimited peacemaking horizons.

- The child's deepest need is to be *seen* and *known*. Simplifying daily life helps that to happen more; as I like to say, "When we overbook, we overlook."
- Kim John Payne's study with children clinically diagnosed with ADHD found that when family life was simplified in three main areas—environment (including what the children were taking in via diet as well as information), screened media, and schedules—well over half of the children (68 percent) tested out of the clinical ADHD range after just four months.[81] No Ritalin, just simplicity.* Definitely with a child younger than six or seven, but also with older kids, the more we can simplify life, the more peace we will have in the home, and thus woven into the fabric of the child's developing brain. It becomes a feedback loop generating a reservoir of inner wealth in your child, available to be spent in myriad peacemaking ways from mastering her moods, to discovering creative solutions, to caressing her loved one.

---

* Along with a reduction in hyperactivity and attention issues, the simplicity intervention also resulted in a significant increase in academic achievement—an outcome *not* seen with medication.

- When seeking to simplify a family environment or routine that has become overly complicated, I suggest beginning with the most basic, recurring events first—eating and sleeping:
  - Sleep is Nature's own simple treasure, offered to us nightly, and we frequently spurn it in favor of all manner of other trivial pursuits. And we suffer for it. Your child needs anywhere between ten and fourteen hours sleep (including naps) depending on her age. Ensuring that our children get the sleep they need means making a sizable commitment to prioritizing it on a daily basis—to serve her dinner early enough to begin the bath-to-bedtime routine means curbing late afternoon errands or activities; throw the afternoon nap in there beforehand and suddenly you're reminded of the earliest days of nursing when it seemed the end of one session practically dovetailed into the beginning of the next, with no "me" time in there anywhere! Clearly, simple doesn't always mean easy. It requires foresight, fortitude, and organization. According to the National Sleep Foundation the sleep needs of various ages are:

Toddlers	12-14 hours
Preschoolers	11-13 hours
School-age children	10-11 hours
Adolescents	9-10 hours
Adults	7-9 hours

  - Make simple, predictable meals (seafood Wednesdays, lentil Thursdays, etc.) that feature limited choices of healthy, child-friendly foods—perhaps including two different vegetables, one he already likes and a newer one that he's free to ignore after one taste. (If you are nonchalant about it, eat it yourself, and keep offering it, he will come around.) Don't enter into negotiations or struggles around food. Don't even begin the slide down the slippery slope of being a short-order cook. Use your calm, loving authority (and the same tranquil conviction with which you buckle her into her seat belt) to make it clear what is on the menu at a given meal. You might keep a fruit-and-vegetable snack center in the fridge that is always available to the child as a reasonable alternative if she's feeling particularly contrary. Cook big batches of things and freeze. Cook dinner in the morning for a simpler afternoon and evening. (I personally think a crock pot in every home would contribute significantly to world peace: twenty minutes

of work in the morning and your dinner awaits you at five—not to mention your home is filled with the heavenly aroma of home cooking!)

- Drastically reduce or banish altogether juices and other beverages from
your kitchen. If I had it to do over again, I'd have gone further than cutting
apple juice with half water; I'd have weaned my children on the delights
of pure, vibrant water, period. Not only are the dangers of high fructose
intake coming to light,[82] inadequate intake of water is a silent epidemic
of untold proportions in most developed countries and is a significant contributor to a long list of physical ailments, suboptimal development and
degenerative diseases. The common belief that juices, soft drinks, coffee,
tea, and other manufactured beverages contribute to the body's need for
liquids is "an elementary but catastrophic mistake," according to F. Batmanghelidj, author of *Your Body's Many Cries for Water*. Yes, they do contain water, but also enough dehydrating agents to cancel it out plus steal
extra water reserves from the body! The book's physician author cautions
that when we give children juice, sodas, and other flavored drinks, we inadvertently (and disastrously) cultivate their innate preference for them,
and "reduce the free urge to drink water."[83]

- Simplify the child's entire sensory field—the environment that is your home,
his room in particular. Reduce the number of things by at least half. Typically,
the number of a child's toys is best reduced by drastic proportions; the fewer
there are, the more meaning each has. It's a great idea to rotate several toys in
and out of her environment every week or two, which injects an element of
novelty and freshness, without having to keep buying. (Of course, you cannot
remove her very precious favorite one or two toys.) The same with books. It
may come as a shock that it's possible for a child to have too many books,
but it is. As with toys, the more select the collection is, the more engaged a
child will tend to become with them. Consider the noise level in your home
as well, listening from inside his new little ears. This may mean installing
double-paned windows to dampen street noise, or laying more rugs down on
your hardwood floors.

- As mentioned earlier, an important aspect of keeping a child's life simple is
in keeping the number of choices per day within appropriate bounds—which
means typically far fewer choices than the average parent offers. Park yourself
in the yogurt aisle at the grocery store and you won't have to wait long to
witness an example, in which a mom launches into an extended negotiation

to placate even the youngest child—three, four—as she reaches for some cartons and her child yells, "No!": "No, not raspberry? Here, how 'bout blueberry, you love blueberry. No? Honey, well [child points]—Oh, you want the vanilla? Okay, we'll get the vanilla…and I'm going to get some blueberry as well [child starts to protest]—No, no, don't worry, you don't have to eat it, it's for Daddy and me." A child freighted with too many choices suffers the anxiety of having too much say in matters that should simply be decided by grownups. There is plenty of time ahead for the empowerment of more choice and greater autonomy, and the more we allow the young child her season of insouciance in which others are in charge, the more fully she can blossom into that next sphere of freedom. My basic rule of thumb for how many choices to offer a child in a day is the same as the classic (though rarely heeded anymore) equation for how many children to invite to his birthday party: the age of the child, plus one. So if he's three, he gets four choices per day on average. Maybe three today and five tomorrow, loosey goosey. And the choices are not open-ended, but a choice between two options (either of which is acceptable to you). And the choice is proffered by you, not demanded by her in the form of a protest against something you've chosen. You can sometimes even say to the child, "Relax, you're not in charge." Calm. Authoritative. Loving. Peace. Ahhhh…

- Speaking of birthday parties, in the words of Thoreau, "Simplify, simplify." Strive to heed the above formula. Steer clear of major productions; homegrown parties are usually the most successful, and most satisfying for the child.
- Here are some ways to both simplify and enrich the very ways in which we interact with our children:
  - Let your discipline mantra be "Imitation, redirection, habituation": be sure you're modeling the kinds of behavior you want to see in your child; when she starts to veer in the wrong direction (like, toward Grandma's priceless vase, or the front door that someone left open), simply redirect her by taking her hand or even literally steering her gently by the shoulders while cheerfully informing her of what's next; the more often you model behaviors and she engages in them, the more habituated she becomes and the fewer kerfuffles and struggles there will be. This notion of habituation goes against the cultural grain, especially since the permissive parenting revolution of the seventies and the idea that children should be allowed to be free to express themselves without such constraints or regimentation.

The fact is, when we begin to learn any skill—carpentry, sculpture, poetry—some regimentation is required. The apprentice must first learn the basic conventions; the more fluent she becomes, the freer she is to then find her uniquely expressive departure from the conventional. A foundational behavioral structure gives the child a safety net so that she may relax.

- If we can recalibrate our own attitude toward misbehavior it brings a lot of simple peace into the family. At this age—certainly until the age of five—it is best to think in terms of your child simply making a mistake rather than breaking rules, misbehaving, or being uncooperative. The brain equipment simply isn't yet in place to retain rules and to restrain their impulses—even though they truly *do* want more than anything else to please you. Would *you* want someone to scold, shame or punish you when you make a mistake, especially if you were trying your best? Making mistakes shows we're risking new growth and exploration. If your child *stops* making mistakes, that's the time to worry; it means she's not feeling safe and secure enough to venture forth into new learning.

- One handy little technique in those moments when you're feeling exasperated is to take a breath and imagine being his *grandmother* rather than his mother. Grandparents have the gift of not getting too bogged down in discipline stuff; their love is just so big and relaxed it kind of blinds them to a child's small infractions. One eight-year-old French boy wrote his description of grandmothers and it included the line, "…and they know how to close their eyes to our mistakes." A variation on this theme is to simply say to the mildly errant child, "When I was your age, I would do that exact thing…" It leavens the atmosphere and lighter is always more peaceful.

- It is often simplifying, especially in cases of repeated "mistakes," to try to suss out the pure impulse behind your child's seriously bad behavior. The future artist might be incorrigible about drawing on the walls; the child who's stealing your jewelry might be having severe separation anxiety and wants to keep you with him. Nancy Jewel Poer tells the story of the little boy who was throwing darts into the wall of the sun porch and when (rather than freaking out and commanding him to "stop that right this minute") a grownup asked why (with sincere curiosity, not as the classic rhetorical ambush), the boy said, "Listen," and then threw another dart. When it landed it made a *booooi-oooi-oooinggg*; this boy went on to become a master mechanic for whom tuning in to those kinds of sounds was essential.

- The more we simplify, the more we embolden ourselves to rely upon and find strength in our own resources. Make no mistake—this is subversive stuff. This book may have innocent little cookies on its cover, but it actually calls for a revolution—an awakening to your own power that comes from within, not from without. And every time your child sees you putting your inner resources to work, even if they are the slimmest of resources, that is a potent education for her. It will come far more naturally to her to do the same.

Resources

Some informative sites on the issue of television:
- "Television and Children": a comprehensive gathering of information from the *YourChild Development & Behavior Resources* of the University of Michigan Health System – www.med.umich.edu/yourchild/topics/tv.htm
- "The Debilitating Effects of TV on Children" – psychcentral.com/blog/archives/2009/09/27/the-debilitating-effects-of-tv-on-children
- "TV & Brainwaves: Published Studies" – www.tvsmarter.com/documents/brainwaves3.html
- "Study Links TV and Depression" – articles.latimes.com/2009/feb/03/science/sci-tv3

Rabbit Ears Entertainment: They have now added illustrations to their repertoire of wonderfully narrated tales, so my suggestion is to play them *just for the audio* to maximize the participation of your child's engaged imagination and forestall the "screen seduction" as long as possible! – www.rabbitears.com.

Chinaberry Books & Other Treasures for the Whole Family: This was one of my most beloved sources of books and audio when my children were young! I encourage you to support this and other dedicated children's bookstores, which are struggling (*a la* Meg Ryan's doomed Shop Around the Corner in *You've Got Mail*) to stay afloat and serve children in the face of giants like Amazon and Barnes & Noble. In Los Angeles we have Children's Book World; see where *your* nearest real children's book store is, and go! Meanwhile Chinaberry has a wonderful selection of storytelling and audio CDs at www.chinaberry.com/cat.cfm/pgc/11400.

Audio Titles I Highly Recommend: See first if you can find them at your local children's bookstore, and if not, yes, they are available from Amazon –

- *Teaching Peace*, Red Grammar (songs)
- *Baby Beluga*, Raffi (songs)
- *10-Carrot Diamond*, Charlotte Diamond (songs)
- *Free to Be You and Me*, Marlo Thomas and others (songs and stories)
- Any storytelling CDs by Odds Bodkin

Videos – A very short list, indeed!
- Episodes of *Mr. Rogers' Neighborhood* and *The Mother Goose Treasury of Sing-Along Nursery Rhymes* Vols. I and II (available on Amazon); it is exactly due to their *un*sophisticated production elements—which seem almost comical to us adults—that these are most developmentally and sensorially respectful.

Step Seven

SHEPHERD THEM INTO THE WORLD—SHAPING AND SHARING PEACE

Sometime around the age of seven, the child takes her first steps into a wondrous world made new by virtue of her awakening powers of cognition. Life forces that have been hard at work completing the vital organs of her body have been freed to animate a whole new layer of life within: her feeling-knowing brain is powering up! Where she has until now related with the world by taking it in through her senses and imitating it, she now engages with her environment through the prism of her imagination and feelings. As educator Henry Barnes sums up this middle childhood stage, "Whatever speaks to the imagination and is truly felt stirs and activates the feelings and is remembered and learned. The elementary years are the time for educating the 'feeling intelligence'."[1]

And indeed, feeling intelligence is central to the qualities envisioned for a generation of peacemakers, so this stage between ages seven and fourteen is of central importance to the endeavor of raising innovative, joyful, socially adept future adults. The rich years of play logged by a Generation Peace child leading up to this stage have enriched his powers of imagination, and now that imagination becomes the lens through which he meets the world in this new way.

This age heralds the onset of mental abilities that genuinely enable children to classify, quantify, arrange objects, symbolize and perform other basic cognitive operations that are needed in order to have a meaningful introduction to math and reading.

Parents who have followed through on the sometimes challenging commitment over the first seven years of tending the bud of their child's intelligence by essentially protecting her ability to fully be a child—enjoying a rhythmic daily life filled with physical and emotional warmth, with play, with a nourishing diet of good food and close relationships; earnestly imitating the adults in her midst; and joyfully following her loving authority figures—are now rewarded with the astonishing metamorphosis she makes, sometimes seemingly overnight! You will have the new delights of seeing your child immersed in a book, in true conversation with a peer, in reciprocal engagement with her world.

The Awakening of Feeling Intelligence

If there were any characteristic to single out as an absolute prerequisite for Generation Peace, it is empathy. And now, between the ages of seven and fourteen, is the time to actively cultivate empathy in a child, the capacity to feel what the other is feeling—in a story, in the street, on the playground, in the classroom. All of the rich play, fanciful stories and close nurturing in Step Six have ripened the child for the blossoming of empathy, why? Empathy is one of the central—and highest—expressions of imagination. Empathy means that I can imagine my way into what you are experiencing—and, that I care about it. Empathy is about feeling the other—a person, a horse, even water or air— and also feeling *for* the other. This requires a vibrant imagination palette, which has ideally been expanding during the first seven years.

We tend to think of imagination as the ability to conceive of what is "far out"—as in fanciful tales or wild science fiction, for example. That is certainly one dimension of imagination, and one that will later serve Generation Peace's innovation and ingenuity, but a more native and vital facet of imagination is that which allows us to go "deep in"—to penetrate the surface of a person, an object, an idea, with what we sense inwardly about them. This connection is designed at the level of our neurobiology to take place naturally—it is how we are meant to be. This book you're reading is not about *changing* humanity, but merely about helping humanity to fulfill its native neurophysiological potential as well as its mandate—to evolve in order to thrive and flourish in new ways!

Every Moment Is the Moment to Begin

One of the most exciting findings of the last couple decades of neuroscience has been that the *plasticity* of our brains persists far longer than we used to think. Plasticity is, quite simply, the ability of the brain to change—its function and even its structure—in response to new circumstances and experiences. Meaning, you *can* teach an old person new tricks—that is, things to *do*. But it's a far more involved task to teach them new social-emotional functioning— ways to *be*.* And wouldn't we rather our children as adults spend that concentrated effort and attention on bringing new fruits of creative innovation to the world, rather than on rewiring in themselves what could have been done beautifully in the first place?

Using home construction as a metaphor, we can think of the scope of circuitry in the child's social-emotional brain as like the framing, wiring and plumbing of a house: it determines the boundaries of how vast that house can potentially be when finished, and how well it will function. Which materials are used for walls, flooring, cabinetry and countertops are choices that come later, and determine important but less foundational details of how this house looks to the world. The critical window of the months and years leading up to around the child's third birthday wires the social-emotional brain for optimal lifelong potential, and the preschool years nourish and strengthen this foundation, readying it for the next layer of optimization.

As anyone who's shopped for homes knows, a house that has "good bones" but is in cosmetic disrepair is a far better investment than one that has been refurbished at surface levels but whose foundation or infrastructure is weak. Child welfare workers know well that if a child has experienced loving, attuned, consistent care in his early years, and then experiences the loss of his parents after the age of six or seven, there is great hope and potential for him—to have

---

* It's important to remain humble on this topic, in light of the fact that we are continually learning ever more astonishing things about how we miraculous humans work, and how vast our developmental potential is. Indeed, the field of energy psychology offers many effective tools—for example, as I've mentioned, EFT, Emotional Freedom Technique—for revising at any age what were thought to be "deeply ingrained" ways of being, feeling and relating.

a solid placement with a new family and to have a successful life. His foundation is solid. By contrast, as child welfare workers unfortunately know even better, a child deprived of that early experience of trust, security, and regulation can later be showered with the finest education, the best enrichment programs, and unlimited amounts of love and attention—yet still struggle well into adulthood, or even lifelong. Her infrastructure is shaky and her center may tend not to hold.

This principle isn't confined to the extreme cases of children in foster care and adoption. To a greater or lesser degree it shows up in cases of regular families in which the children's needs were not tended to, which undercut the optimal development of their foundational psychosocial brain structures and healthy will energies. These may be children who by age six or seven have passed the stage of being "a handful," and now, armed with the cognitive skills that arise at this age, present significant challenges for parents. Parental antennae are then constantly on alert for something about to go wrong, for upsets threatening to happen, for conflicts soon to arise. There is little joy in such negative feedback loop situations.

If that is where you are, take heart. All is not lost—far from it. Step Seven is a valid point of departure for parents seeking a new path—parents for whom these ideas are new, yet curiously inviting. Simplifying and enriching a struggling youth's life with the predictable, secure rhythms prescribed for even the youngest children has proved to be an effective intervention even in the most extreme cases of disordered development or behavior.[2]

Modeling Peace, Passion and Possibilities

It's not too late even at this age to turn things around, provided we stop looking to externals. If parents are prepared to look inwardly, there is always hope. Step Six called for parents to provide their children with an atmosphere worthy of unquestioning imitation, and initiated them into the notion that all discipline ultimately arises from parents' own *self*-discipline. Our children cannot become who we want them to be, or who we tell them to be; they can become only who we strive to be. Note that I didn't say they can become only who we are. If our children's potential was constrained by the limitations of our own accomplishment, we'd be doomed! We'd have to wait until our sixties, seventies, eighties—or maybe never—before we'd feel prepared to be parents. Nature has brilliantly built into the system that our children most powerfully respond to our inner life; thus, it is the ideals, aspirations and earnest striving we engage in that greatly shapes them—our upward striving that assists Life, in theologian John Cobb's words, as it "exert[s] its gentle pressure everywhere, encouraging each thing to become more than it is."[3]

Where the early years were for sheltering your child from many aspects of the outside world, now is the time to become a docent of life, guiding them into the wider world they're eager to meet and prepared to know. If you work outside the home, start talking to them about your work: they really want to know what you do and how you do it. Show them how it all happens, whether you're an accountant, a doctor, a repair technician, a poet. What are the challenges for you, and the rewards? Now is the time when you can tell them in more rich detail how your day went.

If you work as a full-time mother and homemaker, you have an extra challenge facing you (along with, in my experience, extra joys): you need to invest some imagination of your own into mining the satisfying, uplifting aspects of routine tasks. If you do not, you risk the child's perception (and your own) being, "My mother does nothing—she stays at home." Look for ways that your home can be a meaningful expression of you and your family. This is where I love the word *mothercraft*. Seek to bring an aspect of craft and beauty to even the most seemingly mundane aspects—napkins, trash cans, you get the idea. And then try not to let any of it become enshrined and static. (As a child I remember my vague discomfort over the fact that candles in our home always sat untouched, gathering dust, their wicks eternally unlit.) A remarkable treasure of inner strength becomes available to us when we can engage the normal tasks of life with ease, harmony and even delight. The notion of housework shifted for me when I began thinking of it as *caring* for the home that embraced us all so well. Indeed, even today, after caring for my home—especially when I use old-fashioned water, whose negative ions can't be matched by any Swiffer-type of concoction—it seems to sparkle with gratitude.

Do your best to eliminate the destructive word *chore* from your vocabulary. Your children are still learning first and foremost from your example, so now that they are truly capable of setting the table, loading the dishwasher, taking out the trash, feeding the dog, be careful to never make it sound like…that insidious "C" word. Your attitude will carry them naturally along into the uplifted mode of willing service: these are simply things that happen, that need to get done, that everyone pitches in on. "Come help me with…" becomes a handy tool—and as a fringe benefit, conversations while doing the dishes can

I think of the sad story of my friend Ilene's sister-in-law, Estelle, who had descended from a line of women who hated housework and cooking. It was like a curse that had been handed down from generation to generation through the power of example. In a particularly disheartened moment, when the economic downturn had phased out her job and she was "stuck back at home" (children now long grown and gone), Estelle said to my friend, "Ilene, I wish I were like you, you seem to find joy in everything." Not long after that, Estelle committed suicide...at the age of 70.

be such a gift! And if you can strive to always do it with good cheer, even pleasure, you are giving your children a lifelong gift: a little "whistle while you work" attitude goes a long way toward shaping their healthy relationship with responsible stewardship.

Besides pleasure in life's many dimensions, grand and small, parents can also now more explicitly model qualities and principles they envision cultivating in their children. Up until the age of (at least) five it was important that the child experience abundance, and thus be sheltered from many stark realities. Now you can gently begin to introduce him to the idea that others in the world have very different experiences, providing that you help him to make meaning of such human scourges as poverty, starvation, cruelty and the like. The child of this seven-to-fourteen age still needs some sheltering of her emotional life (the *astral body*, which is still in formation)—instead of being exposed too early to the complex realm of grownup emotional turmoil and the extremes of agony, ecstasy and trauma. Yes, some such intense themes turn up in the literature, drama, and history that students encounter at this age, and certainly they are increasingly aware of such themes in popular culture. This is a reasonable time for the child's outer and inner worlds to open to these new layers of awareness *provided that the emotional atmosphere in the child's immediate environment continues to offer the peaceful shelter needed by the newly maturing feeling intelligence.*

One way to invite the beginnings of awareness of the many horizons of human experience is through saying a blessing for humanity before the family meal, or simply sending a shared thought of friendship to those who are suffering—in orphanages or refugee camps, for example. Never mind the old admonition, "Eat all your dinner—there are children starving in Africa." Better to invite children to engage their natural imagination and empathy: "Let us send them our joy...ask that they might know a moment of pleasure and ease today."

Knowing Your Child, Yourself, and Your Discipline Watchword

One of the reasons I promote principles rather than rules, systems, or techniques is that meaningful parenting guidance must allow for everyone's uniqueness. What nurturance looks like to one child will feel like smothering to another; what presence feels like to one mother will feel like imprisonment to another. Principles are meant to be generous in their flexible accommodation while always retaining their essence in application. One fundamental dimension of the parenting journey is being led to ever deeper understandings and appreciation of just who your child is, apart from any other. While the possibilities of uniqueness are infinite, it is sometimes helpful to orient ourselves with the help of various mapping tools. The more we can understand ourselves and what makes us tick—and delight and pout and stress out—the more effective we can be not just as parents but as people in the world. And the more nuance with which we understand our children, the more fluid, harmonious and nurturing the parenting journey becomes.

Three popular personality-mapping tools that prove helpful to many are astrological charts, the Meyers-Briggs Type indicator (which types basic differences in the ways individuals prefer to use their perception and judgment), and the Enneagram (a geometry of nine basic personality types of human nature and how they interrelate). A lesser known yet ancient tool is the four temperaments, which is more focused on traits (inborn tendencies one has) than types (categories of behavior and preferences one fits into). Related to the four elements (earth, air, fire and water), temperaments are used by teachers in Waldorf education in shaping their teaching and discipline approach to best suit individual children.

The most whimsical portraiture of the four temperaments is found in *Winnie the Pooh*'s four main characters: Pooh, the *phlegmatic*; Eeyore, the *melancholic*; Tigger, the *choleric*; and Piglet, the *sanguine*. If the four of them came to a boulder blocking the path, melancholic Eeyore, pulled earthbound with the ongoing search for the meaning of life, would sigh deeply: "That's the story of my life." The organized, consistency-loving, phlegmatic Pooh would complain that "This isn't *supposed* to be here—this isn't how it should be," and the airily light-hearted, sanguine Piglet would cartwheel right over it: "This is fun!" The determined, fiery, choleric Tigger would shove it out of the way so they could all get on with it. As a parent as well as a counselor of parents, I've found the temperaments of great help because they illuminate fundamental

needs (and the flip-side of needs, stressors), which is essential parental information. You can imagine, for example, how knowing a phlegmatic child cannot stand being hurried, while a choleric child thrives on quick results, is a
boon for the ease of daily life!

Until now, parental guidance of the child has focused on limitation and direction. In this seven-through-fourteen stage, when development is centered
upon the feeling intelligence and social-emotional growth, discipline orients
around responsibility, the ability to see others' perspectives, and cooperation.
The mode of discipline evolves from limitation to *consultation*, in which,
stresses Kim John Payne, we listen thoughtfully and openly to their input,
take it into consideration, and then make an authoritative decision. It is *not* a
negotiation. It is a benevolent, reasonable dictatorship, but a dictatorship
nonetheless. Learning obedience is a must until the age of fourteen for the
child's healthy development. It provides a solid anchor when in adulthood he
is met with the strict rules of Life, such as those of his biology or of ethics in
the real world. He shouldn't be burdened with decision-making about shaping
rules right now; the weight of such responsibility will come soon enough.

Right here is where many parents' hands begin to slip off the tiller and
things begin to go off course: they prematurely allow their nine- or eleven- or
thirteen-year-old undue influence in their own discipline. Children at this age
can be brilliantly, doggedly persuasive, but if we give them too much of their
own reins we violate their implicit trust in us. They may make a good show
of it, but they truly don't *want* sole propriety over the daunting responsibility
of being the boss of themselves. When we continue to stand as the final arbiter
in the life of our school-age child, it allows them to relax inside (despite what
their outside might be shouting) and remain in flourishing growth mode.

Seeding Faith

It's fruitful for parents to model their own faithful participation in the hierarchy of life and the natural order of things—the idea that we parents are ac-
countable to higher powers in life and we don't get to just decide willy-nilly
whatever we want. The tenet that children have not been *given* to us, but *entrusted* to us, and as parents we are sacred collaborators with Life, is one of the
most nourishing for us to embrace. It's solidly comforting for the child to
know there's a hierarchy: parents above the child, the higher authority above
the parents. Some democratic-minded parents worry about laying their reli-

gious or spiritual ideas on their children, and think it might be best to convey a somewhat neutral posture regarding the great mysteries of life—so that when the child is old enough, he can decide for himself. It is just the reverse: it will only be through observing his parents' devotion to a faith in something larger than us that he will have the natural capacity to engage in his own explorations and choices. Many young adults whose parents kept their inner lives sequestered (or worse, didn't tend to their inner lives) have found themselves, in their twenties or beyond, experiencing a sort of existential despair—a void in the soul where a model of faith might have resided.

In practical terms, the notion of a hierarchy is of immense assistance during this seven-year stage when so many challenging issues can arise: we can ask for help from the divine realms! Secondly (shhh, don't let it get around), the hierarchical principle can be a boon for maintaining a strong relationship between you and your child when certain hot-button topics come up, which for some parents can become major power struggles. Says one mom, "At eight, Sarah was already tired, it was the middle of the week, and she wanted to have a sleepover. A heated discussion ensued, her insistence was huge and her upset began erupting as she saw my 'No' coming. I told her, 'Life has entrusted you to me; if I let you go have a sleepover when you're already so tired, what would Life think of me?' It seemed she was somehow relieved, as if she was actually seeking the No. She turned to silk immediately, took her bath and went to bed."

Now, there is perhaps no single realm more rife with power struggle pitfalls than that of media: television, movies, video games and the like.

Confronting the Media Hydra

During these years parents enter challenging territory, called upon to make countless decisions about their children's engagement with the wider world via schooling, peers, popular culture and, perhaps most daunting of all, electronic media. It wasn't so long ago—even as few as seventeen years, when our son Ian was seven—that curbing a child's media referred simply to television viewing and Gameboy noodling. Ah, the simple olden days of such quaint technology! Educator and Waldorf parent Helene McGlauflin also began her parenting journey in the mid-'80s, never imagining that eighteen years later she'd write an article in which she admitted that "struggling with screens" had been her most challenging parenting issue. While she agonized over many other serious decisions—day care, learning disabilities, and the dangers of drugs and sex in high school—she realized in retrospect that those had been transient issues, but screened media pervaded their family life without letting up: "Screens are here to stay and an issue for us all."[4]

As I mentioned in the introduction, parenting for peace can be seen as a hero's journey, and one of its most challenging aspects is "taming the media monster," as psychotherapist and Waldorf parent Thomas Poplawski puts it. Greek mythology offers us a fitting image for the proliferation of media aimed at children in the past decade or two—the Hydra, a daunting water creature that begins with nine heads but grows two for every head that is cut off. (For instance, tame the TV screen and up springs a video game and a Sim life; banish those screens and out pops the tiny flickering screen-in-your-pocket Smartphone.) The deadly Hydra, guardian of the entrance to the underworld, was raised by Zeus' wife Hera with the purpose of killing Heracles (Hercules in Roman mythology)—but instead, Heracles summons the will, courage, and ingenuity to survive its deadly vapors, vanquish the exponential regrowth of its heads, and ultimately slay the Hydra.

Corroborated by McGlauflin's struggles, I'm suggesting it will take something on the order of herculean logic, dedication and will to gain confident mastery over the ever proliferating media megapresence. But I encourage you to recognize that aspects of both the dangerous creature and the hero dwell within each of us, and to consider that it isn't part of our journey to kill anything (as in the bumper sticker slogan, "Kill Your TV"), but to *master our relationship with it* so as to minimize its harmful effects. We all definitely reap some important benefits from certain media, used in the right way at the right times. There is much hand-wringing about the ills of media, and for good reason, but whenever we insist on placing a problem *out there*, rather than taking responsibility for how we engage with and manage its influence upon us, we disempower ourselves and are ultimately more vulnerable to the very forces we condemn.

Picking up from last step's discussion of some troubling aspects of the *process* of TV and other screened entertainment, a topic of eternal concern and seemingly endless research is the effect of certain kinds of screened *content* on children's wellbeing—particularly violence. (And keep in mind that *violence* doesn't necessarily assume bullets, blood and gore, but refers to any act of aggression; think *Power Rangers, Superman, Charlie's Angels, Dragonball Z,*

Pokemon, in which the lauded hero uses physical or mental force, coercion or intimidation.)

The National Commission on the Causes and Prevention of Violence first noted in 1969 that there was cause for concern about the effects of television violence. By 1992 the American Psychological Association Task Force on Television and Society concluded that thirty years of research confirmed the harmful effects of exposure to violence in the media (including video games, television, and movies), which fall into three major categories: children may become less sensitive to the pain and suffering of others; they may be more fearful of the world around them; and they may be more likely to behave in aggressive or hurtful ways toward others.[5] The Academy of Pediatrics confirms, "More than one thousand scientific studies and reviews conclude that significant exposure to media violence increases the risk of aggressive behavior in certain children, desensitizes them to violence and makes them believe that the world is a 'meaner and scarier' place than it is."[6]

While researchers, analysts and media producers continue to split hairs over whether the violence *causes* these effects or merely *elicits* them in children who are already predisposed toward these traits due to a variety of other influences, I would propose that this is an academic distinction without much relevance in the trenches for real families. Do we really want to yield up our own children as research subjects in this grand experiment? Now, I suspect that violence-based programming is unlikely to gain much traction in a child raised in accordance with Gen Peace principles; for children possessed of their rightful inner foundation of psychosocial health, disturbing content is likely to be like water off a duck's back. And, screen violence holds little appeal for a youth whose interests are more grounded in the real world, his real experiences, and the real people in his life.

So then, we could reason, as long as we limit media to nonviolent kinds such as the children's fare on countless cable channels, we're okay. But there are degrees of violence, and the subtlety with which of covert acts of aggression take place in most children's programming is staggering upon close scrutiny. So-called family entertainment, including some even bearing the all-hallowed Disney brand, prominently features humor steeped in stealthy deprecation and sarcasm. A quick dictionary search reveals sarcasm to feature mockery, ridicule or derision; indeed, the very term comes from a Greek word meaning "to tear flesh." Sarcasm is poison to the soul of a young child, who cleaves to goodness, kindness and wonder. But even for the older child of school age, witnessing the disrespectful behavior, stereotyping, and sarcastic attitudes that pervade media entertainment is like turning a fire hose on the brilliantly shining flames of the inner virtues you're seeking to tend.

Television as a Neuro-Violent Experience

Producers long ago realized that children require far more novelty incidents (rapid cuts, zooms, pans, etc.) than do adults in order to keep their attention corralled. And one of the most effective novelty incidents is an act of violence. Children's programming features twice the number of violent acts than does primetime adult programming[7]—and Saturday morning cartoons are known to feature up to twenty-five incidents per hour in which animated characters are stabbed, smashed, run over, and pushed off cliffs (but of course, they don't stay dead for long—*huh?*). Last step's discussion of how novelty incidents engage the brain's fight-flight-or-freeze stress response, together with the findings that screened violence make children overall more fearful of the world, offer us one important angle from which to consider the issue of most screened entertainment, including so-called nonviolent programming: the effect they have—not as an accidental side-effect, but as an *intended unconscious process*— is to put the child in a neurological state of protection rather than growth.

It is on this basis alone that I recommend keeping screened media out of the diet of your child's life. I agree with Waldorf parent Karen Livingston when she writes, "It is hard to deny a child something she wants. But, do we really want to hand over our good judgment and parental authority to software programmers, network executives, publishers, and other strangers whose motives are not likely to be altruistic? What if we begin to think about inappropriate exposure to 'media' as a safety issue, as important to our child's health and well-being as eating a balanced diet, having a warm place to sleep, and not playing in the street?"[8]

While most of the focus and concern regarding television is on the troubling possibility of screened violence engendering violence, child psychologist David Elkind poses a chilling notion that I have rarely heard mentioned: what more effective way to provoke someone to aggression and violence than to keep them in a state of chronic fear and anxiety? Especially when they have no conscious awareness of why they feel that way.

Several longitudinal studies have reached the same bleak conclusion: early childhood exposure to TV violence predicts aggressive behavior for both males and females in adulthood. (Now, of course, human violence predates the television era by millennia, so it isn't simply television generating violence. In fact, it's more the reverse: the violence that has permeated human experience in the households of poor and wealthy alike has provided a subliminal breeding ground for today's screened violence to be created in the first place, and then to take hold and lead to such troubling developmental costs and behavioral responses by viewers.) Perhaps the longest and most comprehensive study was one in which the viewing habits of over eight hundred eight-year-olds were tracked, and these children were followed until the age of thirty: children who watched more violent programs were more likely to be identified by teachers and peers as the more aggressive students in school; at age eighteen this relationship persisted, with those children still more aggressive. The follow-up at age thirty was most sobering of all: children who at age eight had watched more violence on TV were more likely to have been arrested for violent crimes including spousal abuse, child abuse, aggravated assault and even murder.[9]

Whenever we must limit or take away something, it's always constructive to focus more on what we're going to fill that void with—which more healthful, life-affirming substance or activity we will choose for enrichment, and why. The child of this age still greatly benefits from engaging in life in a hands-on, three-dimensional manner. A fundamental source of the healthy self-esteem and robust will central to Generation Peace is the intrinsic reward that comes from expending effort—physical, mental, emotional—toward a given experience, and the understanding they feel of the meaningful relationship between their effort and their experience. Big effort, big experience, small effort, small experience.

Author Todd Oppenheimer notes that many Waldorf educators see popular culture, particularly electronic media, as subverting this essential relationship between effort and experience. In his book *The Flickering Mind: Saving Education from the False Promise of Technology*, Oppenheimer makes the compelling case that technology's false promise in schools (and in childhood homes) comes from its sensation of richness, when in most cases the reality is actually superficiality.[10] In a comprehensive *Atlantic Monthly* article on Waldorf education, he wrote:

> As Douglas Gerwin, a Waldorf high school teacher, put it, technology "promises an experience by which we don't have to do anything to make it happen." This is why teachers discourage younger students from watching television and don't generally expose them to computers

until the eighth grade or later. The delay doesn't seem to do much harm. Peter Nitze, who graduated from the Rudolf Steiner School, Harvard, and Stanford, is now a global-operations manager at Allied-Signal, which manufactures aerospace and automotive products. At a recent open house at the Steiner School, Nitze told the audience, "If you've had the experience of binding a book, knitting a sock, playing a recorder, then you feel that you can build a rocket ship—or learn a software program you've never touched. It's not bravado, just a quiet confidence. There is nothing you can't do. Why couldn't you? Why couldn't anybody?"[11]

Oppenheimer points out that when the Information Technology Association of America—a trade group representing a wide range of industries with I.T. positions—polled its members on what skills were most important to them, computer skills did not rank terribly high. Facility in skills like writing, problem solving, and history or sociology mattered much more. "Want to get a job using information technology to solve problems?" the association asked in its report's conclusion. "Know something about the problems that need to be solved."[12]

Aside from the violence aspect—within your child's own neurobiology as well as the statistically greater possibility of him expressing it outwardly in the world—there is another compelling incentive to eliminate or steeply curb your child's exposure to popular media: the preservation of his uniqueness. Recall in Step Five the practice of the forty days of cocooning at home with a new baby, allowing him time to settle into his body, gently orient to brand new sensations, and let his energy field coalesce without undue outside influences that might alter his singular essence. We can see this as another round of cocooning for similar reasons. If we pay attention—especially after the kind of media fast that happens on a camping trip, for example—as teacher Christopher Sblendorio urges, we can see the effects of what he calls "push-button entertainment" on our own originality; just imagine the impact on the far more impressionable eight- or eleven- or fourteen-year-old:

> Carefully observe the effect it has on your inner life of thoughts, emotions, and initiative. You may find that your own self-directed thoughts are replaced by ideas derived from the movie or news broadcast you watched. You may find that your own songs, the folksongs

you sang around the campfire, or the tunes that you hum and whistle, are replaced by the songs and tunes you hear on the radio or in commercial jingles. You may find that you have less initiative to prepare a special dish for dinner, or to write a letter, or to go out for a walk.[13]

Once a child is exposed to an idea, an image, a melody via the media, you can't un-ring that bell. You can't undo the erosion of *wonderment* of which Neil Postman wrote in *The Disappearance of Childhood*. In the life of our own family, I came to regard media as a chorus of clanging bells that could so easily eclipse our children's own unique ideas, images, and melodies, which were organically percolating up over time. The diminishment of any of these, along with the wonder that inspires them, is an incalculable loss when we're seeking to foster a child's own inner forces of creativity, joy and dynamic engagement with life's potent questions.

The Erosion of Childhood

I'll leave you with a compelling final incentive to give this your deep consideration—not simply the impingement upon your own child's uniqueness, but upon the very experience of childhood itself. And without childhood there can be no Generation Peace. Last step I briefly touched upon the notion that media is one of the most adultifying influences on children in an era when growing up fast has become not simply a cultural but a biological reality. In 1850 the average age of a North American girl's first period (menarche) was around 15½; since the 1970s it has remained at around 12½. Obviously there is a complex tapestry of causes for this massive shift; some theorize early menarche as a biologically determined risk factor for a girl's development, while others see it as a positive indicator related to improved nutrition, standard of living, literacy, and less manual labor. There are some crosscultural findings to support the latter: for example, Agta women foragers of Cagayan province, Luzon, in the Philippines, typically experience menarche at 17, and Haitian women at 15.4 years.[14] But other research suggests an explanation that makes the most sense to me—relating early puberty to environmental stress:[15] the body perceives obvious or subliminal stressors—a potent message that "the world is dangerous." Nature responds to this growth-or-protection signal by speeding up sexual maturation, so as to increase the odds of sending genes into the future via reproduction.

I see media as another thread of the maturation-pressure causal tapestry, part of the potent force of popular culture on the delicate unfolding of child and adolescent development. In Postman's compelling history of childhood, he pointed out that childhood is a social construct far more than a biological mandate—and it only came into being in the sixteenth century, as one of the greatest, and most humane, inventions of the Renaissance. He cautioned, "[L]ike all social artifacts, [childhood's] continued existence is not inevitable." He proposed in his chilling book that Gutenberg's printing press created childhood and that electronic media are "disappearing" it:

> Like alphabetic writing and the printed book, television opens secrets, makes public what has previously been private. But unlike writing and printing, television has no way to close things down. The great paradox of literacy was that as it made secrets accessible, it simultaneously created an obstacle to their availability. One must *qualify* for the deeper mysteries of the printed page by submitting oneself to the rigors of a scholastic education...
>
> Television, by contrast, is an open-admission technology to which there are no physical, economic, cognitive, or imaginative restraints. The six-year-old and the sixty-year-old are equally qualified to experience what television has to offer. Television, in this sense, is the consummate egalitarian medium of communication, surpassing oral language itself...
>
> The most obvious and general effect of this situation is to eliminate the exclusivity of worldly knowledge and, therefore, to eliminate one of the principal differences between childhood and adulthood. This effect follows from a fundamental principle of social structure: A group is largely defined by the exclusivity of the information its members share. If everyone knew what lawyers know, there would be no lawyers....Indeed, if fifth graders knew what eighth graders knew, there would be no point to having grades at all...
>
> Children are a group of people who do not know certain things that adults know. In the Middle Ages there were no children because there existed no means for adults to know exclusive information. In the Age of Gutenberg, such a means developed. In the Age of Television, it is dissolved.[16]

Remembering You're a Hero

Holding the technological and electronic invasion at bay in the life of your child is a daunting task that requires commitment, fortitude, and no small amount of humor. McGlauglin's confessional narrative—chronicling the phases of her struggle with screens—highlights that this is messy business with no easy or lasting solutions, even for the most thoughtful, determined parent. For her it was an ongoing process, "involving concern, control or lack thereof, and battles fought, won, and lost. The process has no resolution or end, except that, mercifully for me, my children have grown into young adults and have survived both the screens and my struggle."

In his "Taming the Media Monster" article, psychotherapist Poplawski invokes Elisabeth Kübler-Ross's stages of grief to vividly illustrate the wrestling match with media in a home where parents are devoted to fostering their children's most vibrant health. His examples would be funny if they weren't so painfully true, such as *denial*—"Television isn't a problem in our home. Our children never watch…well, maybe once in a while. Just a little bit during the week and then maybe on weekends a bit more" and *bargaining*—"How about if I limit it to one video on the weekends and give them a little more freedom during vacation times?"[17]

Poplawski notes that holding out against a societal obsession is difficult. It asks more of us as parents, to find alternatives to screens—constructive, engaging activities for our children to do, and for us to do with them. As he says, "The parent's own personal space and time will be compromised." This particular motive for allowing and even encouraging media use in children seems to me to be the most unfortunate of all. I suspect that it's also the most pervasive—our collective dirty little parental secret. Indeed, it is sanctioned as a "wink-wink, you know what I mean" standard in a currently running television commercial, whose plot goes like this: the 15-year-old boy tells us he spends three hours a day on his homework—"At least that's what my mom thinks. With high-speed internet from AT&T I get my homework done fast, leaving me time to download movies and music and chat with my friends."

Mom yells up from downstairs: "How's the studying?" Son: "Uh, it's coming along." His face is less sheepish about the deception than self-satisfied at the deceptive accomplishment. The voiceover announces, "Work fast, play more," and gives the price details. Then we are suddenly downstairs face to face with Mom, on the living room sofa: "Please, I know what he's up to. High-speed internet from AT&T is so fast, we get more done in less time, leaving me time to chat, watch movies, *without* teenage distractions."

Call me a humorless wet blanket, but that is just all kinds of wrong. There's the mutual deception, the unwholesome attitude toward work versus play, the love of downloaded movies above all else—I could go on. But most of all, because I'm familiar with the high stakes of the teenage years, and the need our teens still have for us—our time, interest, engagement—it's the mother's characterization of her son as "teenage distraction" that strikes me as most unfortunate. Her last line is, "…and it's affordable for our family." I wonder if she is aware that the costs of a technologically splintered family are quite likely higher than $14.95 per month. While Poplawski reassures parents like McGlaughlin, who work at reaching reasonable, healthy compromises to total media moratoria, that they needn't endure chronic guilt or fear of impending disaster—especially when there are other wholesome influences in the child's life—his conclusion from years of clinical experience and research is, "Media and commercialism are the most common culprits in stealing the innocence of children in stable families." He finds that when media is present in the home,

> something quite subtle may be compromised in the development of the child. Roberto Trostli is a Waldorf teacher and Waldorf teacher trainer who has taken several classes through the upper elementary grades. He comments that among graduating eighth graders, he can tell which ones still have little or no exposure to media. They are the students with the most capacity for imagination. They are the self-starters and the children in the class with the most initiative.[18]

This speaks directly to Gen Peace qualities, of course, and does also raise the reasonable question of just how long parents should seek to shelter their children from the omnipresent media. Poplawski writes:

> Almost all teachers feel that there should be no media at all before age seven. Some put this at age nine. Many then are willing to countenance judicious use of television between ages nine and twelve, with parents selecting the programs and, ideally, watching along with their children. Many teachers feel that after the onset of adolescence, at

around age thirteen, the young person should have freedom in this area but also the benefit of parental guidance. Individual differences should be taken into account. For a very sensitive child of nine or ten, or older, even relatively benign classic family films like "The Wizard of Oz" or "The Sound of Music" may not be appropriate.

This is where knowledge of your own unique child is invaluable, knowledge you've been cultivating since he began fluttering in your womb or wriggling in your arms. Children at this age are avid for stories, for meaning, for richness of imagination in their activities. Keep the bedtime books, stories and songs coming! For the child of this age, fairy tales are some of the most richly nourishing stories—but the real ones, not the prettied-up, pasteurized ones.

Parents typically recoil when I suggest they read their children Grimm's fairy tales; the idea of regaling their children with stories of orphans and witches, kidnappings and murders—at *bedtime* no less—is daunting, understandably. As parents we tend to want to present something of a Hallmark world to our children, so we naturally gravitate to soothing, sunny, children's books, including denatured versions of fairy tale classics. Wishing to shield them from the darker aspects of humanity, such as anger, greed, anguish, and cruelty, we wean our children on the proposition that people are all good. The problem is that even the youngest child knows differently in her heart of hearts, and the incongruence between what we—the ones they trust to be all-knowing—present them and what they instinctively and intuitively know—that there *are* negative human aspects—breeds insecurity and distrust.

Unlike most contrived screened fare that features gratuitous expressions of violence with little moral context, fairy tales have been carefully honed with meticulous attention to the meaning of every image and act. The early crafters of these tales had the wisdom and vision to know what they were tapping into and accentuating. Fairy tales are universal, and engage deeply with the archetypes of the human psyche. The aim of much of today's media violence is simply to grab the viewer's attention, frequently without much context or resolution, while the confrontation between good and evil in fairy tales is designed to address the knowing children possess within—that there is dark and light within each of us—and to show them the triumph of forces of light, goodness, kindness, courage. And yes, many tales include brutal scenes, but unlike electronic media programmers, a child's own waking mind will not create an image that's intolerable to her psyche.

"Good-day, Little Red Cap," he said.
"Thank you kindly, wolf."
"Whither away so early, Little Red Cap?"
"To my grandmother's."

All children struggle with psychic pressures of various kinds—inner impulses of the soul that are a natural part of growing and developing through each stage of life. The anger and other inner impulses they sometimes have toward us can feel desperately frightening to them, so huge that they don't know what to do with them. If we as parents offer them nothing that suggests that we recognize and sanction these powerful forces, both light and dark, children may expend precious life force repressing them. When we gift our children with fairy tales, we offer them an exquisite mirror in which to meet themselves, material to give "life to the power of imagination lightly dreaming beneath the intellectual layer of consciousness, powers which are already there pressing for development."[19]

> The wolf thought to himself: "What a tender young creature! what a nice plump mouthful—she will be better to eat than the old woman. I must act craftily, so as to catch both."

True fairy tales don't offer a fairy-behind-every-flower sentimentality of life, but rather a highly imaginative, symbolic yet unambiguous world that ingeniously provides a home for the child's deepest soul stirrings, a crucible through which the child, unconsciously, becomes conversant with and gains mastery over inner conflicts. Courage is emphasized, together with growth of the tale's protagonist, and good always triumphs in the end. After hearing her first fairy tale—"Little Red Cap"—one mother's four-year-old daughter, with eyes very wide, declared, "Mommy, this is a very important book." "Why, love?" "Because there is *danger!*"

> And then he said, "See, Little Red Cap, how pretty the flowers are about here—why do you not look round? I believe, too, that you do not hear how sweetly the little birds are singing; you walk gravely along as if you were going to school, while everything else out here in the wood is merry."

Typically, a child will gravitate to her favorite tale and ask for that one on a recurring basis. When this happens you needn't consciously understand what it is about the story that speaks to her—just know that it does, in most nourishing ways! Indeed, it is important, in giving our child the gift of a fairy tale, that we not explain its meaning, which robs the child of the experience of bringing his own soul and imaginative forces to the subliminal task of sussing out its particular relevance to him. Nor that we give him pat, definitive answers ("No, sweet face, there's no such thing as giants or witches or Rumpelstilt-skins") and thereby defuse the tale's power to enchant, and to inspire the child toward weaving individual solutions to her unique dilemmas.

> "Lift the latch," called out the grandmother, "I am too weak, and cannot get up."

Herein lies a fundamental irony in the parenting norms of society today: we profess our desire to protect our children from the vagaries of knowing too much too soon about troubling aspects of the real world (and thus recoil at the idea of Grimm's grim tales) while at the same time hurrying them in myriad other ways into that same adult world! We must not let our parental responsibility as authoritative guides veer toward the wayside as kids press to participate in society's rapid recruitment of children into all things adult, including clothing, media, and bedtimes, using such time-honored lobbying tactics as "But everyone's wearing / doing / getting it!"

Aside from media and other popular culture, perhaps nowhere will your mettle as a hero for your child be called upon more intensely as when you embark on one of the most all-encompassing series of parenting choices ever: school.

The Challenge of Formal Education

Children's immediate environment—which includes their parents—is their primary educational experience, and here they've already learned some of their most foundational lifelong lessons. But second only to home life, school represents the most pervasively influential element in the life of a child from age six or seven, until eighteen (and maybe beyond). Starting then, a child spends more weekly waking hours at school than at home. The goal of any enlightened curriculum should be to educate youth toward becoming confident, effective adults in a rapidly changing world, capable of discernment, independent thinking, and ethical leadership, equipped to creatively adapt and thrive in whatever circumstances the future may hold. To what extent can parents who have been dedicated to nurturing a peacemaker expect that their child's school will pick up the baton—will continue to foster these capacities, skills and qualities needed for socially adept, intelligent, innovative and interested citizens?

To make our way toward a meaningful answer, I'll do what I always told my children when they were tackling a paper on an unwieldy topic, something taught me by one of my professors: start with your reader at the beginning, and tell them an interesting story. I hope to keep this overview a brief but interesting story—and I am indebted to others more knowledgeable than me on the subject for much of what I'm about to relate.

Recall Dotty Coplen's quotation from the introduction, "The more we understand about the future consequences of what we are doing, and the intent that goes with the action, the more successful we will be in caring for our children with our own purposes and goals of parenting in mind."[20] If you replace the word *parenting* with the word *education,* it opens an avenue for exploring what has gone so horribly wrong with education today. What *was* the purpose of universal, compulsory education, and what have been the consequences?

In 1837, American politician Horace Mann accepted the position of secretary of the newly created Massachusetts board of education because it was a good job that paid well. Now widely regarded as the father of American public education, Mann had not had any special interest in education prior to taking that position. But he dove into the job with passion, even spending his own money to travel to Europe and study their schools. It was the Prussian schooling model that most impressed him—particularly the obedience of the children—and Mann was instrumental in importing that model to America.[21] His stated ideals for nonsectarian public education were noble enough—diversity, egalitarianism, the elevation of the citizenry through eliminating ignorance, and social harmony. But one of his primary objectives for education—to turn the nation's "unruly youth" into disciplined, judicious citizens of the republic—truly paved the way for America's emulation of the Prussian model, which featured compulsory attendance, special training for teachers (a totally new concept), national testing of all students (used to classify them for potential job training), national standardized curriculum by grade, and mandatory kindergarten.

This new model that had been devised in Prussia (now roughly East Germany) in the mid-eighteenth century taught citizens the skills (reading, writing, arithmetic) they needed as workers in the emerging industrial age, and also strict rules of ethics, duty, discipline and obedience. The Prussian kings' motives in fostering this first tax-funded education in the world was not only to erode powerful Lutheran influence; it was to shift the locus of political control away from a small group of powerful aristocrats, over to a general population indoctrinated into complete obedience of the state (the King): an illusion of democracy designed to gain complete control. An elite group decided what would be taught, all of it steeped in state ideology. According to legal philosopher Michiel Visser, "Every individual had to become convinced, in the core of his being, that the King was just, his decisions always right, and the need for obedience paramount."[22] The most compliant would be able to climb the totalitarian ladder and get the best jobs in the military or in state bureaucracy. In summer the school children were released to help their parents with the harvest.

Many commentators and critics of modern education have pointed out that this model well served an America on the brink of the industrial revolution: an abundant supply of factory workers were needed, with enough basic skills to perform their tasks, but who had also been trained through eight years of compulsive schooling to willingly, even happily, fall in conforming lockstep as obedient, regimented cogs in the assembly line. Indeed, the image and function of school *as* assembly line has persisted since those early days of Horace Mann and his infatuation with all things Prussian. Education professor Linda Darling-Hammond observes, "...the short segmented tasks stressing speed and neatness that predominate in most schools, the emphasis on rules from the important to the trivial, and the obsession with bells, schedules, and time clocks are all dug deep into the ethos of late-nineteenth-century America, when students were being prepared to work in factories on predetermined tasks *that would not require them to figure out what to do.*"[23]

The Prussian model of regimentation and obedience was further shaped to industrialist America's needs by men not normally mentioned in the lauded histories of egalitarian education, such as human productivity efficiency engineer Frederick Taylor, and the psychologist Wilhelm Wundt, whose research into "how the human machine was best adjusted" laid the groundwork for the behaviorism of Pavlov, Skinner and Watson (as well as such "machine adjustments" as the lobotomy and electro-shock therapy). Writes prominent public school critic (and former award-winning public school teacher)* John Taylor Gatto of Wundt's insidious contribution to the foundations of American education:

> A friendless, loveless, childless male German calling himself a psychologist set out, I think, to prove his human condition didn't matter because feelings were only an aberration. His premises and methodology were imported into an expanding American system of child confinement and through that system disseminated to administrators, teachers, counselors, collegians, and the national consciousness.[24]

Gatto further points out the unsettling premise that since the ideal employees of industrialized America were those who *specialize* their efforts in one aspect of systematized production, "*incomplete people* make the best corporate and government employees....And if that is so, mutilation in the interests of later social efficiency has to be one of the biggest tasks assigned to forced schooling."

Let's stop and just catch our breath for a moment. This is intense stuff. School as we've always known it is a thread so centrally woven into the cultural fabric of American life, that it's largely accepted without notice or question. We haven't really paid it that much mind. Yes, there have been notable surges of government-sponsored reform attempts, such as Bush's No Child Left Behind debacle, and the scourge it delivered upon children and teachers in the name of reform—high-stakes testing. (In a particularly frustrated moment I once ended a letter to the editor with the comment, "Yes, 'No Child Left Behind' is a catchy slogan, but given our bleak youth statistics, *where is it that we're taking them?*")

Before that came the Reagan era's 1983 *A Nation At Risk* report, kicking off a series of education reform efforts at local, state and federal levels, which in hindsight look like frantic, ineffectual tail-chasing. It was this report's bleak assessment of the "rising tide of mediocrity" in our school system that planted

---

* Gatto was named New York City Teacher of the Year in 1989, 1990 and 1991, and New York State Teacher of the Year in 1991 as well. Later in 1991, Gatto famously publicly resigned in the form of a letter published in the Op-Ed pages of the *Wall Street Journal* entitled "I Quit, I Think," saying that he no longer wished to "hurt kids to make a living."

the first seeds of public disenchantment with public education, and the enduring perception that the system is deeply flawed.

Prior to that, the first big educational reform movement of our modern era—after a hundred years of relatively complacent uptake of the Prussian-with-a-side-of-behaviorism model—took place in the 1960s. Tufts child psychologist David Elkind points out that it came in response to two unrelated driving forces: Sputnik and the civil rights movement. The fact that the Russians put a satellite in space before we did sent the U.S. government into a tailspin of humiliated determination: we were going to fix our education system—particularly its coverage of math and science—so we would never be outdone again![25] The curriculum enrichment adjustments took place at mostly college and university levels.

In the same era, the civil rights movement for the first time starkly highlighted the disproportionately poor school performance of disadvantaged children. Frustrated teachers said it was not their fault; these children had missed out on the kinds of learning-readiness experiences enjoyed at home by middle- and upper-middle-class children. This resulted in perhaps the most visible, enduring fixture to come out of the reform movement—Head Start.[26] But notably, this was an enrichment that addressed the other end of the school spectrum—preschool. Primary education was the ignored middle child that persisted unchanged, adrift on the "tide of mediocrity."

Twenty-seven years later, in the same week I drafted these pages, Oprah featured the documentary *Waiting for Superman* and is using her considerable cultural clout to call for America to sit up and take notice of the crisis in our educational system, calling it the most serious problem facing our country right now. So here we are, now in the second year of Obama's Race to the Top, and many of the same old problems are being raised as if they are new—leading historically observant onlookers to recognize this as the doomed Sisyphean task it is. And meanwhile, American students continue to circle the drain.

Our lagging world rank in college graduates and the ominous implications for future U.S. viability as leaders in intellectual, corporate or technological innovation; the ludicrous teacher tenure system that allows egregiously ineffective teachers to keep their jobs forever; heartrending scenes of eager young learners whose educational destinies rely on the pull of a lottery number—these are the top problems being discussed. Meanwhile, two currently proposed approaches to reform are longer school days and shorter vacations. It reminds me of the old joke about the crotchety couple complaining at the restaurant they keep returning to: "The food is so bad," she says, to which he replies, "Yes, and the portions are so small!"

> *It is nothing short of a miracle that the modern methods of instruction have not yet entirely strangled the holy curiosity of inquiry.*
>
> —ALBERT EINSTEIN

There seems to be a stultifying impasse at work: the school system is broken, and has been for at least fifty years, and yet we are somehow convinced that we can remodel it into relevance—at a time when its Prussian roots have become staggeringly irrelevant to our individual and collective needs. What seems to be left out of the discussion is the glaring question, *Is this an education model that is fixable?* (The omission of this question seems all the more disingenuous when leading crusaders themselves often send their children to schools featuring *qualitatively* different models of education.) We might get further in our attempts at reform if we were to embrace the homely truth that, far from being ineffective, *our education system does exceedingly well what it was designed to do*: teach rudimentary basics to the masses, cultivate obedient dependence, and discourage the development of creative, original thought. It is in part the widening chasm between those objectives and the needs of today's students—preparing for tomorrow's world—that makes the crisis all the more urgent. Writes Visser:

> To think that the system of education is doing badly is to miss a crucial issue. Given the general unhappiness with the results of education, the system must be doing something wrong, although many seem to have difficulties articulating just what it is or what should be done about it. But by speaking of crisis, we obscure that the education system *is doing exactly what it was set up to do.* There is a crisis, yet one in the original meaning of the word, "the turning point for better or worse in an acute disease or fever." The education system today is best seen as in a state of acute disease (albeit one inflicted on purpose), the current moment as that point in time where the system must choose between change and collapse.[27]

Before I discuss ideas for parents who cannot wait out this educational impasse, let me add one other dimension of the issue, critical to Generation Peace: not only did America's Prussian-based education system turn out a willing, pliable work force, it also fostered the qualities needed for an eager, compliant *consumer* force. Remember, this was the early- and mid-twentieth century, the heyday of the industrial age and dawn of the television era. We were making stuff, and we needed people to buy it.

Veteran teacher-turned-reformer Gatto writes, "Since bored people are the best consumers, school had to be a boring place, and since childish people are the easiest customers to convince, the manufacture of childishness, extended into adulthood, had to be the first priority of factory schools."[28] He says that the original purposes of education—to make good people, good citizens, and enable each to maximize their particular talents—were long ago pushed to the extreme margins of the education agenda. (Indeed, when those learning experiences happen, for the lucky few, it is through the serendipitous fluke of one extraordinary teacher or the anomaly of one gifted administrator, not as a predictable feature of the system.)

Gatto contends that in meeting the unstated "fourth purpose" of education, school becomes "a servant of corporate and political management," just as it was in Prussian Germany. "The secret of commerce, that kids drive purchases, meant that schools had to become psychological laboratories where training in consumerism was the central pursuit." Gatto, speaking with the inside perspective of someone who taught in New York public schools for thirty years, suggests that this can only be achieved by

> isolating children from the real world, with adults who themselves were isolated from the real world, and everyone in the confinement isolated from one another. Only then could the necessary training in boredom and bewilderment begin. Such training is necessary to produce dependable consumers and dependent citizens who would always look for a teacher to tell them what to do in later life, even if that teacher was an ad man or television anchor.[29]

Indeed, Gatto contends that schools teach children a particularly insidious form of "self-confidence"—one that requires constant confirmation by experts; he calls it "provisional self-esteem." And the consumer issue has become even more glaring and in their faces in the past decade. Alfie Kohn, an outspoken critic of testing, wrote in a 2002 article that there are enough cozy corporate connections—for example, between makers of standardized tests, publishers of texts to *prep* for the standardized tests, and companies that score, evaluate and report on test results—to "keep conspiracy theorists awake through the night." But he suggests that the

> influence is even deeper, more complicated, and ultimately more dis-turbing than anything we might reveal in a game of connect the cor-porate dots. Schools—and, by extension, children—have been turned into sources of profit in several distinct ways. Yes, some corporations sell educational products, including tests, texts, and other curriculum materials. But many more corporations, peddling all sorts of products, have come to see schools as places to reach an enormous captive mar-ket. Advertisements are posted in cafeterias, athletic fields, even on buses. Soft drink companies pay off schools so that their brand, and only their brand, of liquid candy will be sold to kids. Schools are of-fered free televisions in exchange for compelling students to watch a brief current-events program larded with commercials, a project known as Channel One. (The advertisers seem to be getting their money's worth: researchers have found that Channel One viewers, as contrasted with a comparison group of students, not only thought more highly of products advertised on the program but were more likely to agree with statements such as "money is everything," "a nice car is more important than school," "designer labels make a differ-ence," and "I want what I see advertised."
>
> Even more disturbing than having public schools sanction and ex-pose children to advertisements is the fact that corporate propaganda is sometimes passed off as part of the curriculum. Math problems plug a particular brand of sneakers or candy; chemical companies distribute slick curriculum packages to ensure that environmental science will be taught with their slant.[30]

How Then Shall We Educate?

Every parent wants the best for their child, but one of the central problems of the persisting education crisis, as I see it, is agreeing on what *is* the best. At the heart of designing school curricula and ways of engaging children in those curricula, lay fundamental questions: *What do we want to accomplish in the education of our children? Who are our children, at age eight, age eleven, age fourteen? What is education?*

It wasn't until the public school system was firmly embedded in the American experience that the growing understanding of human development and psychology began to reveal ever more insights into those questions. For example, psychologist and philosopher John Dewey promoted progressive ideas on education that influenced many alternatives to the public system, which by his time, the early twentieth century, was a huge machine in full motion: difficult to redirect. Dewey objected to an overly content-centered model of education (the one used in public as well as many private schools), in which the sole focus is on the curriculum to be delivered, without the student being centrally engaged as a participant in the process: "...the child is simply the immature being who is to be matured; he is the superficial being who is to be deepened."[31] I fear that Dewey's characterization—meant to be pejorative—sadly overestimates the state of public education today, in which depth is sacrificed to the meet the breadth mandated by the "tough standards" movement, and superficiality is the means to survive the testing gauntlet.

> *You try to stuff as much information into your brain as possible. Then as soon as you're done with it, out it goes.*
> SAM, STUDENT INTERVIEWED IN *Race to Nowhere*

> *We need to redefine success for kids; it's got to be something we do together, as a society, almost as a movement. We need to really think, "What does it take to produce a creative, happy, motivated human being?"*
> KENNETH GINSBURG, MD, ADOLESCENT MEDICINE
> SPECIALIST INTERVIEWED IN *Race to Nowhere*

Dr. Ginsburg's comment captures a central, knotty problem with the schooling issue: virtually every choice in education rests on such fundamental values as how we define success. For that matter, what is happiness? Creativity? What exactly is meant by the term *potential* as in, "... helping students fulfill their full potential," a buzz phrase that surely appears in every public school's mandate, charter school's mission and private school's brochure? To tease out the values underlying many of the assumptions behind educational goals would constitute a life's work, but the important thing for our purposes is to recognize the very fact that values *are* centrally at work here, in a powerful yet largely invisible way. Ah, the pesky worldview crops up again. Even child development theory is laden with value choices; the theories took their shapes in response to the worldview of those formulating and following them. For example, although I agree with many of his fundamental ideas on education, Dewey was an atheist whose worldview was vigorously pragmatic; his guiding belief was that only scientific method could reliably increase human good. That's good information for me to have if a spiritual worldview is important to me and my child is attending a school with a Dewey-based curriculum.

I've Got Good News and Bleak News

No one has yet fully realized the wealth of sympathy, kindness and generosity hidden in the soul of a child. The effort of every true education should be to unlock that treasure.
                                        —EMMA GOLDMAN

What *should* parents want from education? It is not my aim to make suggestions for how to address this massive problem, but rather offer some thoughts for how parents for peace might proceed to pick their way through the wreckage. There are two central themes I don't hear addressed as of yet in the latest hubbub about the public school crisis, which represent the proverbial good news/bad news scenario for those who are parenting for peace.

The first theme is the critical importance of the years *before* school begins, and the optimal wiring of the young child's brain circuitry that needs to take place in order to truly prepare a child to further flourish through the school-age years and even in preschool. This is the good news for those parents embracing the steps and principles in this book: you are giving your child the gift of robustly developed brain structures, or as U.C. Berkeley professor Marian Diamond puts it, "the nerve cells and dendrites that can respond" to education. This means not only an intellectual responsiveness, but also the vital social and emotional responsiveness central to true learning. They are ready by this current "age of reason"—somewhere in the vicinity of seven, depending on the child— to enthusiastically devote themselves to the adventure of education.

And now the second central unaddressed theme in the uproar about the failure of public school—the question of *meaning*. And here, sadly, is the bleak news. A sure way to frustrate and ultimately alienate a child of any age is to inflict learning that lacks meaning, a fact that consistently remains unaddressed at the heart of our educational crisis. (Along with an apparent unawareness of the biological fact that all true learning takes place in the context of feeling safe, secure and in *relationship* with the teacher, and the subject matter.) Many children suffer having the wind knocked out of their natural learning impulses and affinities when they step into the regimented world of a school intent on imparting a series of facts to them.

Have you ever had a conversation with someone in which you were telling them about an experience that was very meaningful to you, and it was clear that they were simply waiting until you were finished with your story so that they could tell you what *they* wanted to say? That relational hollowness pervades many children's experience of school. It goes to the first of the seven Parenting for Peace principles, presence; the conventional public school curriculum—and by necessity the majority of teachers—aren't present to who children really are and what is important to them. John Dewey saw this problem a century ago, insisting that effective education presents material in a way that allows the student to relate the information to prior experiences and thereby form a deeper, more meaningful connection with their new knowledge.

Even (and perhaps especially) the most engaged, curious children who enter a standard school setting soon discover, as William Glasser wrote in his classic book *Schools Without Failure*, "that they must use their brains mostly for memorizing rather than exploring their interests, expressing their ideas, or solving problems. Even worse, much of what they are asked to memorize is irrelevant to their world."[32] Indeed, John Taylor Gatto's urgent call for reform in *Dumbing Us Down: The Hidden Curriculum of Compulsory Schooling* includes a confessional aspect in which he lists the seven principal (implicit) lessons he (and all other teachers and administrators) taught in public school, beginning with #1, which speaks to this issue of missing meaning:

> Confusion: I teach too much, and everything that I teach is out of context. The orbiting of planets, the law of large numbers, slavery, adjectives, architectural drawing, dance, gymnasium, choral singing, assemblies, surprise guests, fire drills, computer languages, parents'

nights, staff development days, pull-out programs…What do any of these things have to do with each other?

…Fortunately the children have no words to define the panic and anger they feel at the *constant violations of natural order and sequence* fobbed off as quality in education.[33]

For something to be meaningful, it needs to have context—a perceptible way in which facts and ideas relate to each other, and to the student, in order to create a whole picture. Facts, figures, dates out of context hold little meaning for students; thus we see a program introduced in New York City that *pays* fourth-graders to do their homework, so uncompelled are they by the curriculum!

Gatto contends that this disengagement is tacitly encouraged; third on his list of things he was required to teach in public school reads, "Indifference: I teach children not to care too much about anything, even though they may desire to do so."[34] How do students respond to this lack of relevance and meaning? In myriad ways, of course. I imagine that many do as I did years ago, as a model public school student, what I had always done since my earliest days of life—rapidly figured out what I was expected to do and to be, and allowed myself to be lulled into thinking that was indeed me. Glasser mentions another possibility: "Often, their reaction to this is either social withdrawal or destructive anger." Neither of these postures is what we seek for a generation of peacemakers.

> *Ever wonder why we go to school?…It's societies'[sic] way of turning all young people into good little robots and factory workers, that's why we sit on desks in rows and go by bell schedules, to prepare for the real world, cuz "that's what it's like."*
>
> FROM THE JOURNAL OF ERIC HARRIS,
> COLUMBINE SCHOOL SHOOTER

Glasser's observations, written thirty years ago, sadly still hold true today—now abetted by the steroidal impact of high-stakes testing and the so-called accountability movement. Diane Ravitch, one of the nation's most respected education historians and a conservative on education issues, was one of the most vocally enthusiastic supporters of Bush's *No Child Left Behind*. But she wrote in her 2010 book, *The Death and Life of the Great American School System,* that after five years she deemed it a "failure," because it "ignored the importance of knowledge. It promoted a cramped, mechanistic profoundly anti-intellectual definition of education." (Not to put too fine a point on it, but here again, the architects of the Prussian model would be thrilled with such an evaluation; it's exactly what they were after.)

> *The aim of totalitarian education has never been to instill convictions, but to destroy the capacity to form any.*
> HANNAH ARENDT

If there's an upside to the testing debacle, it's that it has thrown into bolder relief central aspects of conventional schooling that have always existed; now they are magnified, intensified, easier for discerning parents to see. The conventional, materialist (where the focus is primarily on the *material* to be conveyed) model has never warmly welcomed the more intangible phenomena of experiential learning—such as the leaping of a child's wonderment at the sight of a shooting star or a starfish. A lucky student might once have happened onto a teacher who took a few extra moments to indulge a child's unique perspective or flight of fanciful imagination. But high-stakes testing eliminated that luxury, and all such organic learning was rendered quaintly irrelevant to "real" education—that which can be quantified, graphed and replicated—which teachers have to install in students under the threat of lost ranking, jobs and district funding if test scores are low. The banking model of education has prevailed, in which we deposit information into young minds, and then withdraw proof of our work with multiple-choice tests. Children (to the anguish of many frustrated teachers) became, more than ever before, widgets on a factory assembly line, to be inspected at regular intervals for quality control. This stressful, dehumanizing approach, if not altogether responsible for, is fueling a crisis in American kids: ADD and other developmental and learning disorders, along with serious behavioral problems, are endemic, and the rates of childhood drug use, violence, depression and suicide keep rising.

Find a Good Lifeboat (or Build One)

In a talk he gave at his daughter's high school commencement, Joseph Chilton Pearce urged the graduates to not waste their time and talents trying to "save the ship of state," but rather to "become really good lifeboats." There is no magic guidance I can offer parents faced with the question of schooling, because circumstances differ so vastly for everyone. The best I can do is present some ideas for building a workable lifeboat for your child, while the ship of public education continues to list badly and take on more water.

Pearce has been at the forefront of optimal human development research for over thirty years, and is a vigorous yet thoughtful critic of education and its hampering impact on the unfolding of children's myriad innate intelligences—and not just public education but most conventional models of education. (Many private schools deliver a similar curriculum in similar ways as the public model, simply with more funds available for more embellishments and grace notes.) He considers Waldorf the best education model available. A quick history of Waldorf is relevant to the objectives of parenting for peace, as it embodies laudable educational principles, and may prove instructive when making choices toward schooling for peace.

In its roots we can see some rather startling alter-ego aspects of the Waldorf system as compared to the Prussian system. The first Waldorf school was founded as a literal factory school—to educate the children of the workers at the Waldorf-Astoria cigarette company in Stuttgart, Germany in 1919. The factory's owner Emil Molt was persuaded by his employees to open a school following a rousing talk that Rudolf Steiner had presented to them. Steiner, a philosopher and scientist, had pointed out to these factory workers that while their own futures were already constrained, those of their children could be vast and unlimited—providing that their schooling addressed their evolutionary potential. With WWI having ended just months earlier, Steiner had spoken of the need for a renewed social order, different ethics and less destructive ways of settling conflicts.

Contrasted with the Prussian kings' objectives of maintaining a proletariat workforce, Molt's goals were to offer his workers' children educational opportunities that could open doors to other, more satisfying life work. Twenty years later, on the cusp of WWII, Hitler shut down the original Stuttgart Waldorf school, along with six others that had since been established. The reason given by the state press was that Germany didn't have room for two kinds of education—one that educated citizens for the state, and another that taught children to think for themselves. Hitler's main objective for his young countrymen was that they be taught to obey.

An Education that Is Present with Students

Waldorf education is centered on the above-mentioned feeling intelligence—animated through the imagination. Steiner wrote, "The need for imagination, a sense of truth and a feeling of responsibility—these are the three forces which are the very nerve of education." Their teacher brings the material to students in a lively presentational way that stirs the imagination and fosters the capacity of feeling *for*.

Before developing his education model, Steiner had devoted himself to developing a penetrating understanding of how humans develop, particularly through childhood—and his insights bear a striking similarity to "new" findings that began coming one hundred years later, from current psychosocial research and neuro-imaging technologies. The Waldorf curriculum was meticulously devised to not only comprise a classical education over the eight primary years (plus four years of high school, available at some schools), but also offer children, at each age and stage, material that strikes a chord of deep recognition and appreciation in their souls as it relates to their own inner development.

For example, when they're in second grade and newly awakening to the positive and negative aspects of people and their foibles (including their own), they study fables from various cultures. The rich imagery of man's animal nature stirs their imaginations to plumb the basic questions of behavior and right and wrong without the morals being given to them. In the third grade children are navigating their first big milestone of individuation since age three, which can bring up fears and insecurities that come from feeling newly separate from a world that up till then they felt at one with. Studying about textiles, house-building and farming instills a timely reassurance in the nine-year-old that stability—shelter and nourishment—is always available, and even within their own power. In the sixth grade, as puberty approaches and they become more aware of their bodies, they study the body of the world in geology. One of the more subtle aspects of the children's changing bodies is a hardening of the bones, bringing a growing awareness of gravity and weight—and an inner affinity for the study of physics. In the eighth grade, everything within and without the student feels like it's in revolt; thus, they study revolutions of all kinds—for example, American, industrial, and social rights.

Students at each age feel met by the curriculum and in response reach out to meet it back. Waldorf families are typically spared those awful homework struggles many parents (and children) suffer through; students at a Waldorf school don't even have homework in the early years, and by the time they do begin bringing work home, they're excited and intrinsically motivated to engage with and accomplish it. (People rarely believe me when I say I never had to tell either of my kids to do their homework!) This is in large part because their education has daily relevance and meaning for them, and it's why Waldorf students have earned a reputation among a growing number of colleges as exceptionally creative and intellectually resourceful, and for becoming adults with a lifelong love of learning.

What I'm presenting here doesn't begin to approach an adequate summary of Waldorf education, which involves nuanced, profound layers and aspects; really understanding it would easily comprise yet another life's work. I've included resources for your own further research. Nor do I want to suggest that Waldorf is a sure-fire panacea. Although I can't really imagine a child for whom the *curriculum* would not be right;* but sometimes the tone and process of a certain class, teacher or school isn't a fit for a student, or perhaps for the student's parents. Waldorf is not without its own challenges, and, just as in the public system or any private school, there are subpar teachers and administrators to be found.

But Waldorf is the fastest-growing independent nonparochial education system in the world, and many Waldorf-inspired charter schools have entered the U.S. public system, suggesting that there is something of value to consider in its curriculum and its approach, especially given the goals of nurturing the creative, flexible intelligences and social adeptness of a future Generation Peace.

Suffering pangs of anxiety over how best to give their child a leg up in this highly competitive culture, parents who choose this education often do so largely in a leap of faith, based in their intuitive response to its countercultural proposition—Waldorf's central acknowledgement that children are not just mental beings to be filled up with facts, but that they are physical beings whose balance, coordination and agility must be fostered; emotional beings whose feeling for and wonder at the material quickens learning at a substantive level; and spiritual beings whose gradually unfolding expression requires more mind-

---

* One common criticism of the curriculum is that it is so heavily Eurocentric; teachers using Waldorf methods in public charter schools revise it to accommodate America's own literature as well as our multicultural population, as do many traditional private Waldorf schools.

ful attention than we typically recognize. For teachers this mindfulness is rooted in their own spiritual life.

The basis of one prominent line of criticism of Waldorf is, for many, one of its central strengths—its vibrant spiritual dimension. Steiner developed highly interdisciplinary guiding philosophies regarding the evolution of human consciousness, from his studies in anthropology, philosophy, psychology, the sciences, and various spiritual traditions, particularly esoteric Christianity.* He called his philosophical framework *anthroposophy*—a term that has been translated as "study of the spiritual nature of man," but which Steiner described simply as "awareness of one's humanity."

These spiritual principles are never shared with students; Waldorf teachers' rules forbid it. Rather, they're meant to inform, enliven, and uplift the teachers so that they can in turn inspire their students with the wonder and curiosity that animates profound learning. School-aged children and young adults respond largely to modeling as a potent (and largely unconscious) learning channel—a fact that is under-recognized in our education culture. As a Waldorf parent I was often moved by the level of attention that teachers devoted to authentically presenting themselves as worthy models for their students.

Educating Toward an Awareness of Humanity

Subjects as diverse as knitting, languages, and music—wind and string instruments, and choral singing—that have been taught for one hundred years in Waldorf education, are just now being recognized to foster aspects of brain development central to Generation Peace capacities. More robust connections between left and right brain hemispheres and increased brain mass support the flourishing of empathy, creativity and high-intelligence "possibility thinking."

Foundations for moral and ethical intelligence are laid through the teacher telling stories that engage the students at each particular stage—in first grade through fairy tales and their archetypal enactment of good and evil; in second grade, animal fables and legends of saints; in third grade, Biblical stories and American Indian stories; and on through Norse, Greek and Arthurian mythologies and historical tales rife with heroes and victims, chivalry and villainy. In his *Atlantic Monthly* article Todd Oppenheimer wrote:

---

* All major religions have *ex*oteric (outer, visible) and *eso*teric form (inner, unseen)—such as Judaism's Kabbalah, Islam's Sufism, and Christianity's Gnosticism.

Waldorf's philosophy of teaching through living out stories may be unusual, but it comes out of a long tradition, from the folkways of ancient cultures to the modern-day theories of child psychologists… such as Bruno Bettelheim and Robert Coles. In his well-known books on the development of a moral and spiritual intelligence in children, Coles stresses an immersion in moral stories. Waldorf teachers go even further.

They believe that when students go through school without such stories, their ability to develop a sense of empathy is inhibited, and that limits their capacity to find meaning in life. Pointing to the psychologist Jean Piaget's famous theories about a youngster's gradual stages of development, Waldorf teachers argue that traditional schools aggravate this problem by imposing intellectual demands on students before they're ready for them. This only discourages youngsters, they say, leaving them prone to become unfeeling but clever cynics or, worse, simply apathetic.[35]

Snapshots of Two Schooling Paradigms

The ideal would be that parents could simply choose an education for their child that aligns with their worldview and values. But that's not always an easy call—certainly financially but also conceptually. I remember when we had first moved out of the city, into a school district that touted some of the highest test scores in the state and an award-winning primary school. Even as we were proudly mentioning this to family and friends, I became vaguely uneasy, as I felt the stirrings of an awareness in me that went something like this: "Even the highest scores on measures that don't mean much to me, don't mean much." That was certainly inconvenient, since we had just made a major commitment to building a house and putting down stakes in a wonderful rural community. I tried not to know what I knew deep down, hoping the whole conflict might all just evaporate!

The descriptions of various approaches to education can be framed in such ambiguous, abstract terms that they all sound wonderful and are sometimes difficult to distinguish from one another. Terms like *child-centered* and *hands-on learning* are ubiquitous and therefore almost meaningless to parents trying to suss out the real deal. One of the most helpful clarifying stories came to me from a friend whose son had been in Waldorf kindergarten but who was hoping that the local public school would work for him. She sat in on the first grade class at both schools on consecutive days in the first week, and through a wonderful stroke of synchrony she witnessed a lesson on the letter M at each school. (This was over fifteen years ago; now, of course, the letter M would be old news by public first grade!) Here is roughly how it went:

At the Waldorf school, the teacher stood before the class and began a story in a voice suggesting big adventure, enunciating each word clearly, knowing that her speech as well as her attitude serves as a strong example for her students' learning. Slowly drawing a big capital M on the board with colored chalk, she said, "Here we have the two tall *mmmm*ountains...with a deep valley in the middle. And then not far away," (as she drew a small m on the board) "are the smaller foothills of the mountains, with the softly rounded *mmm*mounds of soft grass...and the children of the village loved to roll down them..."

In the lesson at her son's public first grade, the teacher said to the students, drawing the M on the board, "Line up, line down, line up, line down—now you try."

Oppenheimer gives an example of Waldorf's "old-fashioned but increasingly rare practice: allowing time for reflection":

> Science classes are an example. In the average school, teachers introduce a concept first and then do a demonstration or an experiment to illustrate it. "It takes the kid out of it," Mikko Bojarsky, the science teacher at the Sacramento Waldorf School, told me. Waldorf teachers turn this process around, doing an experiment before giving the concept much discussion. "Then you let it go to bed for the night," Bojarsky said. "They literally sleep on it. A lot happens in their sleep life." The next day, he said, students generally come in with many more questions than they had the day of the experiment, often including some the teacher never considered. "Nowadays we always push people to think so fast, instead of letting them reflect," Bojarsky continued. The process institutionalizes an important principle that evades many a teacher—to let students struggle toward their answers and individual understanding. "One of the things I had to learn," Bojarsky said, "was to not answer their questions, especially in the twelfth grade. If you give them answers, they'll just shut down. It's amazing what they'll come up with if you wait long enough."[36]

I witnessed a vivid example of the primacy of material over meaning one afternoon in the waiting room at our daughter's orthodontist's office. A mother was working with her young son—maybe age six or seven—in a workbook entitled *Math Made Easy*. The mother read the instructions aloud: "Rank these on the probability scale: 'Impossible' 'Poor Chance' 'Even Chance' 'Good Chance' and 'Certain.' Here's an example: 'It will get dark tonight,'" to which the son accurately answered, "Certain."

Mom: "I'll get a heads when I flip this coin."

Son: "Even chance."

Mom: "Abraham Lincoln will come for dinner."

Son: "Impossible. *Unless* it was back in the time when he lived...*then*—"

Mom (laughing, but cutting him off) "Okay, next one...."

My heart cramped to see this young boy's natural impulse toward curiosity, wonder, and imagination squashed like a pesky gnat, and I wondered how many times this happened to him, and to his peers, every day. If only their parents knew that this causes deep suffering to children, in their soulful need to inhabit knowledge via many pathways—most of all, imagination.

I'm not suggesting that Waldorf is the only viable alternative to a conventional education, public or private—just that its principles and intention trace a visibly worthwhile shape for consideration within a peaceful parenting framework. Its curriculum probably sets the bar for developmental sensitivity at every level—and yet, other schools with developmentally appropriate curricula can certainly be found here and there around the world. Hopefully we will soon begin seeing more such schools within the public charter system, so this isn't so much of a class issue. Despite Waldorf's history of robust tuition assistance programs to reflect their dedication to diversity—like that of so many private schools—the education is still unavailable to huge swaths of middle-class families who cannot afford it and yet don't qualify for scholarships.

Some Thoughts on Alternatives

One type of educational alternative is represented by such schools as the Brooklyn and Manhattan Free Schools,[37] and Sudbury Valley School in Massachusetts. In these schools there is no curriculum (students "explore the world freely, at their own pace and in their own unique ways"), no teachers (through "self-initiated activities, they pick up the basics; as they direct their lives, they take responsibility for outcomes, set priorities, allocate resources, and work with others") and children age five through eighteen are in charge of their own time and their own activities. The fact that there is a long waiting list for the Brooklyn Free School, of students whose parents are desperate for an alternative to the testing nightmare, is testament to the dire need for parents to understand the spectrum of needs of children and teens, and the appropriate role of freedom in their development.

Based on A.S. Neill's Summerhill School in England, these approaches don't address a comprehensive array of children's developmental needs. While this free-school model has its roots in admirably humanistic impulses, including a rebellion against the regimented, conformist British schooling model, and the desire to liberate children from the often abusive realm of adult authority in early twentieth-century England, I suggest that it risks throwing the pupil out with the (admittedly very dirty) bathwater of conventional education. I don't doubt that in the early 1900s Summerhill represented the best—and in some cases lifesaving—alternative for some children to public schooling, but today we have a far more nuanced understanding of child development and a far more sophisticated application of it toward far more fruitful alternatives.

While I embrace John Taylor Gatto's perceptive articulation of the public school disaster, I don't subscribe to his embrace of these schools—which I believe foster the erosion of childhood itself, through what Neil Postman called the "de-differentiation" of children and adults: everyone is equal at Summerhill, five-year-olds and grownups alike. While I'm not exhaustively familiar with the model, and remain open to being persuaded that such an unstructured, self-mediated approach *may* be workable for older students,* I know as a development specialist that structure, predictability, and rhythm impart a level of security to the young child that allows him or her the level of neurobiological relaxation necessary for true learning to take place. I have to wonder if the supposed freedom granted by these free-range learning environments doesn't constrain young students with different kinds of limitation—the anxiety and subsequent defenses that arise *within* when they are left to educationally, experientially, and attentionally fend for themselves.

Also, learning is an *attachment-based process*, grounded in relationship—but much of the learning in these schools is self-directed and self-mediated.

---

* It might take quite a bit to convince me that playing video games all day—if they so choose—would be conducive to the qualities and capacities hoped for in a generation of peacemakers.

The websites of all these schools feature descriptions that would easily impress readers who aren't fluent in these understandings and—equally important—who have not clarified for themselves what their own educational values are for their children.

I also want to mention the option of homeschooling for parents who want to embrace an alternative educational model but for financial or geographical reasons cannot attend such a school. Curriculum materials for myriad alternative educational systems are available for homeschooling use, and the statistics coming out of the growing homeschool movement consistently show homeschooled students at higher levels across many measures of achievement and wellbeing.[38] Of course homeschooling relies heavily upon the teacher—you—but homeschoolers across the country have a growing array of collective resources available to them at the community level; many people establish cooperatives whereby different people serve as teachers for different subjects, for example. Field trips and other group learning experiences are becoming ever more available for homeschoolers.

Aside from his endorsement of Summerhill-based schools, John Taylor Gatto suggests that one remedy to the education crisis is for children to spend less time in school, and more time spent with family and "in meaningful pursuits in their communities"; he also advocates apprenticeships and homeschooling as a way for children to learn—all propositions I would agree with. The key to homeschooling, as with any form of education you choose, is to really do your homework about the conceptual and philosophical underpinnings of the curriculum you want to engage in with your children.

Home Learning

Regardless of where your child goes to school, the home remains a primary wellspring of learning. You have plenty of opportunities to enrich and support your child through the school experience whether or not it's an ideal one; indeed, there are many ways to contextualize, bring more meaning to, and attenuate the stultifying, stressing impact of a conventional materialist curriculum.

Rhythmicity and simplicity – Even as your children grow beyond the early years, let this become a mantra, because at every age—into adulthood—both these principles continue to be great sources of strength, security and center-ing. They're especially important for a child who is feeling the stress of a heavy homework load, together with pressures of extracurricular activities such as music lessons or sports; or a second- or third-grader whose sensory field is overwhelmed by a frenetic playground or the visual bombardment from the typical array of posters, letters, and other wall coverings in many classrooms, or simply the pace of activity.

An ideal curriculum includes a nourishing daily rhythmicity as well as an overall balance of academics, arts, music and physical activity, but if your child's life cannot include all of these due to the high demands of one or an-other of these elements (usually academic), it is best to see to it that the sheer number of the child's commitments are kept manageable—that her life is sim-plified. She may resist you on this; our current culture of overachievement has a certain allure. Many kids today, particularly in high school, load up with in-volvements and responsibilities, partly in response to the intense pressures they feel from parents who want them to succeed in the highly competitive college application gauntlet but also partly because their industrialist culture has taught them to find a kind of high from all that achieving and producing. In-deed, adrenaline and other stress chemicals can (at first) make a person feel so…alive. But as compellingly portrayed in the 2009 documentary film *Race to Nowhere*, too many of America's youth are burning out as the long-term neurotoxic effects of adrenaline and other corticosteroidal stress hormones wreak their havoc on the growth-versus-protection orientation of a child's being: they suffer debilitating stress, anxiety disorders, and depression.

Of course it will be easier to chart a course of balance for our children if we as parents aren't setting an example of overextending ourselves in a whirl of professional, social, charity and school commitments! Setting a calm tone for the day with a few minutes together at the breakfast table can work near miracles; it's worth getting up fifteen minutes early for. Remember, a candle during the winter months when it's still dark in the morning, helps children carry that cozy, soothing atmosphere of nurturance and beauty with them into their school day. Leaving media out of the morning routine also helps to set a healthier, more supportive tone for the day. And if you do spend time in a car going to school with children, embrace that as a chance for conversation and even singing; particularly when you have a carpool with a gaggle of different ages, what a rich time that can be.

Stories and meaning – It is from stories, and the feeling intelligence they stir in the child, that all action of authentic learning finds its genesis. Story is so often missing in most education, so you can become a story weaver at home to fertilize and enliven a topic your child is being taught in school. At this age, it is of key importance that stories include a positive option even in the face of great challenge or peril. Of particular value are stories about the lives of people who've accomplished something outstanding; enriching biographies that would complement world or American history, physics, literature, medicine or mathematics include Copernicus, Galileo, Magellan, Joan of Arc, Jacques Lusseyran, Gandhi, Martin Luther King, Thomas Edison, Marie Curie, Henry David Thoreau, Ralph Waldo Emerson, Victor Frankl, Orville and Wilbur Wright, John Ericsson, Ross Adey and so many more. Consider as a family ritual watching CNN's weekly feature about their hero of the week or ABC's Person of the Week. Here is an example of how television can offer us, if we're mindful, a resource rather than an impediment—to awaken in children of all ages an echo of transcending limitations into vaster possibilities.

To help provide the kind of nourishing curricular continuity and context found in many Waldorf classes (learning history, geography, art and literature in the context of Greek or Norse myths for instance, and in such interdisciplinary high school classes as History through Music), the bedtime story or weekend trip to the museum can be an opportunity to add a bit of thematic connectivity and relevance to the child's world. In his seminal book *Teaching as a Subversive Activity*, Neil Postman wrote, "In order to survive in a world of rapid change there is nothing more worth knowing, for any of us, than the continuing process of how to make viable meanings."[39] Dinner table conversation is always an opportunity to weave cohesion and meaning into what might be disparate subjects your children are studying: "What do you think Plato would say about global warming?" Postman suggested that "the art and science of asking questions is the source of all knowledge. *Any* curriculum of a new education would, therefore, have to be centered around question asking," and in his book are three pages of thoughtful questions rich enough to serve as the basis for years of meaningful learning.[40] In the Waldorf high school curriculum a fundamental cohering question weaves through all the subjects, beginning with "What?" in 9th grade, then "How," "Why?" and finally, "Who?" in the senior year.

Questions and stories can enrich such seemingly straightforward subjects as arithmetic as well. A recent NPR radio story about children and math pointed out that typically a child can readily enough memorize the numbers and learn basic math processes, but when teachers and parents put those numbers in a context—"There are six apples in the basket and four children each take an apple, how many are left?" or counting pebbles or acorns or cars rather that just manipulating the abstract symbol of numbers—their math and associated cognitive skills are enhanced in the moment and also enriched with long-lasting benefits of greater layers of understanding.

Presence and process over product – The mother of two Waldorf school graduates shared her reflections on one aspect she felt made it particularly unique in cultivating a deep inner security and poise in students, from which we might take a helpful cue:

> Waldorf is very process oriented. In most schools, the product is what matters—having reports, projects, and paintings to show the parents is a fundamental part of the mindset. Did you ever see the paintings of our kids in the early grades? Not so much, because it was process, the relationship of color and value that they were experiencing. The teachers never made a big deal about the gorgeous lions they knitted, or bags they embroidered, because that was never the point. Parents of kids in any school might try to hold to that and not focus on the final result of their kids' projects. There's a standing joke amongst public school fifth grade parents about how much work their sugar cube Mission project is. You'd see the architectural creations lined up in the local library or school on parents' night and too many of them were perfect! It would be so helpful if parents could somehow resist that instinct and let the student experience the construction himself (of course the parent should be interested, just not so focused on the end result). Our culture gets so competitive in public and private schools, and it's really hard to buck when that's your world. If children don't have safe mistakes to learn from while they're young, it only gets trickier as they get older. It's just so sad that there's so much peer pressure to present "mistake free" work in this environment.[41]

Care for and feed imagination – Beginning at seven, children flourish in pursuing singing, drawing, painting, dance, so involve them in mindfully structured activities with art. If it appeals to you, and intrigues your child, go for it! In a world of so much technology, it will be ever more important that they a have robust ability to imagine (image-*in*, as opposed to the image-*out* process behind technoscreens of all kinds). Echoing Todd Oppenheimer on the intelligence technology industry, a friend tells me of seeing Lee Iacocca, the legendary industry leader who saved the Chrysler Corporation, interviewed on television in the 1990s, and of her delight in his response to the reporter's question, "When you hire a young professional, what qualities do you look for?" Iacocca answered that he did not care whether his prospective mentees had any technical expertise, because they would be taught and trained at Chrysler. He said he looked for some kind of creativity, imagination, and artistic discipline—that he needed them to be resourceful.

The early tendrils of what may emerge as their affinities for life work are an important aspect of imagination as your child approaches puberty and the teen years. These can be tended through exposure to a spectrum of ways in which people live, work and express their passionate calling. We want to listen to our children with an ear out for the ideals they might wish to embrace— a subtle art that takes into consideration both the egocentric and the altruistic aspects of this age. If your child shows an affinity for building or architecture, be sure she knows the story of Habitat for Humanity; if he's interested in healing arts, introduce him to Doctors Without Borders; if you have any budding entrepreneurs in your midst, regale them with stories of people like Blake Mycoskie and utter cool of his TOMS Shoes One-for-One movement (for each pair sold, a pair is given to a needy child); and a would-be financier or banker should know about such inspiring new-paradigm organizations as Kiva Microfunds.

It's encouraging for idealistic youth (which they naturally are, and need to be allowed to be) to see that there are many ways to use one's beauty and intelligence to the greater good in a sustainable way. It's possible to have a holistic career. They don't have to do it tomorrow, but to know that the possibility exists is of abiding nurturance. The voice and will of the collective is resonating more and more strongly, and those who are ready will listen and find their way to their Generation Peace calling.

With the stakes rising as the teen years loom, few things are more protective in the life of a youth than a high ideal together with passionate interests in the stuff of real life. This is another potent incentive to prolong the media moratorium to a large degree even past puberty. In his article "Push-Button Entertainment and the Health of the Soul," teacher Christopher Sblendorio points out the stark difference between students' real life engagement—which brings a "wealth of the soul" and deep inner peace—and the passive enthrall-ment with electronic entertainment, whereby their emotions are "elicited and manipulated (consciously and cleverly) from the outside." Further he has ob-served, "If we are constantly taking in external images and thoughts and strug-gling to digest them, our imagination, creativity, and capacity for empathy are being dulled."[42]

One great food for the imagination is travel. Up until now the young child's explorations are appropriately limited to the world of home, family and the small outer orbit included in her rhythmic weekly activities. At this age it's fruitful to cultivate the attitude of "One planet, one humanity—it's yours, discover it!" This can certainly be done through books or videos (another con-structive application of media), but a certain amount of actual travel is like a tonic. Travel can mean a simple camping trip, a road trip or a deluxe excur-sion—across the world or across town. We all live in or near cities rich with textural diversity we rarely take the time to explore. If this seems a daunting proposition, consider your inner work to be creating a shift, from "Let's be afraid" to "Let's be curious." Curiosity will define effective peacemakers, and as parents we need to model it.

Warm them up – I see a coolness epidemic hitting families everywhere, phys-ically, emotionally and relationally. One fairly straightforward way to add ease, comfort and security to your child's life is through warmth of all kinds. Aside from hot summer months, of course, keep your home warm. Along with invisible forced air from the furnace, burn candles, get the fireplace going and simmer something deliciously fragrant on the stove. (Never un-derestimate the powers of soup!) Make sure your child has soft, natural fiber shirts and sweaters she's inclined to put on; if you've been tending to her warmth by dressing her in layers all these years, she may carry on this whole-some habit. Either way, getting her a sweater or jacket she loves is a good in-vestment in her wellbeing.

Think in terms of warming up your child with the enveloping quality of your presence, your embracing tone of voice, the loving expressions on your face. Remember the power of touch. Learn the footbath ritual, and use it often. Whenever my daughter or I were feeling peaked, like we might be coming down with something, we'd take a footbath. (Much better than a whole body bath if you're feeling under the weather; it spares the body the cooling that happens after a bath or shower—and the energy drain of warming it up again—while warming the entire body.)

One of the most positive daily influences you can weave into the life of your child(ren) is the family's evening meal. Quite a bit of research has revealed dinners together to be one of the strongest predictors of everything from better school performance to fewer eating disorders to lowered risk for engaging in risky behaviors like drugs and alcohol;[43] when scrutinized further, it's not merely dinner together, but dinner together featuring vibrant conversation.[44] Earlier I mentioned saying a blessing before meals as one way to invite the child's dawning awareness of the vastness of our human family. It is also a way to add extra warmth to the experience of the family meal. A book such as *A Grateful Heart: Daily Blessings for the Evening Meal from Buddha to the Beatles* can offer you many choices regardless of your spiritual orientation. Here's a favorite of our family that Eve learned in the Waldorf kindergarten:

> *Before the flour the mill,*
> *before the mill the grain,*
> *before the grain,*
> *the sun, the earth, the rain:*
> *the beauty of God's will.*

Finding Peace in Extracurricular Activities

Brace yourself for one of the most countercultural points in this book: the organized competitive sports so popular today aren't necessarily the most nurturing choice parents can make for school-aged children (and certainly not younger—the truly appropriate time for team sports like soccer, softball, basketball and the like is high school). We're looking at the child's development as an organic and gradual series of unfolding intelligences—with the "feeling intelligence" center stage during these years. The guiding feeling principle behind organized children's sports programs can be seen as *ambition*, and it has an adultifying influence (except in the rare cases of those that are truly flexible and organically play-based, and keep the focus on the kids). Yes, the body wants and needs to move—to run, kick, throw, spin—and in freer forms of playful physical activity, or "less organized" organized games programs, the guiding feeling principle is joy at work—a healthier scaffolding for subsequent Generation Peace development.[45]

Many fine lines need to be navigated in making the choice to involve one's child in organized sports; thus, as with most every other aspect of parenting, it becomes an issue of our own self-discipline and inner mastery. If it's our motive to foster and support our child's natural impulse to develop physical skills and coordination, and to have fun, let's play with her! Kick and throw, play tag or Capture the Flag. If it's our motive to foster the kind of discipline, attention, and cooperation associated with team sports, it's helpful to recognize that these brain-based capacities emerge according to a biologically based timeline, are shaped through appropriate experiences and engagement with the environment, and don't come meaningfully into the picture until the child is entering adolescence. Individual music lessons—provided the child feels engaged and relates well to the teacher—are a more constructive extracurricular activity during the school-aged years for nurturing myriad important neurological connections as well as the will development fostered through daily practice.

If you're worried that *not* involving your child in a formal sports program will cost him or her an invaluable learning experience, let yourself off that hook. Get a few kids together in a safe location (hurray for the cul-de-sac!) and play games. During the seven-through-eleven years, the self-confidence, teamwork and inner mastery we wish for Generation Peace are fostered through informal play and games whose organization, rules and process is controlled by the kids themselves. This prepares them to more richly benefit in adolescence from organized team sports, which feature formal rules and strategies controlled by adults.[46] When a client of mine was trying to decide between horseback riding or soccer as an activity for her eight-year-old daughter, the girl's teacher pointed out that riding features the *relationship* with the horse— as well as the private instructor, whereas at that age children typically play "beehive soccer," swarming frantically around the ball rather than engaging in the spread-out team strategy with which the game is designed to be meaningfully played. She also pointed out the differences in the fluid coordination of the entire body when learning to horseback ride, and the abruptly segmented, percussive kicking gestures in soccer—and how those gross motor movements play a shaping role at this formative age in the patterns of circuitry wiring in the brain.

Looked at through an unsparingly sharp lens, organized sports programs for children follow an adult model that we've co-opted, downsized, and loaded up with supposed "self-esteem building" frills. In this way it's not unlike student government—another adult model and experience we've decided would be good for children to...practice?

Another popular extracurricular choice for parents of even the youngest children is martial arts, whose guiding feeling principle is *fear*. This also imposes an adultified inner path on the child. Many such programs, especially for children, have separated out the physical conditioning, agility and fighting aspects from the cultural and spiritual dimensions of martial arts, which is its source of inspiration and purpose. This not only strips it of essential meaning, it actually serves as a metaphor for what we're trying *not* to have happen in the development of the brain's integrative capacities: to have the impulsive, defensive circuitry operate without the participation of the higher, meaning-making centers.

In the traditional past of the martial arts, masters waited until the student matured from adolescence to adulthood before moving into the true teaching, beyond conditioning basics. Only then did the young adult have the faculties and the ability to understand and control the special energy and power that he was subsequently taught to develop. Equipping children with these powers before they have the maturity to deal with them is one of the more dangerous aspects of modern martial arts: it can turn a meek child (who is perhaps a victim of bullying) into a bully, and a bully into an even more powerful bully.[47] Even if the child doesn't become proficient, he may still develop an aggressive stance toward problems, which will permeate his social aptitudes in other arenas of life.

And While That Precious Window Is Still Open...

One of the most important books I've encountered about parenting during early adolescence is poignantly and aptly titled *Our Last Best Shot*. As she embarked on the book's two years of research into what influences at this life stage (age ten to fifteen) are most strongly associated with psychosocial well-being and success, author Laura Sessions Stepp "wanted to minimize the significance of parents and emphasize the importance of other adults." While she discovered the important role other adults do indeed play in the healthiest outcomes for adolescents, Stepp declares at the book's conclusion, "The kids themselves kept leading me back to their families."[48] We remain—ideally but not automatically, as we'll soon see—their central polestars and their templates. Given that fact, what do they need from us during this time when our window of potent influence is so soon to close?

Our championship and love – Can you think of another word in the English language that so reliably, so unanimously, elicits the rolling of eyes and groans of fear, contempt and disgust as *teenager?* The teenage years are comically derided as a parental purgatory, dismissed as a stage to be survived with as little collateral damage as possible to us adults—our sensibilities and sanity, our social status, our homes and automobiles. Stepp highlights a national survey that found more than three of five Americans believe that today's kids will either make the world a worse place or make no difference at all. She cautions, "[Y]oung adolescents are sponges, able to comprehend fully for the first time what people think of them....Our expressions have the potential to provoke the very kind of behavior we expect; in fact, some might say they already have."[49]

Stepp wisely points out a fact that should reassure parents heeding the steps and principles in this book: "The majority of adolescents do not turn into some unrecognizable Jekyll and Hyde monster. They just become more of who they are. If we liked them most of the time when they were three, four, and five, chances are we'll like them when they're thirteen, fourteen, and fifteen—most of the time."[50]

I'm reminded of something I once heard: you either walk the floor nurturing them when they're small, or pace the floor worrying about them when they're older. Parenting for peace is definitely a frontloaded process, in which you sow the seeds for healthy development early on, provide the nurturance and culture in which those seeds can best flourish, and then...*enjoy the harvest!* The fruits of conscious early parenting are indescribably delicious, almost sinfully so. You may find yourself feeling like you harbor a shocking secret, unspeakable in civilized company: *My teen is really interesting and enjoyable to be with.* (That's right up there with "I can eat all I want and not gain weight" as a popularity winner.)

While it merits a book of its own, understanding some things about the adolescent will make it easier to reap this sweet harvest. Neurologically speaking, the teenager's development is at a crossroads as fragile as during infancy and toddlerhood, when an attuned attachment relationship was called upon to lay the template for the optimal wiring of her orbitofrontal cortex. Now, a most explosive brain development since she was in the womb renders the teen supremely dependent upon the environment and a use-it-or-lose-it principle as her cerebellum and prefrontal cortex undertake their second great expansion, with the potential to uplift her into new realms of maturity, capacity and achievement.

In the ongoing discussion of the brain's development I have focused most on the prefrontal cortex because of its essential role in elevating the human species into unprecedented levels of higher ordered reasoning, empathy and creativity. The cerebellum has gotten short shrift, as it has for years in the neuroscientific world, often lumped in with the brainstem and seen as primarily related to motor coordination. I mean, we all want to be graceful as we move through our world, but hey, Generation Peace can afford to be clumsy more than callous—or can they?

A couple of intriguing things about the cerebellum: it's the part of the brain that changes the most during the teen years, still in the flux of maturing until the early twenties; and it's a brain region that is minimally governed by genetics. Identical twins' cerebellums are no more alike than those of other siblings—which tells us that its development is highly susceptible to environmental input. That is, *what the teen is engaged in and surrounded by has a huge impact on the massive developmental spurt of the cerebellum.* And while it has always been seen as primarily the mediator of motor coordination, neuroscientists now understand the more expanded role of the cerebellum— its critical function in social intelligence.

According to NIH neuroscientist Jay Giedd, "We now know it's also involved in coordination of our cognitive processes, our thinking processes. Just like one can be physically clumsy, one can be kind of mentally clumsy. And this ability to smooth out all the different intellectual processes to navigate the complicated social life of the teen and to get through these things smoothly and gracefully instead of lurching, seems to be a function of the cerebellum."[51] Giedd suggests that the traditional view—that physical activity most influences cerebellum development—is probably still the most valid, and points out the concern that today's society is "less active than we ever have been in the history of humanity," aside from our texting thumbs and gaming wrists. The evaporation of running, jumping, throwing—playing!—from the lives of American students concerns him with regard to healthy cerebellum development, and he emphasizes its integrated role in all of the brain's capacities needed by Generation Peace.

"One analogy that computer people use," Giedd explains, "is that [the cerebellum is] like a math co-processor. It's not essential for any activity. People can get by quite well without large chunks of it. But it makes many activities better. The more complicated the activity, the more we call upon the cerebellum to help us solve the problem. And so almost anything that one can think of as higher thought—mathematics, music, philosophy, decision-making, social skills—seems to draw upon the cerebellum."[52]

Between the higher-ordered prefrontal cortex and the coordinating cerebellum, the use-it-or-lose-it mandate of this expansive phase of adolescent brain development is clear: to the extent that a teen is richly engaged in intellectual and physical activities, connected relationships, and meaningfully creative pursuits; that she has the support and backstopping presence of caring adults; that she receives healthy nourishment and enough sleep, is the extent to which she may arise to the heights Nature has planned for her!

Giedd gives voice to the irony that the impossibly sophisticated technology that now can peer into the "black box" of the teen brain to reveal its secrets ends up pointing us back to very basic tenets—that "with all of the science and with all the advances, the best advice we can give is things that our grandmother could have told us generations ago—to spend loving, quality time with our children." Noah Williams IV—fondly known as "Quatro"—one of the most beloved and gifted veteran teachers at Highland Hall Waldorf high school in California, is often asked by perplexed parents of young teens how best to deal with them. "Just love 'em," he replies.

"Just love 'em."

Our optimism, for them and for the world – As in all of nature and certainly in human development, we see in the adolescent an echo of an earlier stage of emergence: the negativism of the third year returns in the thirteenth, as he is disappointed by the realities of his world, the foibles of the formerly invincible adults around him, and his shaken surety about himself and his place in the order of things. This has the optimal potential to be followed by the resounding *Yes* of the sixteen-year-old's embrace of the world (just as it was at age five)—*if* the dejected early adolescent finds the models around him that he needs to support this new intelligence of idealism to engage and open fully. Adults around him who model integrity, passion, courage, engagement, and their own dedication to an ideal and to possibilities for the world—this is what the child at this age so dearly needs.

Instead, as our child begins to look and act so grownup, and can carry on sophisticated conversations, we tend to lay on her our wearied, disheartened outlook on the world, our pessimism, our complaints. I heard educator Jack Petrash tell the story of going camping with his teenaged son, who could finally no longer abide his father's doomsday litany. His son told him that he needed him to not complain about the state of the world, its questionable leaders, the environment, etc.; he needed to feel his dad's hope for the world he is about to inherit. It was a game-changing moment for Petrash, who suggests that parents "strive to be lighthearted and buoyant on a regular basis."

Joseph Chilton Pearce writes of "a trinity of great expectations" in the adolescent.[53] The first is "a poignant and passionate idealism" arising in early puberty. Pearce reminds us that with each new opening in brain growth—which now happens again around age eleven—comes the opening of a new level of intelligence. The "Anything is possible" exuberance of the eleven-year-old reflects this idealism sailing upon her newly emerging powers of abstract thought. One of the ongoing sorrowful stories of our culture, bemoans Pearce—and thus one of the great areas of opportunity in consciously parenting for peace—is how a child's sense of power, optimism and idealism at age eleven can become so shattered by age fifteen.

Due to the tender open door that neurological and hormonal biology provides at this critically fragile juncture in development, culture can deal a sharp blow to the adolescent's formerly exuberant sense of self. Writes Friday of late childhood, "[S]pontaneity is king as it will never be again, not with this unique freedom from judgmental eyes, slotting us. Just around the corner waits adolescence with its ironclad rules of behavior, a straightjacket compared to the leisured informality of the noncritical world of the nine-year-old."[54]

The more we can demonstrate optimism about life, and be unflagging, sunny champions for our adolescents in the face of their inner tumult, the better we serve them and our broader intention toward peace. A recent study of 20,000 teens found that many adolescents believe they're going to die before their thirty-fifth birthday; moreover, teens who carry this hopeless sense of fatalism are more likely to engage in dangerous behavior, including drugs and alcohol, violence, unprotected sex, and suicide.[55] Writes Betty Staley, "Some adolescents never recover from their initial disappointment in the world. As adults, they feel justified in abusing other people to compensate for the previous hurts and disappointments they have suffered."[56]

The sureness of our own center – The adolescent is an exuberant, passionate, pinball bouncing off the newly expanding borders of his life. The sheer intensity of his emotions, his explorations, his confusions, his delights can be unsettling to a parent who may no longer feel he or she has access to those rich veins of life energy. The teen is driven by the big questions—*Who am I? Is life worth living? Is there a meaningful future for me?*—and one of the biggest challenges to us in staying closely connected is hearing bittersweet echoes of our own adolescence. We are confronted with self-assessment: how far have we come in our own development around these basic existential questions? (Being open to this inquiry will actually help draw our adolescents to us; they no longer seek for us to be wellsprings of authoritative answers but rather partners in exploring questions.)

If you aren't beset by at least the passing contemplation that you're not up to the task of parenting an adolescent, then you're not paying attention. Life is about to turn high-octane. The contact highs and lows of staying connected to your adolescent can be intense indeed, and it's the lows that get the most press. Apart from the disillusionment that comes with ever expanding powers of cognition and perception of reality, the basis for some of the adolescent's negativity is their growing self-consciousness. We can see their perception that everyone is watching and noticing and caring what they do (which David Elkind refers to as "the imaginary audience") as a recapitulation of the intense (and normal) self-orientation of the three-year-old. We didn't berate or try to talk them out of it then, nor should we ridicule or scoff at it now, but rather, have compassionate understanding for their tenderly emerging newness. One primary focus of their volatile self-consciousness is related to their changing bodies (or, in the case of late bloomers, bodies that aren't changing as quickly as they would like).

If parents understand adolescent negativity as a normal hallmark of the stage, they can hopefully feel less shut out and insulted by their child's supposedly diminishing interest in them, and occasional outright rejection. You have been preparing for this since before your child was born. All of the presence practices, the cultivation of self-mastery, the enrichment of your inner life have been like an extended rehearsal and now hopefully you can say, "I'm ready for my close-up," because your close-up is ready for you! Indeed, paradoxical to her seeming disinterest in all things parental, you will be subjected to the most unsparing scrutiny by your child, your child who no longer looks up to you, literally—but rather, eye to eye with you. She so recently saw you as perfection personified but is now trained on you like a heat-seeking scope, watching for you to contradict your ideals, your word, your integrity, and hoping more than anything that you don't. One of the supreme tests in parenting adolescents lies in their need for the adults around them to be steady, strong and sure in who they are and what they stand for, and for their actions to line up with their words.

But there's one small restriction—the embarrassment factor. It's one of the greatest examples of Nature's sense of humor, this cosmic, catch-22 gotcha: just when parents of pubescent and adolescent kids are reaching the stage in their own development (forties, fifties) of finally feeling at home in their own skins and secure enough to be themselves without inhibition or apology, their children have reached an age when they are mortified by any behavior of ours that is the least bit "weird" or in any way even noticeable. Ah, the hilarity that ensues…

Our availability as their off-board brain – The famously mercurial nature of the young teen's emotionality, and the questionable judgment that marks their sometimes infeasible plans and outrageous behaviors, can now be largely explained by our current understanding of the brain at this age. While teens are capable of extraordinary intellectual and creative achievement, areas of the brain that moderate emotion and mediate measured, critical thought…planning and strategies…assessing possible consequences…go "offline" for a time as children enter adolescence, a time of massive neurological growth and reorganization.[57] As your teen literally comes undone at the neurological level—as evidenced by fMRI scans—your service is required to augment his curtailed brainpower.

Here again we revisit the time in infancy and toddlerhood when your neural structures of state regulation served to regulate his fluctuating states. And again, a reprise of *function projected into the periphery until the structure is built inside*. While the brain structures that govern what one researcher calls the "sober second thought" are under major construction and remodeling, he again needs you to be a locus of calm, reasoned, loving stability until his newer, more mature structure is built inside him.

It's at about age fourteen, when the child's powers of thinking have begun their next big leap and they're forming these inner resources to manage choices in the wider world, when Kim John Payne's discipline watchword changes from consultation to *collaboration*. With our teen we discuss plans, alternate plans, fallback plans; boundaries and restrictions; and agree *in advance* on consequences for violations.[58] Despite all evidence to the contrary ("Mom, puh-leeze!"…"Dad, really, I got it…"), he needs you to do the most intricate tightrope walk imaginable: to be available, yet inconspicuous; nonjudgmental, yet strong in your convictions; interested in his life, yet respectful of his autonomy. And always at the ready with a sober second thought.

It is at this moment right here, as the teen years unspool, that even the most well-meaning parents often veer off course. A common and dangerous misconception is that the teenager—so capable, so independent, so grown up!—no longer needs close tending by parents and other adults. The fact that the adult-looking adolescent is as developmentally tender as the infant is ignored, trammeled by the ubiquitous media portrait of the sexually sophisticated, mentally adept, socially adroit teen. A treacherous mistake for raising Generation Peace, made in our culture in epidemic proportions, is to "drop" our teens and leave them to their own devices.

The largest ever crosscultural investigation into the root causes of violence found two overarching factors: lack of nurturing during infancy, and parental disapproval or rejection during adolescence.[59] As much as they seem to push us away, the insecurity they experience if we let them do so results in a protection-not-growth posture and undermines the remarkable potential brain growth Nature intends at this stage. Writes Joseph Chilton Pearce in *The Biology of Transcendence*, "Because the secondary stage of prefrontal growth is the highest evolutionary movement within us, it is the most fragile....This means that the emotional nurturing received at that mid-teenaged period serves as a major determinant in the success or failure of this latest opening of intelligence."[60] Teens need us as they never have, to shepherd their spirited explorations into the world, to provide a solid home base from which they may draw guidance as their passion and longing lead them, ideally, to formulate myriad fundamental questions emanating from the most fundamental one of this stage, *Who am I and how do I fit in the world?*

Our continued, connected involvement – Make no mistake—media, coarse culture, and peers wait at the ready to replace your central role as the child's compass if your understandable hiccup of confidence or constitution causes you to "drop your teen," as is so common. So don't—just simply don't do it. You're in this together and there is still so much journey remaining!

The second of Pearce's "trinity of great expectations" is a sense in the teen of a hidden greatness within—a secret knowing that he or she has some unique, extraordinary purpose. But rather than models to reinforce the noble truth behind this elusive knowing, and to support teens in finding their way to their unique paths of service and contribution to the world, they are offered counterfeits: stuff to buy, substances to take, buttons to push—to numb their unmet need for models of greatness. With too little inspiring them inside, and too little occupying them outside (such as meaningful, family- and community-centered—and centering—daily work), they emulate adult role models in breathlessly pursuing the diversions of materialism and "culture as anesthetic."[61] Given the sobering statistics on teenage ennui, many still feel an emptiness. Remember George Leonard's acute observation about the bait-and-switch trap of materialism, "You can never get enough of what you really don't want."[62]

Trying to get enough of what you really don't want is the poignant basis of addiction: what addicts of all stripes are seeking is the activation of the brain's pleasure and reward circuits that are unresponsive from not getting what they really do want, and did want years earlier, and have wanted all along—human connection, meaning and joy. The largely unrecognized mainspring of addiction is steeply imbalanced circuitry in the brain's self-regulating structures, which weren't adequately developed through secure attachment relationships. Oxytocin did not flow freely and frequently enough for the stress-and-pleasure system to attain its intended capacity for maintaining inner balance. This leads the individual to rely on *external* soothing and regulation to (ultimately unsuccessfully) make up for the *internal* capacities for such centering that weren't internalized when they should have been. We now know that this circuitry continues to be shaped, through relationships with adults, into adolescence and beyond.[63]

This reaching-outside-yourself for self-regulation is something most of us do to some extent and in some situations ("What a day—I just want to veg out with some TV!"…"I'd love a martini"…"I need a good workout"). It's a question of how essential the external substance or behavior becomes, how compulsively we pursue it, how insufficient we feel without it, and how negative its consequences are in our lives. Gabor Maté's eye-opening book about the relational basis of addiction, *In The Realm of Hungry Ghosts*, takes its title from the Buddhist concept of a realm in which people feel empty and seek solace from the outside, from sources that can ultimately never nourish. And because they cannot truly nourish, the activation they trigger in the pleasure axis is flaccid and prone to rapid extinction: the addict is compelled to seek ever more of it for an ever diminishing pay-off in good feelings. By contrast, as Maté points out, brain circuitry that has been adequately bathed in oxytocin and other chemicals of connection through experiencing relational richness is impervious to addiction.[64]

Maté uses the extreme example of drug addiction to shine a light on the less obvious compulsions rampant in society—some of which are culturally sanctioned, such as workaholism and perfectionism. While they differ in degree and desperation, they all spring from the same lack—feeling empty, inadequate, disconnected. This lack is not a moral failing, nor the result of too little will power—it is the result of missing human connection, a void that has become inscribed in a person's brain circuitry.

A study just released as I write this finds that teens engaged in "hyper-texting"—sending more than 120 texts per day—are far more likely to be sexually active, abuse drugs or alcohol, smoke cigarettes, and cut school.[65] The study authors emphasized that the connection is *correlational* and not *causal*—meaning that rather than hyper-texting *causing* these other behaviors, there are factors present for kids doing that much texting that also go along with multiple risky behaviors. Nowhere in the media feeding frenzy did anyone seem to consider that texting, especially with that frequency, has a character of compulsiveness to it—exactly the kind of reaching-outside-yourself attempt at self-soothing I'm talking about. Other kinds of typical adolescent attempts at self-regulation indeed include substances, sex, and the high of such adventurous acts as cutting school.

The same study found that "hyper-networkers"—those spending three hours or more on social networking websites—are the same teens who are at higher risk for stress, depression, and suicide. Remember the central risk factors for addiction are feeling empty, inadequate, disconnected. A telling statistic that jumps out to me from the numbers in that study is the 94 percent increased likelihood in these kids to be involved in a physical fight—a sure marker of steeply inadequate internal self-regulation—and the prevalence of permissive parenting reported by these kids. Our teens need us to stay close, so they can continue to download and internalize balance, security and "enoughness" for their optimal unfolding.

The third of the adolescent's great expectations, according to Joe Pearce, is the passionate expectation, arising in the middle to late teen years, that "something tremendous is supposed to happen." It is as if Nature has imbued them with a deep-seated inkling of the magnificent leap that is possible if everything goes to plan. Writes Pearce, "In fact, the development of these new prefrontal additions should ideally result in a mind that is so remarkably different from the one we operated with before that it would present to us in full the biological possibility of transcendence."[66] Something tremendous, indeed.

But once again—as with so many of the developmentally sensitive windows of transcendent evolutionary potential—our sociocultural circumstances and practices have led us to thwart "something tremendous" and settle for far less. Teens today suffer a double whammy. On one hand, everything in today's culture challenges them to navigate an edgy world of sex, smokes, weed, booze, blow, porn, LBGT, cutting, huffing, texting, sexting...and to always appear cool, sexy, and unfazed while doing so. At the same time, epidemic numbers of them no longer feel the reassuring security of emotional connectedness with the important adults in their lives.

In *Hold on to Your Kids*, his must-read book about the developmental importance of adult connectedness throughout adolescence, psychologist Gordon Neufeld starkly outlines lifelong social-emotional costs to teens when their primary attachment orientation shifts from parents to peers. The *invulnerability* that peer-oriented teens must cultivate to shield themselves from possible ridicule or attack by their equally immature home base carries drastic consequences for maturation and learning—and thus, of course, for peacemaker potential. In an atmosphere of such protective bravado, growth is curtailed (since, as you by now know by heart, growth and protection are mutually exclusive postures): "In such an environment," writes Neufeld, "genuine curiosity cannot thrive, questions cannot be freely asked, naïve enthusiasm for learning cannot be expressed. Risks are not taken in such an environment, nor can passion for life and creativity find their outlets."[67]

Ironically, these tough-acting children are far more vulnerable and fragile, deprived of the powerful social-emotional shield conferred when a parent or other adult is still the child's polestar, since it is their consistently encouraging, eyes-of-delight appraisals that provide the adolescent with a secure bedrock of self-perception—a healthy source of actual diminished peer vulnerability. Neufeld points out, "as long as the child is not attached to those who belittle him, there is relatively little damage done." On the other hand, disapproval by peers who are her everything threatens to evoke such overwhelming feelings of vulnerability that her emotional brain makes defensive adjustments as a protective measure, resulting in what Neufeld calls "emotional stiffening."

Research finds a strong connection between peer orientation and childhood aggression, whose driving force Neufeld points out is (usually unconscious) frustration over a missing or unsatisfying attachment—meaning, one that doesn't do what Nature intends: to provide safe harbor and emotional succor, particularly during this singularly stormy period of development that is adolescence. Neufeld astutely notes:

> Peer relationships can rarely withstand a child's true psychological weight. The child must edit herself constantly, being careful not to reveal differences or disagree too vehemently. Anger and resentment must be swallowed if closeness is to be preserved. There is no secure home base, no shield from stress, no forgiving love, no commitment to rely on, no sense of being intimately known in the peer relationship....Children who are stuck with frustration seek opportunities to attack and are highly engaged by attacking themes in music, literature, art, and entertainment.[68]

The culture of bullying, while a perennial issue, has emerged in recent years as a virulent danger to adolescents. Neufeld notes that while it has always been true that "children can be cruel," it has not been true in our recent modern history that so many of them are adrift without secure emotional, relational ties to adults—a fact that is consistently overlooked in our hand-wringing rhetoric over bullying. "Our failure to keep our children attached to us and to the other adults responsible for them," writes Neufeld, "has taken away their shields, but put a sword in the hands of their peers. When peers replace parents, children lose their vital protection against the thoughtlessness of others."[69]

Research on adolescent risk and resilience consistently turns up the finding that the most protective factor is strong attachment with an adult. Stepp points to a landmark national survey showing that *a caring relationship with teachers* was the strongest predictor of school success; psychologist Carol Gilligan suggests that this effect is even more pronounced in adolescent girls, who depend more than boys do on the assessment of others.

Underlying the constellation of stunted emotional development, premature sexuality, aggression, engagement in drugs, alcohol, self-mutilation and other numbing agents we see in peer-oriented adolescents, is a most poignant counterdevelopmental process with sobering Generation Peace implications: what Neufeld calls the "crushing of individuality." The precious bloom you have been tending all these years, that pure light within your child whose undimmed radiance you have been sheltering—his individuality —is, as Neufeld characterizes it, "the foundation of true community because only authentically mature individuals can fully cooperate in a way that respects and celebrates the uniqueness of others."

There is a brutal intolerance among adolescent peer groups for any signs of budding individuality among its members, which effectively arrests their emotional development inside its shell. In the absence of later dedicated psychospiritual exploration and work, this arrested development persists lifelong and expresses itself in a constellation that can include chronic frustration and feelings of victimhood; covert aggression; the inability to feel fulfilled; and the inability to reveal themselves in an authentic, intimate or truly connected way in later relationships, including with one's spouse and children. Generation Peace begins in the home and, after our children venture into the world, must continue to weave back through the home, with connectedness and joy, if it is to radiate into the world with healing and hope.

This sounds so hopeless, so daunting given the peer-saturated world of our adolescent! What's a parent to do? As hinted at above, the answer is so simple as to be almost laughable, given the millions of dollars devoted to research on youth violence; programs to teach inclusion and nonviolence; interventions aimed at empowerment, self-esteem, and resilience. One of the largest resilience studies turned up the primary finding that "teenagers with strong emotional ties to their parents were much less likely to exhibit drug and alcohol problems, attempt suicide, or engage in violent behavior and early sexual activity."[70] Neufeld refers to the work of psychologist Julius Segal, noted for his pioneering research on youth resilience. After reviewing studies from around the world, Segal concluded that the single factor that most strongly protects children from being overwhelmed by stress is "the presence in their lives of a charismatic adult—a person with whom they identify and from whom they gather strength."[71]

Writes Neufeld, "For parenthood to fade before the end of childhood is disastrous for both parent and child. When we are stripped of our parenthood, our children lose the positive aspects of childhood. They remain immature, but are deprived of the innocence, vulnerability and childlike openness required for growth and for the unfettered enjoyment of what life has to offer. They are cheated of their full legacy as human beings."[72]

Our Children, Ourselves

And so too are we parents cheated if we allow our irreplaceable role to be supplanted by cultural counterfeits. Writes Stepp, "The early adolescent years are not only our last best shot at guiding our children, they're our last best shot at being guided by our children before we lose them to the world."

Whether children are inspired or disappointed, what they find during this seven-year period of stunning metamorphosis will shape their morality and ethics, direct their will to power or to service, and define the breadth of their humanity. Let us inspire them on this cusp of adulthood, this last best shot at raising peacemakers to share with the world.

———— **PRINCIPLES TO PRACTICE** ————

Presence – I once heard Joseph Chilton Pearce say that all the "spiritual jocks" who publish best-selling books write about the same essential thing, the age-old guidance to *Be here now.* One classic esoteric tenet says that spirituality can be distilled to "presence, or lack of presence"—at all levels. For instance, whatever we do in life, we're either present to the moment, or not. We're also either present to our higher self, or not. And a basic principle from the Kabbalah states, "According to what I'm doing, and how I am doing it, I'll attract the attention of higher energies, or not."

- Harness presence to mind your own ways of being—the pace of your schedule, the flux of stress, your moods and modes. Are you present to what you do, to your own ideals? And to what are you devoting your time? Your life is now under close scrutiny by your child, more and more as he or she approaches puberty. Walk your talk; you'll be challenged and sometimes interrogated.

- Without yielding your role as the authority and the decider, strive to make your presence to your child nonjudgmental and understanding—one that says, "I've been there." Especially in adolescence, one thing that will erode your child's goodwill faster than almost anything else is you expressing judgment about their friends. One helpful approach can be to ask questions rather than making declarations—but let your questions be open-ended, open-hearted and open-minded. Interrogator mode is a no-go. Even what feels to you like the gentlest observation can be taken by the adolescent as a judgment.

- Cultivate an inviting atmosphere that makes your home a welcoming place for your children's friends and your kitchen a place for many a cozy conversation, about simply everything.

- As puberty unfolds and it can be more challenging to corral your child's presence, the car is sometimes your greatest friend. Consider those chauffeuring moments as golden opportunities for important conversations. Preteens and adolescents *do* care about what their parents think, so making it clear to them what you think is important. While modeling continues to be a fundamental means of conveying your values, explicit words are now also very important.

Awareness – Here again, your parenting will be more enjoyable and effective if you're attuned to the developmental lay of the land for these years, and some of the key turning points. One mother says of this stage (and it sounds like she meant it as self-preservation), "Be aware of everything you can." Because your child now is aware of everything (or at least thinks he is) and doesn't want to be more aware than you!

- The gradual process of the child's individuation hits a pivotal moment in the ninth year: the sunny, carefree atmosphere of his early childhood gives way to a more sober, sometimes somber, sense of the gravity of life. Melancholy, self-consciousness, and fear can arise as the child for the first time really, truly recognizes and deeply feels his separateness from the rest of the world. Rudolf Steiner saw it as such a decisive moment that he gave it a name: The Nine-Year Change. It's a time for the first pangs of loneliness, but also the first conscious joys of solitude. The true reality of death can now be understood for the first time, and in a kind of existential death process, the child begins to question all that was previously taken for granted. Thomas Poplawski entitled an article on this stage "Paradise Lost," and included lines from U.S. poet laureate Billy Collins' poem "On Turning Ten," which poignantly captures it so well: "It is time to say good-bye to my imaginary friends, / time to turn the first big number. / It seems only yesterday I used to believe / there was nothing under my skin but light. / If you cut me I would shine. / But now when I fall upon the sidewalks of life, / I skin my knees. I bleed."[73]
- Attune your awareness to many details of who your child is, relishing and celebrating his likes. His favorite foods, favorite colors, favorite musical groups or songs—these are all joys for you to participate in, and a wonderful way to meet your child's most profound need to be seen and understood.
- Cultivate a kind of awareness I call *previewing peace*, enabling you to envision two steps ahead at key moments. This can enhance your own inner stability, which is a boon for your child. Whenever we're caught unawares by our children's on-the-spot requests—and thus we're less prepared to give a thoughtful response—it tends to go less well than when we've mentally previewed the

scenario. These are moments that tend to happen in stores (for example, in the cereal aisle or the checkout line candy gauntlet at the grocery store) or during transitions of all kinds. For instance, arrive Friday afternoon to pick your daughter up from school aware of the likelihood she'll ask if her girl-friend can sleep over. If you have previewed possibilities of how you might answer her—allowing for the tide of the current moment to have its impor-tant influence, of course—you can remain centered and grounded even if your answer is not what she was hoping for. It also helps you to have the next move at the ready: "I know you really wanted Betsy to come over, and she will another time. Right now we're on our way to the plant store and I would like your help in choosing the best colors for planting by the front door." I'm aware that this previewing aspect of awareness seems like the antithesis of presence ("be all here right now"), and yet when well developed, this capacity actually fosters your ability for presence in heated situations that tend to rattle you away from the moment, from your center, and from your child.

• Also, strive not to answer your child's request in a kneejerk or autopilot man-ner—because it is important that you stand by that response. Rudolf Steiner said that one of the most harmful things for a child is to give him directions about what he is to do, and then reverse those directions; children's confusion from unclear adult thinking lies at the heart of many behavioral and other problems. The keynote inner capacity children need to develop in these seven years is to respect and obey wise authority. We need to model that, respecting our own authoritative decrees. So keep this little slogan in your awareness: *What you say will have to stay!* Repeat after me: "Let me think about that, and I'll give you an answer soon." Use it often, together with its handy partner, "If you're demanding an instant answer, the answer will be 'no'." Always said kindly, and with loving compassion. (And of course, as with every rule there are exceptions; there will and should be those *occasional* instances in which you also model reasonability, thoughtfulness and flexibility, when it is con-structive to say, "You know, sweetheart, I gave this more thought and I think I answered too quickly. Your point made a lot of sense and I'm sorry I didn't hear it quite well enough in that moment. So I'm revising my answer to yes.")

Rhythm – Daily and weekly rhythm remains a potent source of internal strength and steadiness for children at these ages, even though we now see more different tempos introduced, adding textural variety to their life and ours. Perhaps the most vividly noticeable shift will come in the child's internal rhythms in the last few years of this step, as he or she moves into adolescence with its tidal surges of hormones.

- Your parenting journey has been marked by the ebbing and flowing of energy levels—for some, the tiredness of early pregnancy, the exhilarated energy of the second trimester, the sometimes wracking exhaustion of the early post-partum weeks. The appearance of the child's first permanent tooth marks the withdrawal of one aspect of the energetic dependency he has on you, and while far subtler than earlier fluctuations, you may notice a surge of new energy within you now that this level of his maturity has been achieved. (Sometimes it's most noticeable in the form of a rise in libido!)

- In Step Two you explored the attitudes you gathered as a child toward a woman's reproductive functions, particularly menstruation. Now comes an echo of that inquiry as you come full circle—your attitudes, comments and behaviors are shaping your son's or daughter's such attitudes. Remember, your children's most potent childbirth preparation is taking place right now! Without loosening the boundaries of appropriate modesty, allow the "sacred normalness" of your period, and your approach to womb ecology, live in the atmosphere of your home.

  - As your daughter's period begins, reassure her that Nature's rhythms are idiosyncratic and to be ridden like waves, not figured out according to timetables. (It can take years for a girl's periods to become regular, and sometimes they never do; this can create anxiety for them, depending on their temperament and other individual circumstances.) A friend of mine recently posted from her visit to Fiji that the morning's high tide was over five hours behind schedule—so even Nature herself has irregular cycles!

- A natural part of the preteen and adolescent stage is that they gravitate toward a complete lack of moderation and routine. Everything is about extremes and exaggeration at their age, so as mentioned above regarding serving as their "off-board brain," they need our help to add some external regulation to their lives. It is good to keep some basic rhythms in place—breakfast, dinner, perhaps a new "wicked" tradition, such as one family I know has midweek: pizza and a well-chosen Netflix movie. But keep in mind that these cannot be too rigid, nor can they be accompanied by lots of cajoling and explanations; carefully choose those things you're going to the mat for, and then simply assert your authority to see that they participate.

- Parents of preteens find themselves especially bombarded by a near-constant pressure—from the tweens and the culture itself—to subvert the natural maturation rhythm of their children's awakening sense of worldliness, awareness of adult themes of fashion, materialism, sexuality, and general sophistication. One of the handiest answers to become fluent with is "Not yet." You can find many personalized variations on this alternative to "No"—such as "Not right now," "Not quite yet," and so on.
    - Here is one surprisingly effective tack to take in responding to a significant milestone request—such as to start wearing make-up…or go on a first date…or attend a party where (they're honest enough to disclose to you) there will be alcohol, which they promise they won't drink. It employs one of the most effective parenting strategies—authenticity. Tell your child that while *they* may feel very ready for it, *you* simply aren't quite ready, but you'll work on getting there.

- Discover for yourself the rhythms that soothe *you* the most, and, without much discussion or fanfare, enrich their lives with these rhythmic aspects. Maybe it's a soothing warm bath on Sunday night to warm up for a reasonable bedtime for meeting Monday morning refreshed and energized; maybe it's a time preserved for reading a few pages of a favorite book or magazine; maybe it's a cup of hot water to begin each day; maybe it's a candle lit at the breakfast table. They may not say much, but if you fill it or light it or set it out for them, they will likely come.
- Having said so much about the importance of rhythm, one of the greatest gifts of a consciously rhythmic family life is the delightful refreshment of breaking the rhythm; your teen especially will be enchanted when you're willing to exit the sameness.
    - Be unexpected: "Let's forget about homework and go to a double-feature!" Now, this works well in a homeschooling situation, but don't be surprised if, after all these years of tending his will forces—and especially if he finds school meaningfully engaging—he'll balk and explain why he cannot do that. See the point above about being aware of his life: you'll need to attune to and assess when the right moment for such a treat would be!
    - Infuse novelty: "Instead of picking up dinner from the restaurant, let's spend that money on flowers for all over the house and have PB&J sandwiches for dinner." Aim on occasion (once every month or two?) for something impromptu, unexpected, whimsical—and if it's absurd or

outrageous, so much the better! Remember, your inner experience of being a teenager is being awakened by virtue of living with one, so conspire with your inner teen.

Example – Until now your child has been fully receiving whatever you express through your living example. Now you can speak about it as well—your ideals, experiences, dreams, sorrows—inviting them to see and hear your joy in it all at a more explicit level.

- Model for them the richness of finding resources inside oneself. So much of what they learn today is that everything we need, every solution, comes from the outside. (*I have a headache, so what should I do? Take a pill, rather than think about the past three days and ask what I have done to stress my liver.*) When we continually turn to the extrinsic intervention or external resource and don't use our inner resources, they atrophy; when we don't appeal to our inner strength, that muscle doesn't develop.
- Now is the time to become more verbal about your passion—engine repair or orchids or Joni Mitchell, whatever it is for you. Now you not only model it but you can talk about your knowledge of and passion for it, tell stories about your adventures with it, how you came to adore it—that is all now ripe fruit for your child's eager feeling intelligence.
- Let your child see how you are a citizen of the world, how your own world-view inspires you. One couple obtained beautiful photographic portraits of an individual from each of the four continents and hung them in their dining room, as an expression of their ideal that all the world be fed—in the future with actual food, yes, but also in the moment, with the joy and gratitude their family feels at each meal.
- Demonstrate your dedication to an ideal, through which the child will absorb to a great degree an implicit understanding about the power of an idea to or-ganize (or disorganize) one's inner life. This is about a purpose-filled life, yes, but also purpose-filled days and hours. The esoteric side of today's popular power of intention tells us that when we dedicate our day to an ideal—or our glass of water, our errand to the market, our anything—with mindfulness, it organizes the energies within us and confers strength and resilience. There are innumerable ways of doing this, as in, "I dedicate this shower to all those around the world who don't even have running water"...or "I dedicate my

joy of walking in today's sunshine to all of those who are stricken by illness or injury and cannot leave their beds."

- This is the age at which children are developing the ability to take the perspective of others, to try on different worldviews. Plays, movies and stories—especially when we discuss them together afterward—are a great way to help them flex this blossoming capacity. And, children at this age are soon to enter a world of responsibility for their *choices*. Whenever you share such a story together, or even a current events item, engage them in identifying the choices people made that changed the course of the story.

  - Mystery stories are wonderful for kids at this age, as they foster a pleasurable interest in solving Life's puzzles, provided that an avenue for resolution is present. In fact, this is one important criterion for discerning the quality of a movie or story for your child: is there an avenue of sane possibility running through the plot? This works like an organizing bass line in a piece of music. There needs to be a way out in every confrontation between good and evil—which isn't the case in a lot of children's fare. For example, stories in the *Goose Bumps* book series always begin innocently, and then there's the discovery of a skeleton/monster/horror—but not one adult or other resourceful circumstance through which the child(ren) can find a solution. Any story—the funniest, saddest, scariest—must have a voice of sanity in it.

- Perhaps because of how it typically deals with timeless themes in perceptible, often exaggerated ways, theater in particular offers portraits of certain traits and choices of the inner life, and the consequences they bring. Take Shakespeare—King Lear's suspicion, Macbeth's brutal ambition, Shylock's mercilessness. Go see *Othello* and you can almost hear the Bard whisper, "Let me show you where jealousy leads," and as you watch the play it's as if you board the engine of jealousy and try on for size where it takes you. So many of his plays are as if designed for the preteen and adolescent since they don't preach but show by vivid example; in all these stories, the point is: "If this choice is made, these are the consequences."

- When you encounter conflict, disappointment, confrontations and the like (such as during family visits with your own parents!), strive to reach inside yourself for extra resources—to be self-restrained and magnanimous. Meaning, don't lose it! It can actually be of help to recognize the lasting implications of having your child noticing you, giving you perhaps that extra nudge toward following your better angels in trying moments. This offers your child a living example of fortitude and wisdom, which are taking root in them.

- Last step I cautioned about the ease and pleasure with which we can find ourselves speaking critically about others. If I had a do-over with my mothering journey, this is one area I would truly do over in a big way: I allowed myself to participate in the cultural norm that suggests we somehow appear smart and savvy when we notice and articulate flaws—in other words, criticize. Not only does this set an example that children will internalize, but now at this age it also dangerously undermines their trust: if they hear you badmouthing others behind their backs, they'll easily assume you also badmouth *them* behind *their* backs.

  - The notion of *judgment* has gotten a bad rap in our culture, for many good reasons. But there is certainly a place for discernment and noticing aspects about people. There are times when it's reasonable to say something negative about someone, and in this case it is important to close with a comment about some good quality about that person.

- When your kid really messes up, you always have a choice—attack in some way, or respond more compassionately. Unlike when they were younger, we don't want to simply overlook mistaken, unwise, or risky behavior. But we need to keep in mind that they are their own worst judges right now, and *that* is a most effective discipline. If we come down on them on top of that, it negates their own developing inner self-monitoring—and ultimately undermines our peaceful parenting intentions. Don't look the other way, but use a light touch—adopt a curious stance to see what his thoughts are on the matter; use humor; share your own such peccadilloes at his age. We adults also screw up—we forget to turn off the oven, we leave the door open and the dog gets out, we dent the car—things we can be so quick to hammer our kids for! So don't jump on their backs in righteousness when they goof up; be *with* them instead of against them. In the later teenage years, when the famous "I forgot my notebook at home" phone call comes, bring it to school for her; if you get (as I once did) the dreaded "Everyone's fine, but I just had a car accident" call, most important of all is to hold in your mind and heart the image of your child's pure essence. Of course you'll be annoyed, or worse—but in the interest of the bigger picture, find a way to have compassion, perspective, and even a sense of humor about it. (But, of course, don't laugh *at* them, or else you're digging your own grave!) We're modeling that supreme social intelligence capacity of *response flexibility*; we don't waver from our principles and rules, but we allow for suppleness, space, and creative thinking. We model peacemaking.

Nurturance – Beginning even before pregnancy, whatever nurtures you nurtures your child. This seventh step brings a balance of reciprocity to that equation: whatever nurtures your child also nurtures you! Yes, you derived pleasure from your toddler's joy on the swing—but wow, when you go with your eleven-year-old to the old-growth forests up north and share his awe...or feel her exhilaration as she delves into the next in her series of *Nancy Drew* books... or thrill in unison as you paddle together down a whitewater river! *That* is nurture all around.

- *Now* is the time when all of your own fascinated interest in how things work—inside flowers, out in space, up in airplanes, including all the details—is of great nurturance to your child. As with so much in the parenting process, so much is about *timing*: too soon and it undermines their gathering will energies; now it feeds them!
- Continue to nurture your child with stories of all kinds, including about yourself from your childhood onward, about your perceptions of your life and of his. Relish together the true communication that is now possible.
- Demonstrate your interest in everything that interests her. We typically grow up with the absence of that, which is a certain kind of neglect. If I'm a girl who goes horseback riding every weekend, year after year, and my parent never comes, that's *antinurturance*. This can call for an observant eye if your child has yet to find any intense interests; it may require noticing the subtlest signs of affinity in your child for a particular topic or activity and then finding opportunities for him to engage with and explore it to see if it really grabs him.
- As children spend more time away from home at school, the "global cooling" aspect can often be felt strongly. Continue to foster warmth wherever possible. Cuddle them if they'll still let you! One way that some older children will happily accept warm physical affection is through a foot rub or back massage at bedtime; add wonderful oil warmed between your hands (Weleda's Arnica massage oil is great).
- Rather than shying away from the confrontation of disciplinary moments, consider them as opportunities for nurturance: every course-correction you offer your child is deeply imprinted as a growth-or-protection template for

how constructively he or she will orient to mistakes in the future. (And since we learn far more from our mistakes than our successes, Generation Peace will need to have a really friendly rapport with mistakes!) When your clear, unwavering words of correction and redirection are called for (sometimes unfortunately referred to as "scolding"), if you can feign sternness or even anger while being filled inside with love for your child in that moment—that is, with a huge smile in your heart—this can perform an alchemy within them whereby their psyche may warmly associate constructive failure with positive growth.

- An essential form of nurturance is the shelter we offer to our child's still-maturing feeling intelligence. Of particular importance is the quality of the interactions between the child's parents, which will imbue him with a lifelong template for how men and women treat each other and how they carry out their respective societal roles. When there is constant strife, arguing, and mutual lack of regard, it predisposes the child to reenact this pattern in her own adult relationships; more immediately, it drastically erodes the level of respect and trust she is able to feel for her parents. If your child sees you and your partner in frequent discord, you can be sure she will not come to you for advice in her life, and a golden opportunity will be lost. On the other hand, when parents treat one another with kindness and respect, this parental harmony offers the child a level of security that allows him to feel safe to experiment with life's new dimensions in a playful and innocent fashion, as he develops his inner resources for managing their complexities.

- As mentioned earlier, a milestone in the feeling life and overall psychospiritual development of children is the nine-year change—the time when, cosmically speaking, they've really come to earth and they're not always happy about it. This is the age when you may hear, "Everyone's *mean*." "*Nothing* good happened today." Nurturance at this tender turning point in your child's life means recognizing the existential fall from grace he's experiencing, while affirming for him in myriad ways that life is full of wonderful reasons for being; indeed, this is the moment when his developmental task is to incorporate ("put inside his body") that the world is good. This requires your own self-awareness in how you perceive, filter and comment upon events large and small. We can take helpful cues from the Waldorf third-grade curriculum for ways of providing nurturance specific to the nine-year-old's angst. For example, they study stories from the Old Testament ("crossing the desert to find salvation") as one way to address their inner experience, which can feel like being suddenly alone in a desert. Learning to make textiles, build shelter and grow food reassures the child that they can work with the world to generate abundance and comfort. Playing stringed instruments, on which there are no absolute notes, requires that the student continually come out of herself and relate to her fellow players, listening for whether the note she is bowing is correct, and blending with those of the others, which adds a gentle dissuasion away from the tendency the nine-year-old can have to withdraw into herself in response to her newfound sense of separateness.

- Family time together is a great source of family nurturance, and it's so efficient—everyone gets nurtured at once! As mentioned above, family dinner is a big-bang-for-the-buck way to enrich your life with this principle. Games are another way to gather together. A fantastic, world-class game for ages seven to seventy is Wise and Otherwise—it fosters an awareness of mulicultural lore, skills of imaginative thinking and writing, self-possession in speaking aloud, and a lot of laughter.

- As they move into adolescence, with their feeling intelligence more ripened, they gradually become able to face the challenges of a more complicated emotional and social life (and often dive into that complication with gusto!). Virtually all traditional cultures have recognized the spiritual reality of this aspect of maturation through coming-of-age ceremonies. Our modern culture doesn't have that for this age, aside from the religious rites of bar and bat mitzvah and confirmation. So you're left to weave ways in which you can note and bless the gravity of this momentous time—around age thirteen—when they are rounding the bend toward young adulthood. One way to do this is to think in terms of passing the torch.

  - Fathers, let your boys be by your side, seeing you be strong, and heartily engaged in whatever is your true, deep thing, with the intentional unspoken attitude of, "I pass this torch on to you." It isn't a ritual, which can so easily become emptied of true meaning when we don't inhabit it anew with each doing. You simply have activities together, as an embrace of this passage. You're simply passing the torch of your truest, strongest male self to your boy, now becoming a man. In the summer of our son Ian's thirteenth birthday, he and his father went on a road trip through Oregon, where they fly-fished together (and Ian caught—and then released—the biggest steelhead their guide had yet seen that season) and then headed to Washington where they summited Mt. Adams together with Ian's cousin and uncle.

- For girls, it's a bit different. Hopefully, mothers, all along you have been sharing that which is most deeply yourself with your daughters. Now there is a shift that is more subtle than the "doing-ness" of the male torch-pass: it doesn't involve an action so much as a *look in your eye*, that's a mixture of admiration and approval: "I see your budding womanhood and I enjoy the woman you are becoming."

- Extended family members can also play an important part in this process. A boy who was foundering a bit in his thirteenth year—no organizing interest or passion had yet taken root for him—saw a sailboat he loved, and his grandfather helped him with the year-long project of building one. This cultivated a sense of mastery that permeated to his core—a central basis of authentic self-esteem.

- Nature continues in this stage to be an essential source of nurturance for children (and the entire family)—perhaps even more now that children's inner and outer lives are getting busier with assignments, scheduled activities and friends. Hiking; swimming in the ocean, a lake, or a pond (if you're blessed enough to be near one); even sitting beneath the stars at night or on the grass during the day to listen to the birds and the breeze—these are essential forms of nourishment for us all.

- Traveling with your child brings a unique form of nurture. Take her somewhere you know well and love dearly. See the leaves turn in New England, or the geese returning to Canada, the natural monuments in Utah or Arizona, the Midwest plains. Children now have the capacity to speak about their own perceptions, which enhances both their pleasure and yours.

- Continue to keep the kitchen stocked only with healthy foods and snacks so you don't have to become the junk food police inside your own home. The healthy habits you've been establishing with and for them all these years will serve them well—even though they may seem to often take leave of them during adolescence! One mother's sanity solution to the tween and adolescent junk food issue was to make their home a haven for enjoying healthy, wholesome food...and to completely relax all rules or prohibitions related to anywhere else. Her daughter (and for that matter, husband) was free to have chips and pizza and McDonald's outside the borders of their home and her loving nutritional dictatorship.

  - If you drive children to and from school, one nutrition-protective idea is to have a snack basket for the car. They are hungry after school, and they'll eat whatever is available. String cheese, nuts, bite-sized veggies, apple slices, dried fruit—the car ride home is your guaranteed opportunity to get these inside your child!

Trust – One fundamental of parenting for peace is the fostering of trust and hope in your child from the very beginning, onward in an unending arc of faith—in herself, in you, in her fellow humans, in Life. While you've been promoting growth mode in your child's neurophysiology and physical structure, so you've been nurturing trust mode in her psychospiritual structure (as contrasted with the protection mode of suspicion or cynicism). Insecurity, an antithesis of trust, carries a scent akin to fear—it repels and undermines the connection and collaboration required for peacemaking. By contrast, trust is the great attractor, and it is possible to tame the most powerful forces simply with deep and abiding trust. (Marshall Rosenberg catalogs many astonishing examples of how seemingly life-threatening confrontations were transformed when one person held abiding trust in the nonviolent roots of the other's violent posture.)[74]

- Certainly at this age of preteen years giving way to teen years (which will be followed after that by driving and increased autonomy outside your sphere of direct influence), trust becomes a big issue for many parents. Practicing these principles from the beginning can be a tremendous help—just like undertaking a training regimen years before a demanding hiking trip. Body-mind pioneer Louise Hay reminds us that the level of trusting surrender that we bring to our breathing is the level of trusting surrender we can bring to every aspect of life: most of us don't fret or even give a thought to whether there will be a breath waiting to come in after we exhale! Just as our lungs, guided by intricate mechanisms in our brainstem, breathe without us controlling them, so too our lives very often breathe along better without our meddling attempts at direction. This is certainly true of parenting, in a paradoxical way: of course we need to make plans, have structures and boundaries in place, and have goals and visions, certainly. And then we let those intensions breathe us—we can "live out of pure trust," in the words of Rudolf Steiner, "without any security in existence—trust in the everpresent help of the spiritual world. Truly, nothing else will do if our courage is not to fail us. And let us seek the awakening from within ourselves, every morning and every evening."

- Trust that everything your child has been living these many years with you has taken firm root in his soul, and while it may seem obscured for some years by the normal excesses and swings of adolescence, it will rise again to be the foundation of his ongoing choices and behaviors.
- You will almost certainly have this principle used against you sometime during your child's adolescence when he or she pushes back against a rule with a remark that can really throw you if you're not prepared: "You don't *trust* me!" But trust needs to be reasonable and not blind—based on realistic expectations of the child's capabilities, and cultivated through experiencing the child's trustworthy behavior. Along these lines, not trusting your fourteen-year-old daughter to spend time alone behind closed doors with her boyfriend is as reasonable as it was to not trust her to go drop a letter in the corner mailbox when she was three! In neither case is there sufficient judgment, maturity, or experience to safely navigate the territory, so not only need you not feel guilty for your lack of trust, trusting her would be a form of parental negligence. "You shouldn't trust your preteen or teenager to manage his behavior beyond his capacities or always to tell you the truth about it," writes adolescent parenting specialist Jean Walbridge.[75] In the boyfriend example, you can make it clear that while you don't doubt her intentions or her essential goodness, "...of *course* I don't trust you to be able to manage a situation like that, that is so hard for *anyone* to manage, let alone someone who has no experience, and so many strong feelings whose power you don't yet fully grasp." The more tranquil (that is, less guilty or distressed) you can be in taking such a stand, the more the child will perceive your clear distinction between her essential goodness and her admittedly limited capabilities. In yet another developmental occurrence of *projection of function outside before internalizing the capacity*, this helps her to begin exercising this kind of gauging discernment of her own capacities within herself.
- It builds trust (for us and our children) to name the giants on whose shoulders we stand—the philosophers, educators, scientists and artists—the great benefactors of humanity whose contributions have paved the way for us to thrive here on earth. Open a refrigerator or turn on the light and mention a gratitude to Edison; turn on the faucet or shower and thank the brilliant engineers of the nineteenth century; flush a toilet and offer a thanks (with a chuckle) to John Crapper who first mass produced them. (It's interesting and paradigm-informative to note that the two major innovations that transformed public health in the nineteenth century did not come from the all-hallowed world of medicine, but from engineering: pipes whereby clean water could

come into homes and excrement could leave them without contaminating the water supply, and the preservation of food allowed by refrigeration, radically changed the course of life.)

- Especially around the nine-year-change, this reassurance about what extraordinary feats have been accomplished and what forces can be mastered helps children cross that essential bridge to be able to trust Life.

- Trust in the stirrings of your child's affinities toward a possible vocation; your preteen may already know what his calling is. Help him enrich his understanding of his interests, while remaining true to yourself. (For example, if she wants to sing rock and you cannot stand rock, find someone else to introduce her to that world.) Assist her in meeting people and going places that coincide with her preferences; don't automatically assume it's childish or that it's a phase. Let us not dismiss their enthusiastic interests with a figurative pat on the head: "That's nice, sweetheart."
- Coming full circle from the early steps of your child's formation in the womb, trust the forces of life still very much at work in your son or daughter. Count on the fact that she will do many things that make you groan (to yourself, of course), "Will this kid *ever* grow up?!" Also trust that the answer is *Yes*. Not so very long from now this very child of yours will be treating you to *your* favorite concert and inviting you to dine at *your* favorite restaurant!

Simplicity – This is the age at which life can become so complicated: atop the school day itself there is homework, class projects, extracurricular activities, and the gravitational pull of friends, parties, and sleepovers. This principle is perhaps your greatest ally in continuing to parent for peace, as illustrated by the subtitle of Kim John Payne's book—*Using the Extraordinary Power of Less to Raise Calmer, Happier, and More Secure Kids*. Concerned about them getting caught up in the treadmill of consumerism? Simplicity. Determined that they be human beings rather than human doings? Simplicity. Worried that the family is splintering into separate units of technological consumption? Simplicity. It's not possible to hold back the river, so the best way is to discover and turn to the alternative pleasures found outside the fray. Simplicity always has the ring of truth. It is unencumbered. It is freeing. It brings joy.

- If you've been heeding simplicity all along, it will be natural (though maybe not always easy) to continue to simplify schedules, clothing, spending, the family diet, and the home's atmosphere.

- We can even simplify at the level of discussion. If you have developed a familiarity with the needs framework of nonviolent communication, this is a great help in getting to the heart of an argument (which can become more commonplace with children entering adolescence). In all of your conversations with your child as this stage unfolds, delve into the essence and the marrow—the rest is cumbersome.

- There is something magic in the humbly simple statement, "I don't know." It can open doors into your child. Jack Petrash points out that especially as they enter their teens, our children don't want us to be *knowers*, they want us to be *learners*. Thus, the wise parent during this stage performs a rather deft maneuver—a seemingly seamless transition from the loving, all-knowing, authority figure to the loving, always-learning, authority figure! Whenever possible with your child—particularly at eleven or twelve and beyond—when discussing stories, friends, and family, joys and sorrows, give of yourself in this most intimate, inviting, simple way: "I don't know"…"I don't understand"…"I wonder." Show your child that you, too, are a student of Life.

- Harness one of the simplest all-purpose virtues, which can serve as a connector, an impasse-smoother, a love booster, a joy bringer—*humor and play.*

- When you find wealth in ideas, you equip yourself and your child with the strength to weather the most trying challenges.

- If you are in my club—the Present Past Perfectionists—there is always the tendency to relapse into this culturally encouraged addiction. While practicing presence helps prevent slippage back into this "production and evaluation" aspect of the industrial worldview, simplicity is your greatest ally. Let "I'm letting myself off the hook" become a mantra. Choose where you'll let your high bar stand (the quality of presence with your children and partner) and where you'll let it relax to formerly unknown humble levels (the color coordination of your bedding). If this means buying salad in a bag once or twice a week, or using beans from a can rather than cooking them yourself…use the energy you might have spent beating yourself up over it, and instead bless the lettuce and the beans— along with those who prepared it so that you might simplify this moment.

- I'll close this step with gorgeous words from Kim John Payne: "Why simplify? The primary reason is that it will provide your child with greater ease and wellbeing. Islands of being in the mad torrent of constant doing. With fewer distractions their attention expands, their focus can deepen, and they have more mental and physical space to explore the world in the manner their destiny demands."[76]

Resources

Personality and Temperament Typing: www.myersbriggs.org, www.enneagraminstitute.com, fourtemperaments.com/whatistemperament.htm.

World Prosperity: www.world-prosperity.org/index.html. Great source of excellent information on the school reform movement; site is "dedicated to ascertaining and alleviating the root causes of social dysfunction."

Association of Waldorf Schools of North America: www.whywaldorfworks.org.

Race to Nowhere: www.racetonowhere.com. Not just a compelling film about "the dark side of America's achievement culture," this is "a movement about change as individuals, as school communities, as a country and as a global community. Our goal is to use the strength of numbers to influence change at many levels. We all have influence on our schools, communities, policy makers and culture." Many tools and practical ways to get involved in this healing movement.

Wise and Otherwise: I'm such a fan of this game as a family treasure that I'm including it here, with a "Highly Recommended" thumbs-up. It may seem pricey (around $42) but look at it this way: that's less than you'd spend on a movie for three with popcorn, and this game will provide you with *dozens* of hours of enriching, interactive fun.

EPILOGUE

How wonderful it is that nobody need wait a single moment
before starting to improve the world.

ANNE FRANK

There is a parable in which three villagers are strolling along the bank of their community's river, and suddenly to their dismay they see a child, then another, then many children, being swept past them in the water's swift current. One villager without hesitation dives in to try to save at least one or two; another dashes up the street to a shop in order to call for rescue help. (There are no cell phones in this parable.) The third villager simply runs away, which shocks her companions. They are stunned by her insensitivity and apparent apathy to this tragedy. But she is neither insensitive nor apathetic; she runs her heart out up-river to see how she might prevent the children from falling into the river in the first place.

Parenting for peace in the ways described in this book may very well lead you to sometimes feel uninvolved in "right now" approaches to social renewal, political or policy reform, environmental activism, and efforts toward spreading peace. But hopefully I have made the case for what an imperative, long-view healing approach it really is: like FDR said, "We can't build the future for our youth, but we can build the youth for our future."

While living these seven parenting steps and principles certainly does not preclude participating in more short-term progressive activism, it does call for restraint in spreading yourself—time, attention, energies—so thin that it erodes the impulse to which you have dedicated yourself at home. Tendrils of guilt may arise as you delete email after email inviting you to join this coalition or send that letter or make just a single phone call in the name of any of countless worthy causes. But your worthy cause is finishing her popsicle-stick castle and needs your technical support. Of course as children grow older and spend days at school…teens spend evenings at play rehearsal…our own time and energies become freer to take up action on projects that align with our ideals. And indeed, this is the embodiment of the example principle, a potent means of guiding our children's affinities toward intentionality in life—a central dimension of the peacemaker.

Mother and Child Communion

If you've read this far, then what I'm about to say won't likely shock, surprise or even disturb you. I unapologetically and politically incorrectly declare what I know to be an irreducible truth about human development: *Children need their mothers.*

Nature set it up this way, and it's based on psychobiological realities that we ignore at our collective peril. Of course one doesn't say this in polite company, at least if you don't want to be branded an antifeminist seeking to overturn women's rights. Yes, fathers are irreplaceably important and can indeed be the primary caregiver, as can any consistent, loving, attuned adult—eventually. But in those early weeks and months, it is the mother whom the child knows from his nine months of prenatal communion, it is the mother whose body, voice, smell, heartbeat and essence is perceived as an extension of his very being, and it is indeed the mother in whose sphere he will experience the most unperturbed, healthy unfolding of his *self.*

But the topic of whether mothers should be with their children is a political and philosophical landmine, fenced off from scrutiny by a "cultural code of silence," notes Mary Eberstadt in her bracing *Policy Review* article "Home Alone America." In it she quotes columnist George Will's point that "we are far advanced in a vast experiment in mother-child separation that is essentially off-limits to public debate."[1]

The past fifty years of social and human-rights evolution have flung open doors and choices to women. And yet, the past fifteen years of advances in brain and developmental science have given us information that should—if we're paying attention—make those choices harder: *relationship with a consistent, stable, attuned, loving adult, within a predictable, stable environment, is what builds a healthy brain and develops a successful human, period.* In addition to the serious neurodevelopmental implications of infant/child-mother separation—and despite massive amounts of propaganda to the contrary—statistics show that the more time infants and children spend per week in institutionalized day care, the more likely they are to exhibit aggression, cruelty, noncompliance, lack of impulse control, and other precursors of the joyless, low-peace adult.[2] Their social brain develops differently.

These findings indicate an *association* and not *causation* between day care and these developmental trajectories, with the possibility that other features of these children's environments contribute to such outcomes. Highlighting the complexities of this tough issue, which belie blanket solutions, is the fact that this finding does not necessarily hold true for children of low-education mothers; in this circumstance research has found the reverse may be true— that the time *away* from home in day care can reduce aggression in children.[3] Several such studies have replicated the finding that "family characteristics are generally stronger determinants in physical aggression problems than participation in daycare." Indeed, central to our intentions of parenting for peace is that "the strongest predictor of how well a child behaves was a feature of maternal parenting that the researchers described as sensitivity—how attuned a mother is to a child's wants and needs."[4] There it is again, that beautiful word *attuned*. Higher maternal education and family income also predicted lower levels of children's problem behaviors.

I'm probably really asking for it by suggesting that educated mothers stay home with their young children. Especially when the prevailing cultural atmosphere is expressed in blog entries like this: "I love my son, but I was losing my mind staying home with him. We finally put him in day care part-time; I reasoned that I could spend $100 a week on a therapist, who would tell me to put him in day care, or I could send him straight to day care for the same price."

Due to what Eberstadt calls "the reluctance of many academics and opinion leaders to be seen as hostile to the social advancement of women," this mother-child conundrum is either ignored or reduced to a polarizing, overly simplistic "Mommy Wars" caricature. But women's lib isn't the culprit; it has been the choice of mothers in eras long before feminism to contract out the "drudgery" of childcare to others. The loss here is deep and pervasive: no ruling class in human history has a collective positive memory of the endeavor of raising children. Those who are equipped to really enjoy being with their children, and who find full-time mothering an enriching experience, are still a cultural anomaly! It is no wonder then, in a society where social programs are driven by consumer demand of the economic majority, that we don't have family leave, career flexibility, and other policies that would support mothers and children being together for the critical first three years. We wish we wanted them, but do we really?

No doubt Erica Jong (most famous for conceptualizing the *zipless fuck* in her best-selling 1970s sexual liberation manifesto *Fear of Flying*) expressed the feelings of many when she decried attachment parenting in a recent *Wall Street Journal* editorial, saying it's "a prison for mothers, and it represents as much of a backlash against women's freedom as the right-to-life movement."[5] My book is not designed to convince those who, like Jong, would actually say with a straight face, "Our cultural myth is that nurturance matters deeply." If you feel truly and irretrievably imprisoned by motherhood, then by all means find someone freer to raise your child; according to all of the neurobiological principles I have shared in this book, and the shaping power of your example, you would likely raise a child who also feels imprisoned, and who might naturally seek to imprison. This book is not to proselytize but to invite: if the ideas I share resonate somewhere inside you, wonderful. Try them on, see if and how they fit. It is my intention that on the foundation of these principles, your own intuitive and inner knowing, in collaboration with Life, will emerge and engage as you journey through the steps.

I myself was the most unlikely image of the woman who would fall for that "cultural myth" that nurturance would matter deeply to my children—and indeed, to reconceive my career, my priorities, and ultimately, my very self. I had a Golden Mike trophy on the piano, a Perma-Plaqued Emmy nomination on the wall, and a bright future in documentary television production. Who knows what I might have produced? But behind my hyperachieving, always-gleaming façade, which shone with "higher-than-average self-esteem," there were essential aspects of myself I had unknowingly tucked away in order to live my tidy and ultimately somewhat superficial life. Something in my soul knew that to answer this call to mothering—*really* mothering, not hiring it out like my own mother had—would enrich me in unimaginable ways. No one was more surprised than me that I decided to stay home and do the hard work of motherhood.

Mothering broke me open and then urged me toward wholeness. The first mother profiled in Step Five was me. I was adopted when I was five days old in one of the first open adoptions in California. Mom (my adoptive mother, who died when I was twenty-one) was a charismatic, energetic, powerfully attractive woman with exquisite taste in everything, and a keen business sense. She wasn't home much, but there was always some caring housekeeper around to attend to me, and to do the cooking. Many hands attended to me but never the ones that felt like home. My shining high self-esteem was a fragile sham to keep my profound experience of "not-enoughness" hidden.

While inside I struggled, outside I strained to present a status-quo face. I wore J. Crew, prepared organic baby food, went to Mommy & Me, clenched my teeth, and tried to keep it together. I was living what Clarissa Pinkola Estés calls *the grinning depression*. My mounting inner conflict made me feel like an alien in a world of seemingly happy mothers-who-adored-mothering. One day, I drove alone to a scenic canyon overlook and in the cocooned privacy of my car screamed, "*I hate being a motherrrrr!*" It is clear to me now that my torment would have been tremendously eased had I not been so firmly entrenched in the production-and-evaluation-focused industrial worldview, had I situated myself in a context in which the halting process of my own inner development would have been more compassionately held and valued. As it was, I had summoned up Lisa Reagan's recipe for hell—trying to be the "perfect holistic mother" without redefining what perfection really is: *being present to whatever is authentically presenting itself in this moment.*

A big part of mothering my children involved reparenting myself, rewiring my brain. I am not the woman I was when I watched that first pregnancy test stick turn positive. Life intends that along with our children, we too become new people by allowing parenthood to remodel us from the inside out.

Long before I dreamed of the term…or the book…I discovered by living it that the miracle of parenting for peace is profoundly reciprocal: if we allow ourselves to fully enter that riotously flowing river of chaos, striving toward consciousness and connection, not only are our children raised into people of peace, we are also remade…reborn…rekindled by Life.

It is the ultimate joy ride.

On the other hand, it may be that you find yourself right now feeling sadness or regret because you are reading this "too late." You missed the boat. You already parented children, so your chance to try all this has passed. Or, you *were* already parented, and didn't receive these things that children need. As I said in the opening pages, my intention is not to provoke blame, regret, or, most of all, guilt. With new awareness comes an understandable tendency to veer in that direction. I invite all of us who missed those many boats to heed an admonition from the renowned psychiatrist and Holocaust survivor Viktor Frankl, who wrote, "What is to give light must endure burning." Let us be willing to feel the burn of what we missed, and light the way for those to come.

Raising Human Nature

Research has found that people who possess an internalized sense of trust and security express a whole range of what we would call human virtues: altruism, compassion, the willingness to forgive. One study, encouraged by the Dalai Lama, reveals that Buddhist monks' mindfulness and meditation practice changes brain circuitry to enhance compassionate response to suffering; the scientist behind that research says the message he has taken away is that virtues can actually be considered as "the product of trainable mental skills."[6]

Psychologist Michael McCullough suggests that we all have the neural equipment for both revenge and forgiveness, and that which we choose to use is largely dependent upon our life histories. "By the time I'm an adult," he says, "my history of being betrayed, violated, having my trust broken—or their opposites—pushes me toward a strategy *tuned to the circumstances of my development.*"[7]

I italicized that last line because in the same week I'm writing this, a huge media hullaballoo is unfurling over Amy Chua's new book about so-called tiger mothering— stereotyped by her as Chinese—which details a severely authoritarian parenting model featuring shame, judgment, and withering performance demands. She suggests that as a guiding principle, Chinese parents (as contrasted with American) "assume strength, not fragility."[8] While *Parenting for Peace* does not fit the simplistic stereotype of the American parenting model Chua maligns (which includes permissiveness, indulgence, and oversaturation with self-esteem-building praise—all of which I also decry), it is at fundamental odds with Chua's central principle. I would suggest that instead of *assuming* strength rather than fragility, our role is to *allow for the development of* strength and the diminishment of fragility. In that difference may very well lie the future of our species.

I also want to point out that it is possible to be intellectually or artistically accomplished yet virtually devoid of the kinds of social intelligence that characterizes the peacemaker. Two examples: Seung-Hui Cho, the perpetrator of the Virginia Tech massacre (the deadliest peacetime shooting incident by a single gunman in U.S. history, on or off a school campus), was noted for his excellence in English and math, and held up by teachers as an example for other students; and Amy Bishop, who killed three (and wounded three other) fellow University of Alabama professors who had voted against her tenure, was considered a brilliant biologist. When she called her husband from jail, Bishop asked if their children had done their homework. It was soon uncovered that she had shot and killed her eighteen-year-old brother in 1986 (deemed accidental in a ruling police were "never comfortable with") and was the prime suspect in a 1993 pipe bombing attack on a Harvard professor from whom Bishop was anticipating a poor evaluation.

In their exquisite book *A General Theory of Love*, Thomas Lewis and his fellow child psychiatrist coauthors warn, "In humans, the neocortical capacity for thought can easily obscure other, more occult mental activities. Indeed, the blazing obviousness of cogitation opens the way to a pancognitive fallacy: *I think, therefore everything I am is thinking*. But in the words of a neocortical brain as mighty as Einstein's: 'We should take care not to make the intellect our god; it has, of course, powerful muscles, but no personality. It cannot lead; it can only serve.'"[9] We're well advised to follow Rumi's admonition: "Sell your cleverness and purchase bewilderment."

Raising Humanity

Martin Luther King warned, "Our scientific power has outrun our spiritual power. We have guided missiles and misguided men." So how to have well-guided men, and women? In their remarkable book *Spontaneous Evolution: Our Positive Future*, Bruce Lipton and Steve Bhaerman note that civilization today more accurately represents inhumanity than humanity, and suggests that the "indifference, intolerance, cruelty, spitefulness" and other inhumane traits so prevalent in today's world are largely the result of developmental programming—i.e., the beliefs, attitudes and behaviors with which we are raised as children and unquestioningly carry into our adulthood. They write:

From an evolutionary standpoint, we can no longer point to the best among us as evidence of our fitness. As we find our civilization precariously perched on the Endangered Species List, our biological imperative is unconsciously driving us to adopt humane traits so that humans may fully evolve into the life-sustaining organism defined as humanity.[10]

There is a beautifully perfect storm gathering for us to do just that. Lipton and Bhaerman (along with others, such as philosopher Ervin Laszlo, in his *Chaos Point: 2012 and Beyond*) trace the upside of the breakdown of virtually all of our current systems—such as our economy, our environment, our politics. It is precisely when systems groan under the burden of pressures they cannot withstand, and decay toward collapse, that the opportunity for transformation presents itself. A new worldview can then ascend: breakdown paves the way for breakthrough. Lipton and Bhaerman also see us on the cusp of the next in a historical series of shifts, from our current reductionist worldview—a matter-centric model of reality in which everything can be explained, experienced or fixed by reducing it to its component parts—to a holistic worldview, which values matter and spirit in balance and embraces what the quantum physicists have long known: everything interacts with everything else, and individual consciousness is the agent of change. Laszlo envisions how the ascendant worldview, which he terms *holos*, will open humanity to higher planetary values and priorities—"the expansion of human consideration beyond its own needs into the universe of wisdom and compassion of which it is part."[11] He sees that cultivation of consciousness lies at the heart of this monumental shift.

Even though he wrote almost sixty years before them, Teilhard—who framed evolution as "an ascent towards consciousness"—sounds like a contemporary of the above futurists, envisioning that when we can finally use our sophistication to "harness for God the energies of love," for the second time in our human history, we will discover fire. We're currently at the point where lots of people are rubbing lots of sticks together and some sparks are starting to glow. Lipton and Bhaerman stress that we not wait for change to flow from even the most enlightened people in positions of power—that this change isn't going to come from "individuals who lead from the top. The emphasis in on the awakening of all cellular souls who create a coherent loving field so empowered leaders can be attuned to the healthy central voice of the super-organism that is humanity."[12]

We are the ones we've been waiting for.

We are the fire-makers and the sparks.

With doomsday looming ever larger in our viewfinder, can we truly consider the humble endeavor of raising children as a viable contribution toward planetary transformation? I fail to see how we cannot! Lipton, Bhaerman and Laszlo agree that an urgent metamorphosis requires that a critical mass of people like you and me take an active role in the shift, by changing their fundamental belief systems. Why not also go up-river and keep people from falling into the waters of a faulty worldview in the first place?! And at the same time raise a generation whose neural circuitry is natively wired, rather than retrofitted, for the new world we hope to usher in?

There are a mere handful of notable writers who acknowledge the importance of healthy child development to our viable future, such as child psychiatrist Bruce Perry's mention in *Born for Love: Why Empathy is Essential—and Endangered* that "raising children in a way that fully expresses empathy may be the key to cultural productivity, creativity and security."[13] Likewise, Lewis and his coauthors conclude:

> The thick marble walls of libraries and museums protect our supposed bequest to future ages. How short a vision. Our children are the builders of tomorrow's world—quiet infants, clumsy toddlers, and running, squealing second-graders, whose pliable neurons carry within them all humanity's hope. Their flexible brains have yet to germinate the ideas, the songs, and the societies of tomorrow. They can create the next world or they can annihilate it. In either case, they will do so in our names.[14]

But psychiatrists don't typically wield much muscle in the arena of social development goals and policymaking. I find it astonishing that amidst the many current books by acclaimed futurists who engage brilliant levels of imaginative thinking toward strategic, intentional planning for a more sustainable future for humanity, *nowhere does anyone mention children or parenting!* Despite what seems like a most obvious strategy for reforming the future—introducing a fundamentally reformed style of future citizen—the so-called visionaries seem to suffer a gaping blind spot—a sobering reflection of our powerful, collective forgetting of childhood and its pivotal role in our shared fate. This forgetting is so strong that these visionaries even invoke powerful images related to life's beginnings seemingly without noticing they've overlooked a most significant dimension of change potential. In Laszlo's book alone, not only is there a chapter entitled "The Birthing of a New World," but in the foreword Barbara Marx Hubbard invokes a delivery room metaphor in which our new, sustainable world is coming down the birth canal but it is not clear whether the midwife (us) will be able to ensure a safe birth.

One exception to this deafening silence is Raffi Cavoukian's *Child Honoring: How to Turn This World Around*, an exceptional collection of chapters by renowned experts in many fields, addressing the novel concept of orienting ourselves around a worldview that meets the needs of its children—"the untapped power of our species." Cavoukian, who has transformed from a beloved children's troubadour into a "global troubadour and advocate not only for children but also for a viable future we all might share," conceived Child Honoring as "a global credo for maximizing joy and reducing suffering by respecting the goodness of every human being at the beginning of life, with benefits rippling in all directions." He emphasizes that "effective strategic planning must embrace—as a priority—the universal needs of the very young. Their wellbeing will comprise the true test of all our efforts."[15]

But do our efforts come too late? Can we parent for peace with any sense of tranquility that it is enough, soon enough? Despite the urgency of the crises we face, Teilhard counseled that we are wise to maintain perspective and sidestep discouragement:

> After all half a million years, perhaps even a million, were required for life to pass from the pre-hominids to modern man. Should we now start wringing our hands because, less than two centuries after glimpsing a higher state, modern man is still at loggerheads with himself?…To have understood the immensity around us, behind us, and in front of us is already a first step.…Let us keep calm and take heart.[16]

If you have chosen the path of parenting for peace, most likely feeling like a salmon swimming upstream against the tide of the status quo, you may encounter countless moments of doubt. There will be times when it will be easy to lose sight of the fact that you are contributing powerful leverage toward the worldview shift on which will turn planetary transformation. On those days, find encouragement in the words of Neil Postman, who wrote so eloquently about what he saw as the inexorable erosion of childhood and what parents might do to resist this devolution—such as controlling the flow and influence of media in the lives of their children. He called for "conceiving of parenting as an act of rebellion against American culture," and admitted that it requires "a level of attention that most parents are not prepared to give to child-rearing."

> Nonetheless, there are parents who are committed to doing all of these things, who are in effect defying the directives of their culture. Such parents are not only helping their children to *have* a childhood but are, at the same time, creating a sort of intellectual elite. Certainly in the short run the children who grow up in such homes will, as adults, be much favored by business, the professions, and the media themselves. What can we say of the long run? Only this: Those parents who resist the spirit of the age will contribute to what might be called the Monastery Effect, for they will help to keep alive a humane tradition. It is not conceivable that our culture will forget that it needs children. But it is halfway toward forgetting that children need childhood. Those who insist on remembering shall perform a noble service.[17]

Parenting for peace has its own paradoxical wave-particle nature: it is something lived for the richness it brings in each moment—the human connection, the joy, the growth—and also a profoundly important investment in the well-being of our global family. It is the ultimate Now and Later proposition.

Farewell and Fair Winds

And now it is later. Fourteen came and went…sixteen…eighteen. Joy flowed, along with some tears. The milestones of driving and graduation passed. Your baby bird grew wings and flew away. Now the world is his nest, and his canvas. Where did the years go, you wonder. Those molasses days of her infancy and toddlerhood, days that stretched on and on and felt like they'd never end, when did they become the steady march of childhood and then overnight the unstoppable blur of her teens? What in the beginning felt like an infinite reach of time stretching out before you—your child's childhood—today feels like a handful of quicksilver that shimmered for a moment and then was gone.

Unless you're reading this after your child is grown, you won't believe me. You'll think I'm overly sentimental, or a terrible exaggerator, like those annoying people who, when they see you with your baby or toddler, warn you *It goes so fast*. Really? Goes so fast? Do you know how long I waited while he sat on the potty chair this morning and did nothing? And then he went in his pants five minutes later! Do you know how long I waited for her to unlock her door after storming in there because I insisted she finish her sophomore project before she could drive to the mall? Part of the miracle and the mystery is this wave-particle aspect of life: both are true, depending on where you stand. The parenting journey is at once interminably long and achingly brief.

I should qualify that: the *residential* portion of the parenting journey can feel like a marathon in the moment and a sprint in retrospect. The silver lining of the so-called empty nest is that you never stop being a parent and your child never stops needing you. Your grown children indeed need you to be solidly there for them in new ways, so the seeds you've sown and tended all these many years can unfurl into vibrant maturity. Life is now their teacher, but you are still needed as an unwavering source of love, counsel, friendship, and enthusiastic support as they experiment with myriad dimensions of being in the world.

This is when you as a parent for peace are graced to witness your child's emergence as a fully flourishing global citizen with emotional, intellectual and social intelligence and a reverence for both humanity and nature—a peacemaker, poised to make a positive difference in a challenged world.

Awe is exceeded only by gratitude in the soul of a parent who knows that this is because he or she answered Life's invitation to learn, stretch and grow as their child's parent. Because you answered that call with a resounding yes, there are no regrets and no what-ifs.

And there is no peace like that peace.

NOTES

INTRODUCTION

1. National Institute of Mental Health. "The Numbers Count: Mental Disorders in America." nimh.nih.gov, www.nimh.nih.gov/health/publications/the-numbers-count-mental-disorders-in-america/index.shtml.

2. WHO, World Mental Health Survey Consortium, and Ronald C. Kessler. "Prevalence, Severity, and Unmet Need for Treatment of Mental Disorders in the World Health Organization World Mental Health Surveys." *JAMA* 291, no. 21 (2004): 2581-90; Van Dusen, Allison. "How Depressed Is Your Country?" In *Forbes*, 2007.

3. Paul, Pamela. "Can Preschoolers Be Depressed?" *New York Times*, www.nytimes.com/2010/08/29/magazine/29preschool-t.html; Healy, Melissa. "Labeled: Are We Too Quick to Medicate Children?" *Los Angeles Times*, November 5 2007, F1.

4. National Institute of Mental Health. "Suicide in the U.S.: Statistics and Prevention." nimh.nih.gov, www.nimh.nih.gov/health/publications/suicide-in-the-us-statistics-and-prevention/index.shtml.

5. Science Daily. "Teen Suicide Rate: Highest Increase in 15 Years." www.sciencedaily.com/releases/2007/09/070907221530.htm; Pfeffer, Cynthia R. "Suicide in Children and Adolescents." In *Textbook of Mood Disorders*, edited by Dan J. Stein, David J. Kupfer and Alan F. Schatzerg, 497-507. Arlington, VA: American Psychiatric Publishing, 2005.

6. Liptak, Adam. "U.S. Prison Population Dwarfs That of Other Nations." *New York Times*, www.nytimes.com/2008/04/23/world/americas/23iht-23prison.12253738.html.

7. Rudin, Mike. "The Science of Happiness." BBC News, news.bbc.co.uk/2/hi/programmes/happiness_formula/4783836.stm.

8. Reinberg, Steven. "U.S. Life Expectancy Drops Slightly." BloombergBusinessweek, www.businessweek.com/lifestyle/content/healthday/647200.html.

9. Colman, Ronald. "Measuring Genuine Progress." In *Child Honoring: How to Turn This World Around*, edited by Raffi Cavoukian and Sharna Olfman, 163-73. Vancouver, BC: Homeland Press, 2006, 2010.

10. Reagan, Lisa. "When the Shift Hits the Fan." In *Freedom for Family Wellness Summit: Celebrating Our Shift to Conscious Choice*. Washington, DC, 2010.

11. Institute of Noetic Sciences. "The 2008 Shift Report: Changing the Story of Our Future." Petaluma, CA: Institute of Noetic Sciences, 2008, pg. 14.

12. Grille, Robin. *Parenting for a Peaceful World*. NSW, Australia: Longueville, 2005.

13. Cavoukian, Raffi, and Sharna Olfman, eds. *Child Honoring: How to Turn This World Around*. Vancouver, BC: Homeland Press, 2006, 2010, pg. xx.

14. Penn, Mark, and E. Kinney Zalesne. *Microtrends: The Small Forces Behind Tomorrow's Big Changes*. New York: Twelve, 2009.

15. Coplen, Dotty. *Parenting for a Healthy Future*. Gloucestershire, UK: Hawthorn House, 1995.

16. Human Genome Project Information. "How Many Genes Are in the Human Genome?" genomics.energy.gov. Counting genes isn't like counting beans, and this count is still a somewhat theoretical estimate. In any event, with each recalculation of the original finding of somewhere between 35,000 and 50,000 genes, the total has continued to drop!

17. Lipton, Bruce. "The Wisdom of Your Cells." www.brucelipton.com/articles/the-wisdom-of-your-cells/.

18. Carmichael, Mary. "A Changing Portrait of DNA." *Newsweek*, 2007, 63-67.

19. Duke University Medical Center. "'Epigenetics' Means What We Eat, How We Live and Love, Alters How Our Genes Behave." *Science Daily*, www.sciencedaily.com/releases/2005/10/051026090636.htm.

20. Lipton, B. *The Biology of Belief*. Santa Rosa, CA: Mountain of Love/Elite Books. 2005.

21. Radin, D. (1997). *The Conscious Universe*. New York: HarperSanFrancisco; Goleman, Daniel, Gary Small, Gregg Braden, et al. *Measuring the Unmeasurable: The Scientific Case for Spirituality*. Boulder, CO: Sounds True, 2008; Therapeutic Intent/Healing: Bibliography of Research; Compiled by Larry Dossey, M.D., and Stephan A. Schwartz, www.stephanaschwartz.com/distant_healing_biblio.htm.

22. Jensen, Derrick. "The Plants Respond: An Interview with Cleve Backster." In *The Sun*, 1997.

23. O'Leary, Brian. *Exploring Inner and Outer Space: A Scientist's Perspective on Personal and Planetary Transformation*. Berkeley, CA: North Atlantic, 1989.

24. Dossey, Larry. *Reinventing Medicine: Beyond Mind-Body to a New Era of Healing*. San Francisco: HarperCollins, 1999.

25. Jahn, RG, and BJ Dunne. *Margins of Reality: The Role of Consciousness in the Physical World*. New York: Harcourt Brace Jovanovich, 1988; Radin, Dean. *The Conscious Universe*. New York: HarperSanFrancisco, 1997.

26. Schlitz, Marilyn, and William Braud. "Distant Intentionality and Healing: Assessing the Evidence." *Alternative Therapies* 3, no. 6 (1997): 62-73.

27. Schwartz, Jeffrey M, and Sharon Begley. *The Mind and the Brain: Neuroplasticity and the Power of Mental Force*. New York: HarperCollins, 2002.

28. Teilhard de Chardin, Pierre. *The Phenomenon of Man*. New York: Harper & Row, 1959/ Perennial reprint 2002, 1959.

29. Ibid, pg. 251.

30. Biologist Alister Hardy, quoted in Barbour, Ian G. *Religion and Science: Historical and Contemporary Perspectives*. San Francisco: HarperCollins, 1997, pg. 223.

STEP ONE

1. Lewis, Thomas, Fari Amini, and Richard Lannon. *A General Theory of Love*. New York: Random House, 2000.

2. Siegel, Daniel J. "Emotional Trauma and the Developing Mind." Paper presented at the From Neurons to Neighborhoods: The Effects of Emotional Trauma on the Way We Learn, Feel and Act, Mt. St. Mary's College, Dept. of Psychology, March 2-3 2002.

3. Pearce, Joseph Chilton. *The Biology of Transcendence: A Blueprint of the Human Spirit.* Rochester, VT: Inner Traditions, 2002.

4. Lodge, Henry S., and Chris Crowley. *Younger Next Year.* New York: Workman, 2007. Coauthor Henry Lodge, a Columbia Medical School internist, points out that while this isn't entirely accurate, "it's very close."

5. McCraty, Rollin, Mike Atkinson, and Dana Tomasino. *Science of the Heart: Exploring the Role of the Heart in Human Performance.* Boulder Creek, CA: Institute of HeartMath, 2001. A free download of this monograph is available at www.heartmath.org/free-services/downloads/free-download-library.html.

6. Lewis, Thomas, Fari Amini, and Richard Lannon. *A General Theory of Love.* New York: Random House, 2000.

7. Harmon, Amy. "Researchers Find Sad, Lonely World in Cyberspace." In *New York Times*: New York Times Company, 1998. This article details the first such study; many have been done since, and they have reached similar conclusions—that the more time someone spends online, the less happy and more depressed he or she is likely to be. Just two hours of surfing the net *per week* was associated with various forms of anxiety and depression, leading to reclusiveness and feelings of alienation. And, they were passionate consumers!

8. Goleman, Daniel. *Social Intelligence: The New Science of Human Relationships.* New York: Bantam/Dell, 2006, pg. 7.

9. Wallis, Claudia. "The New Science of Happiness." *Time*, Jan. 17 2005, A3-A9.

10. Pearce, Joseph Chilton. *The Biology of Transcendence: A Blueprint of the Human Spirit.* Rochester, VT: Inner Traditions, 2002. I recommend this very readable and riveting book for a thorough explanation of the triune brain—and many other processes involved in parenting for peace.

11. Lipton, Bruce. *The Biology of Belief.* Santa Rosa, CA: Mountain of Love/Elite Books, 2005.

12. Dispenza, Joe. *Evolve Your Brain: The Science of Changing Your Mind.* Deerfield Beach, FL: Health Communications, Inc., 2008.

13. DiCarlo, Russell E., ed. *Towards a New World View: Conversations at the Leading Edge.* Erie, PA: Epic, 1996, pg. 164.

14. Pert, Candace B. *Molecules of Emotion: Why You Feel the Way You Feel.* New York: Scribner, 1997. Mine is a vastly simplified description that suggests one mechanism to explain the long-observed role of emotions in susceptibility to illness. One of the aspects of the unmentioned complexity of this example is that norepinephrine serves different functions in different circumstances and in varying concentrations, including playing a role in the famous "fight, flight or freeze" stress response.

15. Weaver, Jane. "Can Stress Actually Be Good for You?" msnbc.com, www.msnbc.msn.com/id/15818153/ns/health-mental_health/#.

16. Leonard, Brian E., and Klara Miller, eds. *Stress, the Immune System and Psychiatry.* West Sussex, England: John Wiley & Sons, 1995.

17. Begley, Sharon. "The Depressing News About Antidepressants." In *Newsweek*: Harman Newsweek LLC, 2010, www.newsweek.com/2010/01/28/the-depressing-news-about-antidepressants.html.

18. Odent, Michel. "Womb Ecology: New Reasons and New Ways to Prepare the Prenatal Environment." *Journal of Prenatal & Perinatal Psychology and Health* 20, no. 3 (2006): 281-89. Also available at www.wombecology.com/newreasons.html.

19. Chavarro, Jorge E, Walter C Willett, and Patrick J Skerrett. "Fat, Carbs and the Science of Conception." *Newsweek*, 2007.

20. Payne, Niravi. *The Whole Person Fertility Program*. New York: Three Rivers Press, 1997.

21. Jameson, Jamie. "Properties of Water: The Miraculous Wonder of Water." Yahoo, www .associatedcontent.com/article/2627571/properties_of_water_the_miraculous.html?cat=58. Water violates several basic laws of physics regarding liquids, in ways that allow individual and planetary life to be sustained.

22. Schwartz, J. M., & Begley, S. (2002). *The Mind and the Brain: Neuroplasticity and the Power of Mental Force*. New York: HarperCollins, page 334.

23. Siegel, Daniel J., and Mary Hartzell. *Parenting from the inside Out: How a Deeper Self-Understanding Can Help You Raise Children Who Thrive*. New York: Jeremy Tarcher/Putnam, 2003, pg. 1.

24. Payne, Niravi. *The Whole Person Fertility Program*. New York: Three Rivers Press, 1997.

25. Siegel, Daniel J., and Mary Hartzell. *Parenting from the inside Out: How a Deeper Self-Understanding Can Help You Raise Children Who Thrive*. New York: Jeremy Tarcher/Putnam, 2003.

STEP TWO

1. Baker, Jeannine Parvati, and Frederick Baker. *Conscious Conception: Elemental Journey through the Labyrinth of Sexuality*. Berkeley, CA: North Atlantic Books, 1986, pg. 48.

2. Relier, Jean-Pierre. "Influence of Maternal Stress on Fetal Behavior and Brain Development." *Biology of the Neonate* 79, no. 3-4 (2001): 168-71.

3. Khashan, AS et al. "Rates of Preterm Birth Following Antenatal Maternal Exposure to Severe Life Events: A Population-Based Cohort Study." *Human Reproduction* 24, no. 2 (2009): 429-37.

4. Kolata, Gina. "Picture Emerging on Genetic Risks of IVF." *New York Times*, www.nytimes.com/2009/02/17/health/17ivf.html.

5. Relier, Jean-Pierre. "Influence of Maternal Stress on Fetal Behavior and Brain Development." *Biology of the Neonate* 79, no. 3-4 (2001): 168-71.

6. Radin, Dean. *The Conscious Universe*. New York: HarperSanFrancisco, 1997.

7. Emoto, Masaru. *Messages from Water*. Tokyo: Hado Kyoikusha Co., 1999.

8. Huxley, Laura Archera, and Piero Ferruci. *The Child of Your Dreams*. Rochester, VT: Destiny Books, 1992, pg. 31.

9. Maté, Gabor. *Scattered: How Attention Deficit Disorder Originates and What You Can Do About It*. New York: Penguin, 1999.

10. Carmichael, Mary. "A Changing Portrait of DNA." *Newsweek*, 2007, 63-67.

11. Bustan, M.N., and A.L. Coker. "Maternal Attitude toward Pregnancy and the Risk of Neonatal Death." *American Journal of Public Health* 84, no. 3 (1994): 411-14; McNeil, TF et al. "Unwanted Pregnancy as a Risk Factor for Offspring Schizophrenia-Spectrum and Affective Disorders in Adulthood: A Prospective High-Risk Study." *Psychological Medicine* 39 (2009): 957-65; Asarnow, Joan Rosenbaum, and Michael J Goldstein. "Schizophrenia During Adolescence and Early Adulthood: A Developmental Perspective on Risk Research." *Clinical Psychology Review* 6, no. 3 (1986): 211-35.

12. Roe, K.V., and A. Drivas. "Planned Conception and Infant Functioning at Age Three Months: A Cross-Cultural Study." *American Journal of Orthopsychiatry* 63, no. 1 (1993): 120-25.

13. Hallet, Elizabeth. "How I Stumbled across a New Frontier." Tony Crisp, dreamhawk.com/pregnancy-childbirth/knowing-baby-before-birt/.

14. Aïvanhov, Omraam Mikhael. *Education Begins before Birth*. 1990 ed. Frejus, France: Prosveta, 1938, pg. 13.

15. Pesso, Albert. "The Effects of Pre- and Perinatal Trauma." *Hakomi Journal*, no. 8 (1990), pg. 35.

16. Sonne, John. "Magic Babies." *Journal of Prenatal and Perinatal Psychology and Health* 12, no. 2 (1997): 61, 65.

17. Pert, Candace B. *Molecules of Emotion: Why You Feel the Way You Feel*. New York: Scribner, 1997, pg. 143. "These recent discoveries are important for appreciating how memories are stored not only in the brain, but in a *psychosomatic network* extending into the body, particularly in the ubiquitous receptors between nerves and bundles of cell bodies called ganglia, which are distributed not just in and near the spinal cord, but all the way out along pathways to internal organs and the very surface of our skin."

18. House, Simon. "Primal Integration Therapy—School of Lake: Dr. Frank Lake Mb, Mrc Psych, Dpm (1914-1982)." *Journal of Prenatal and Perinatal Psychology and Health* 14, no. 3-4 (2000), pg. 221.

19. I'm indebted here to the embryological insights of Michael Shea and Guus Van der Bie. Shea, Michael. *Biodynamic Craniosacral Therapy, Vol. 1*. Berkeley, CA: North Atlantic Books, 2007; Van der Bie, G. *Embryology: Early Development from a Phenomenological Point of View*. Netherlands: Louis Bolk Institute, 2001.

20. Steingraber, Sandra. *Having Faith: An Ecologist's Journey to Motherhood*. New York: Berkeley, 2001, pgs. 24 and 17.

21. Zou, Kang et al. "Production of Offspring from a Germline Stem Cell Line Derived from Neonatal Ovaries." *Nature Cell Biology* 11 (2009): 631-36.

22. Mozurkewich, Ellen, Deborah R Berman, and Julie Chilimigras. "Role of Omega-3 Fatty Acids in Maternal, Fetal, Infant and Child Wellbeing: Fetal Brain Development and Early Childhood Iq." *Expert Review of Obstetrics and Gynecology* 5, no. 1 (2010): 125-38.

23. Mayo Clinic staff. "Pregnancy and Fish: What's Too Little—or Too Much?" In *Pregnancy week by week*: MayoClinic.com, 2009.

24. Odent, Michel. "Primal Health Research: Mercury Exposure During the Primal Period." *Journal of Prenatal and Perinatal Psychology and Health* 18, no. 3 (2004): 212-20.

25. Rose, Amanda. *Rebuild from Depression*. California Hot Springs, CA: Purple Oak Press, 2009.

26. Gibbons, Ann. "In Mice, Mom's Genes Favor Brains over Brawn." *Science* 280 (1998): 1346.

27. Moore, T., and D. Haig. "Genomic Imprinting in Mammalian Development: A Parental Tug-of-War." *Trends Genet* 7, no. 2 (1991): 45-9; Iwasa, Y. "The Conflict Theory of Genomic Imprinting: How Much Can Be Explained?" *Curr Top Dev Biol* 40 (1998): 255-93.

28. Lipton, Bruce. personal communication with author, January, 2002.

29. Gibbons, Ann. "Solving the Brain's Energy Crisis." *Science* 280 (1998): 1345-47.

30. Personal communication, January 2002.

31. Lipton, Bruce. "Nature, Nurture and Human Development." *Journal of Prenatal and Perinatal Psychology and Health* 16, no. 2 (2002): 167-80.

32. Adey, W. Ross. "Electromagnetic Fields, the Modulation of Brain Tissue Functions: A Possible Paradigm Shift in Biology." In *International Encyclopedia of Neuroscience*, edited by B.

Smith and G. Adelman. New York: Elsevier, 2003. By leading the development of this new model, Ross Adey antagonized authorities whose reputations are based on preserving the status quo, as well as powerful groups with vested financial interests in not rocking the boat. Yet because of his unassailable credentials, integrity and other (i.e., more acceptable status quo) research streams, he wasn't impeded by the kinds of reputation-undermining personal attacks and funding cutoffs that have plagued others trying to investigate EMF effects.

33. Morter, M.T. *The Healing Field.* Rogers, AR: Best Research, 1991, pg. 57. Morter developed the renowned Bio Energetic Synchronization Technique (B.E.S.T.), used by energetically aware healthcare practitioners worldwide.

34. Uplinger, Laura. "A Cosmic Collaboration." In *The Marriage of Sex & Spirit*, edited by Geralyn Gendreau. Santa Rosa, CA: Elite Books, 2006. It bears noting, relative to that blind spot I mentioned earlier, that in an anthology containing forty-five essays from brilliant visionary leaders on the intersection of sex and spirituality, Uplinger's is the sole chapter that mentions the creation of a baby.

35. Quoted in Cobb, J.J. (no relation). *Cybergrace: The Search for God in the Digital World.* New York: Crown, 1998, pg. 56.

36. Braun, Joe M, Amy E Kalkbrenner, Antonia M Calafat, Kimberly Yolton, Xiaoyun Ye, Kim N Dietrich, and Bruce P Lanphear. "Impact of Early-Life Bisphenol a Exposure on Behavior and Executive Function in Children." *Pediatrics* doi: 10.1542/peds.2011-1335 (2011).

37. Walker, Matt. "Rape—an Evolutionary Strategy?" Paper presented at the Human Behavior and Evolution conference, London, UK, 2001.

STEP THREE

1. Paul, Annie Murphy. *Origins: How the Nine Months before Birth Shape the Rest of Our Lives.* New York: Free Press, 2010.

2. Diamond, Marian. "Enriching Heredity: How the Environment Impacts Brain Development." *Touch the Future*, no. Spring (1997): 7-11.

3. Liu, Jianghongh. "Early Health Risk Factors for Violence: Conceptualization, Evidence, and Implications." *Aggression and Violent Behavior* 16, no. 1 (2011): 63-73.

4. Profet, Margie. *Protecting Your Baby-to-Be.* New York: Addison-Wesley, 1995.

5. Scheibel, Arnold B. "Embryological Development of the Human Brain." Johns Hopkins University School of Education, education.jhu.edu/newhorizons/Neurosciences/articles/Embryological%20Development%20of%20the%20Human%20Brain/index.html.

6. March of Dimes. "Smoking During Pregnancy." March of Dimes, www.marchofdimes.com/pregnancy/alcohol_smoking.html.

7. March of Dimes. "Drinking Alcohol During Pregnancy." March of Dimes, www.marchofdimes.com/Pregnancy/alcohol_indepth.html; WebMD. "Alcohol Effects on a Fetus—Topic Overview." www.webmd.com/baby/tc/alcohol-effects-on-a-fetus-topic-overview.

8. Karr-Morse, Robin, and Meredith S. Wiley. *Ghosts from the Nursery: Tracing the Roots of Violence.* New York: Atlantic Monthly Press, 1997.

9. E.g., Davis, Elysia Poggi et al. "Prenatal Exposure to Maternal Depression and Cortisol Influences Infant Temperament." *J. Am. Acad. Child and Adoles. Psychiatry* 46, no. 6 (2007): 737-46; Glover, Vivette. "Maternal Stress or Anxiety in Pregnancy and Emotional Development of the Child." *British Journal of Psychiatry*, no. 171 (1997): 105-06; Glynn, Laura M., and Curt A. Sandman. "The Influence of Prenatal Stress and Adverse Birth Outcome on Human Cognitive and Neurological Development." *Int'l Review of Research in Mental Retardation* 32 (2006):

109-36; O'Connor, Thomas G. et al. "Maternal Antenatal Anxiety and Children's Behavioural/ Emotional Problems at 4 Years." *British Journal of Psychiatry* 180 (2002): 502-08; Wadhwa, PD. "Prenatal Stress and Life-Span Development." In *Encyclopedia of Mental Health*, edited by H Friedman, 8-10. San Diego: Academic Press, 1998.

10. Selye, Hans. *The Stress of Life*. New York: McGraw-Hill, 1976, pg. 460.

11. Hepper, Peter G. "Fetal Psychology: An Embryonic Science." In *Fetal Behavior: Developmental and Perinatal Aspects*, edited by Jan G. Nijuis. New York: Oxford University Press, 1992.

12. E.g., Janus, Ludwig. *The Enduring Effects of Prenatal Experience: Echoes from the Womb*. Northvale, NJ: Jason Aronson, 1997; Paul, Annie Murphy. *Origins: How the Nine Months before Birth Shape the Rest of Our Lives*. New York: Free Press, 2010; Piontelli, Alessandra. *From Fetus to Child*. New York: Tavistock/Routledge, 1992; Verny, Thomas, and John Kelly. *The Secret Life of the Unborn Child*. New York: Delta, 1982.

13. Share, Lynda. *When Someone Speaks, It Gets Lighter: Dreams and the Reconstruction of Infant Trauma*. Ne Emerson, William. "The Vulnerable Prenate." *Pre- and Perinatal Psychology Journal* 10, no. 3 (1996): 125-42.w Jersey: Analytic Press, 1994.

14. Emerson, William. "The Vulnerable Prenate." *Pre- and Perinatal Psychology Journal* 10, no. 3 (1996): 125-42.

15. Sonne, John. "Abortion Survivors at Columbine." *Journal of Prenatal and Perinatal Psychology* 15, no. 1 (2000): 3-22.

16. Verny, Thomas, and John Kelly. *The Secret Life of the Unborn Child*. New York: Delta, 1982.

17. House, Simon. "Primal Integration Therapy—School of Lake: Dr. Frank Lake Mb, Mrc Psych, Dpm (1914-1982)." *Journal of Prenatal and Perinatal Psychology and Health* 14, no. 3-4 (2000): 213-35.

18. Pearce, Joseph Chilton. "The Biology of Trancendence: Shaping Your Life in a Radically Changing World." Santa Barbara Graduate Institute, September 20-21 2002.

19. Odent, Michel. "The Function of Joy in Pregnancy." *Primal Health Research Quarterly* 14, no. 3 (2006).

20. Sandman, Curt A et al. "Psychobiological Influences of Stress and Hpa Regulation on the Human Fetus and Infant Birth Outcomes." *Annals of the New York Academy of Sciences* 739 (1994): 198-210.

21. Barker, DJP. "Fetal Origins of Cardiovascular Disease." *Ann Med* Apr; 31, no. Suppl 1 (1999): 3-6.

22. Beversdorf, David. "Stress During Pregnancy Linked to Autism." In *Society for Neuroscience Annual Meeting*. San Diego, CA, 2001.

23. Barbazanges, A et al. "Maternal Glucocorticoid Secretion Mediates Long-Term Effects of Prenatal Stress." *Journal of Neuroscience* 16, no. 12 (1996): 3943-9; Stratakis, CA et al. "Neuroendocrinology of Stress: Implications of Growth and Development." *Hormone Research* 43 (1995): 162-67.

24. Insel, Thomas et al. "Prenatal Stress Has Long-Term Effects on Brain Opiate Receptors." *Brain Research* 511 (1990): 93-97; Sandman, CA. "Persisting Subsensitivity of the Striatial Dopamine System after Fetal Exposure to Beta-Endorphin." *Life Sciences* 39 (1986): 1755-63.

25. Sandman, Curt A et al. "Psychobiological Influences of Stress and Hpa Regulation on the Human Fetus and Infant Birth Outcomes." *Annals of the New York Academy of Sciences* 739 (1994): 198-210.

26. Sandman, Curt A, et al. "What the Maternal Heart Tells the Fetal Brain." Poster presented at the Developmental Origins of Health and Disease, Portland, OR, September 2011.

27. Santa Barbara Graduate Institute. "The Very First Relationship." In *Trauma, brain and relationship: helping children heal*: HealingResources.info, 2004. www.healingresources.info/ emotional_trauma_online_video.htm#1. There are some indications that regulation disorders such as ADD/ADHD and OCD may have their beginnings in the womb, when this basic neural regulatory wiring is laid down.

28. Levine, Peter. "When Biology Becomes Pathology." Paper presented at From Neurons to Neighborhoods: The Effects of Emotional Trauma on the Way We Learn, Feel and Act, Mt. St. Mary's College, Los Angeles, March 2-3 2002.

29. Barker, DJP, ed. *Fetal and Infant Origins of Adult Disease*. London: British Medical Journal, 1992. The kind of fetal programming studied by Barker and a growing number of other researchers is distinguished from the processes of conditions such as fetal alcohol syndrome, for instance, where the effects of the toxic uterine environment are noticeable at birth or early in life. These findings refer to relatively more subtle suboptimal conditions in the womb, which by directly contributing to fundamental weaknesses in fetal physiology program an individual with tendencies and vulnerabilities toward disease that may not show up until the latter half of life. Barker's research and theory features in—and indeed provides the title for—Annie Murphy Paul's 2010 book, *Origins: How The Nine Months Before Birth Shape the Rest of Our Lives*.

30. Docker, Sophie. "Brain Function Linked to Birth Size in Groundbreaking New Study." EurekAlert, www.eurekalert.org/pub_releases/2011-02/uos-bfl021811.php.

31. Nathanielsz, Peter W. *Life in the Womb: The Origin of Health and Disease*. Ithaca, NY: Promethean Press, 1999.

32. Stratakis, C.A., P.W. Gold, and G.P. Chrousos. "Neuroendocrinology of Stress: Implications of Growth and Development." *Hormone Research* 43 (1995): 162-67.

33. Nathanielsz, Peter W. *Life in the Womb: The Origin of Health and Disease*. Ithaca, NY: Promethean Press, 1999.

34. Sandman, Curt A, Elysia P Davis, and Laura M Glynn. "Prescient Fetuses Thrive." *Psychological Science* (In press).

35. Barker, DJP, ed. *Fetal and Infant Origins of Adult Disease*. London: British Medical Journal, 1992. There seems to be a diabetes domino effect taking place in the Western world whereby the rise in the incidence of diabetes far outstrips the ability of diabetes genes to account for the epidemic. Some experts account for it with this mismatch between the fetal environment of poorly nourished newly pregnant women, and the nutritional overabundance into which their babies are born and live their lives.

36. Odent, Michel. "The Function of Joy in Pregnancy." *Primal Health Research Quarterly* 14, no. 3 (2006).

37. Hall, Mitch. *Peacequest: Cultivating Peace in a Violent Culture*. Sausalito, CA: Peacequest, 2003, pg. 25.

38. Paul, Annie Murphy. "The First Nine Months Shape the Rest of Your Life: The New Science of Fetal Origins." *Time*, October 4 2010, 50-55.

39. DiPietro, JA et al. "Fetal Antecedents of Infant Temperament." *Child Development* 67 (1996): 2568-83.

40. Personal communication, 2/17/11.

41. Hepper, Peter. "Unravelling Our Beginnings." *The Psychologist* 18, no. 8 (2005): 474-77.

42. Oates, John, and Andrew Grayson. *Cognitive and Language Development in Children*. 2nd ed: Wiley-Blackwell, 2004, pg. 66.

43. Hepper, Peter. "The Behavior of the Human Fetus." In *13th Int'l Congress of APPPAH*. Los Angeles, 2007.

44. Cheour, M et al. "Psychobiology: Speech Sounds Learned by Sleeping Newborns." *Nature* 415, no. 6872 (2002): 599-600.

45. Diamond, Marian. "Enriching Heredity: How the Environment Impacts Brain Development." *Touch the Future*, no. Spring (1997): 7-11. Diamond's research, which rankled her biology peers by upsetting the then prevailing notion (this was the 70s) that DNA alone determines brain structure, revealed thicker neocortexes in the pups of rats whose mothers when pregnant lived in an enriched environment, as compared to those living in an impoverished, stressful environment. Her finding that is of greatest import for the purposes of Generation Peace is one that she never published because it was simply too controversial and might have tanked her UC Berkeley standing, but she did report it orally at some conferences in the 80s: the gains in brain volume enjoyed by the pups of pregnant mothers in enriched environments *persisted into the next generation, regardless of the circumstances of those next pups' pregnant mothers!*

46. Sandman, Curt, Pathik D. Wadhwa, Manuel Porto, Thomas J. Garite, and Aleksandra Chicz-DeMet. "Maternal Corticotropin-Releasing Hormone Levels in Early Third Trimester Predicts Length of Gestation in Human Pregnancy." *Am J Obstet Gynecol* 179, no. 4, Oct. (1998): 1079-85.

47. Personal communication, August 2007.

48. Abrams, Douglas Carlton. "The Making of a Modern Dad." *Psychology Today*, March/April 2002.

49. March of Dimes. "Drinking Alcohol During Pregnancy." March of Dimes, www.marchofdimes.com/Pregnancy/alcohol_indepth.html.

50. Gaskin, Ina May. *Ina May's Guide to Childbirth*. New York: Bantam-Dell, 2003.

51. Ziskin, M. C., and S. B. Barnett. "Ultrasound and the Developing Central Nervous System." *Ultrasound Med Biol* 27, no. 7 (2001): 875-6.

52. Mentor, Steven. "Witches, Nurses, Midwives, and Cyborgs." In *Cyborg Babies: From Techno-Sex to Techno-Tots*, edited by Robbie Davis-Floyd and Joseph Dumit, 67-89. New York: Routledge, 1998, pg. 81.

53. Davis-Floyd, Robbie, and Joseph Dumit. "From Technobirth to Cyborg Babies: Reflections on the Emergent Discourse of a Holistic Anthropologist." In *Cyborg Babies: From Techno-Sex to Techno-Tots*, edited by Robbie Davis-Floyd and Joseph Dumit. New York: Routledge, 1998.

54. Odent, Michel. "The Function of Joy in Pregnancy." *Primal Health Research Quarterly* 14, no. 3 (2006).

55. Aïvanhov, Omraam Mikhael. *Education Begins before Birth*. 1990 ed. Frejus, France: Prosveta, 1938.

56. Uplinger, Laura. "I Know a Planet." Wonders of the Womb, www.wondersofthewomb.com/i-know-a-planet1.htm.

57. Huxley, Laura Archera, and Piero Ferruci. *The Child of Your Dreams*. Rochester, VT: Destiny Books, 1992, pg. 149.

58. Lipton, Bruce, and Steve Bhaerman. *Spontaneous Evolution*. Carlsbad, CA: Hay House, 2009, pg. 5.

59. Uplinger, Laura. "Womb Service." Wonders of the Womb, www.wondersofthewomb.com/womb-service.htm.

60. England, Pam. *Birthing from Within*. Albuquerque, NM: Partera Press, 1998, pg. 96-97.

61. Beeber, Linda. "Maternal Depressive Symptoms: More Than the Baby Blues." Paper presented at the Smart Start National Conference, Greensboro, NC, May 2007.

62. In Black, Shirley Temple. *Child Star*. New York: McGraw Hill, 1988, pg. 4-5, appears this enchanting explanation: "One summer day in 1927, in her 34th year, [Gertrude, my mother] announced her intention to produce a baby girl....Pregnancy was only a starter for Gertrude, who believed devoutly in self-determination. The female sex and artistic interests of her own child must be established long before birth. Her scheme involved preempting the name Shirley for no particular reason, with Jane added to honor her paternal grandmother. To endow her unborn child with a sense of self-discipline, she switched from beloved chocolates to raw carrots. Marshaling her array of feminine instincts, although unable to carry a tune herself, she kept the radio blaring out classic orchestral programs, read good literature aloud, toured local museums, purposely pausing to admire architectural beauty along the way, bathing herself in color, form, and aesthetics. Occasionally she attended a local movie, exposing her unborn child to sounds and sensations of romantic films such as Janet Gaynor's *Seventh Heaven* and *Street Angel* as she dabbed away her sympathetic tears. She walked down to the ocean, remarking on the natural beauty in flowers, and listened to the rhythmic thump of sea turf, the rustle of palm fronds in the Pacific wind, and the happy babble as she passed public playgrounds. It was her mystical, Teutonic conviction that noble thoughts, beautiful sights, and pleasant sounds could somehow imprint themselves directly on her child, a prenatal blitzkrieg. On the twenty-third of April 1928, her basic plan reached a major milepost. I was indeed a baby girl..."

63. Côté-Arsenault, Denise, Davya Brody, and Mary-Therese Dombeck. "Pregnancy as a Rite of Passage: Liminality, Rituals and Communitas." *Journal of Prenatal & Perinatal Psychology and Health* 24, no. 2 (2009): 69-87.

64. The store at your nearest Waldorf school is a good place to look, or online at Toy Garden.

65. Caddis, Dana. "Prenatal Ultrasound Safety: What Parents Should Know About Diagnostic Fetal Scans." Suite101, www.suite101.com/content/prenatal-ultrasound-safety-a78544.

66. Gaskin, Ina May. *Ina May's Guide to Childbirth*. New York: Bantam-Dell, 2003, pg.

67. Steiner, Rudolf, quoted in Salter, Joan. *The Incarnating Child*. Gloucestershire, U.K.: Hawthorne Press, 1987, pg. 14.

STEP FOUR

1. E.g., Emerson, William R. "Birth Trauma: The Psychological Effects of Obstetrical Interventions." *J of Prenatal and Perinatal Psychology and Health* 13, no. 1 (1998): 11-44; English, Jane. *Different Doorway: Adventures of a Caesarean Born*. Point Reyes Station, CA: EarthHeart, 1985.

2. Smith, Roger. "The Timing of Birth." *Scientific American*, March 1999, 68-75.

3. Sandman, Curt A., Laura Glynn, Pathick D. Wadhwa, et al. "Elevated Maternal Cortisol Early in Pregnancy Predicts Third Trimester Levels of Placental Corticotropin Releasing Hormone (CRH): Priming the Placental Clock." *Peptides* 28 (2006): 1547-63; Sandman, Curt, Pathik D. Wadhwa, Manuel Porto, et al. "Maternal Corticotropin-Releasing Hormone Levels in Early Third Trimester Predicts Length of Gestation in Human Pregnancy." *Am J Obstet Gynecol* 179, no. 4, Oct. (1998): 1079-85.

4. Norwitz, Errol, R., Julian N. Robinson, and John Challis. "The Control of Labor." *New England Journal of Medicine* 341, no. 9 (1999): 660-66.

5. Leboyer, Frederick. *Birth without Violence*. Rochester, VT: Healing Arts Press, 1974, pg. 31.

6. Cheek, David B. "Prenatal and Perinatal Imprints: Apparent Prenatal Consciousness as Revealed by Hypnosis." *Pre- and Perinatal Psychology Journal* 2, no. 2 (1986): 97-110.

7. Jacobson, B, and M Bygdeman. "Obstetric Care and Proneness of Offspring to Suicide as Adults: A Case-Control Study." *Journal of Prenatal and Perinatal Psychology and Health* 15, no. 1 (2000): 63-74; Jacobson, B, G Eklund, L Hamberger, et al. "Perinatal Origin of Eventual Self-Destructive Behavior." *Pre- and Perinatal Psychology Journal* 2, no. 4 (1988): 227-41.

8. Leboyer, Frederick. *Birth without Violence*. Rochester, VT: Healing Arts Press, 1974, pg. 49.

9. Datablog. "Maternal Mortality: How Many Women Die in Childbirth in Your Country?" Guardian.co.uk, www.guardian.co.uk/news/datablog/2010/apr/12/maternal-mortality-rates-millennium-development-goals. The U.S. ranks an abysmal 41st on the World Health Organization's list of maternal death rates, behind South Korea and Bosnia—yet we spend more money on maternity care than any other nation; Friedman, Danielle. "Why Are So Many Moms Dying?" Daily Beast, www.thedailybeast.com/blogs-and-stories/2010-03-24/why-are-so-many-moms-dying.

10. Adams, Alice E. *Reproducing the Womb: Images of Childbirth in Science, Feminist Theory, and Literature*. Ithaca, NY: Cornell University Press, 1994.

11. Goer, Henci. *The Thinking Woman's Guide to a Better Birth*. New York: Perigee, 1999;

12. Raine, A, P Brennan, and SA Medink. "Birth Complications Combined with Early Maternal Rejection at Age 1 Year Predispose to Violent Crime at 18 Years." *Archives of General Psychiatry* 51 (1994): 984-88.

13. Prentice, A. "Fetal Heart Rate Monitoring During Labour: Too Frequent Intervention, Too Little Benefit?" *The Lancet* 330, no. 8572 (1987): 1375-77.

14. Cartwright, Elizabeth. "The Logic of Heartbeats: Electronic Fetal Monitoring and Biomedically Constructed Birth." In *Cyborg Babies: From Techno-Sex to Techno-Tots*, edited by Robbie Davis-Floyd and Joseph Dumit. New York: Routledge, 1998, pg. 243-244.

15. Ibid, pg. 249.

16. Goer, Henci. *The Thinking Woman's Guide to a Better Birth*. New York: Perigee, 1999.

17. Klaus, Marshall H., John H. Kennell, and Phyllis H. Klaus. *Bonding: Building the Foundations of Secure Attachment and Independence*. New York: Addison-Wesley, 1995.

18. Davis-Floyd, Robbie, and Joseph Dumit, eds. *Cyborg Babies: From Techno-Sex to Techno-Tots*. New York: Routledge, 1998.

19. Roan, Shari. "C-Sections on Rise as View of Risks Changes." *Los Angeles Times*, January 29 2001, A-1.

20. Davis-Floyd, Robbie, and Joseph Dumit. "From Technobirth to Cyborg Babies: Reflections on the Emergent Discourse of a Holistic Anthropologist." In *Cyborg Babies: From Techno-Sex to Techno-Tots*, edited by Robbie Davis-Floyd and Joseph Dumit. New York: Routledge, 1998, pg. 257.

21. Cohen, Nancy Wainer, and Lois J Estner. *Silent Knife: Cesarean Prevention and Vaginal Birth after Cesarean*. New York: Bergin and Garvey, 1983.

22. Goer, Henci. *The Thinking Woman's Guide to a Better Birth*. New York: Perigee, 1999.

23. Safranski, Misha. "CDC Says Cesarean Triples Neonatal Death Risk." Yahoo, www.associatedcontent.com/article/1980192/cdc_says_cesarean_triples_neonatal_pg2.html?cat=25.

24. Childbirth Connection. "Best Evidence: C-Section." Childbirth Connection, www.childbirthconnection.org/article.asp?ck=10166#babies; BBC News. "Caesarean Increases Asthma Risk." BBC, news.bbc.co.uk/2/hi/health/7755439.stm.

25. Henkart, Andrea Frank. "On the Cutting Edge." In *Trust Your Body! Trust Your Baby! Childbirth Wisdom and Cesarean Prevention*, 179. Westport, CT: Bergin & Garvey, 1995, pg. 16-17.

26. News-Medical.net. "Epigenetic Modulation at Birth - Altered DNA-Methylation in White Blood Cells after Caesarean Section." In *The Medical News*, 2009.

27. Davis-Floyd, Robbie, and Joseph Dumit, eds. *Cyborg Babies: From Techno-Sex to Techno-Tots*. New York: Routledge, 1998, pg. 9.

28. Goer, Henci. *The Thinking Woman's Guide to a Better Birth*. New York: Perigee, 1999.

29. Leverant, Robert. "Ruminations on Being Labor Cesarean Born." *Pre- and Perinatal Psychology Journal* 14, no. 3-4 (2000): pg. 311.

30. The Guardian. "Maternal Mortality: How Many Women Die in Childbirth in Your Country?" In *Datablog*. London: Guardian, 2010.

31. March of Dimes. "Nation Scores a 'D'." March of Dimes, www.marchofdimes.com/padmap.html.

32. Henkart, Andrea Frank, ed. *Trust Your Body! Trust Your Baby! Childbirth Wisdom and Cesarean Prevention*. Westport, CT: Bergin & Garvey, 1995.

33. Block, Jennifer. *Pushed: The Painful Truth About Childbirth and Modern Maternity Care*. New York: Da Capo, 2008, pg. xvii.

34. Johnson, Kenneth C, and Betty-Anne Davis. "Outcomes of Planned Home Births with Certified Professional Midwives: Large Prospective Study in North America." *British Medical Journal* 330 (2005).

35. Maternal and Newborn Health/Safe Motherhood Unit of the WHO. "Care in Normal Birth: A Practical Guide." Washington, DC: World Health Organization, 1996.

36. Sandman, Curt A et al. "Psychobiological Influences of Stress and Hpa Regulation on the Human Fetus and Infant Birth Outcomes." *Annals of the New York Academy of Sciences* 739 (1994): 198-210.

37. Odent, Michel. *Birth Reborn*. Medord, NJ: BirthWorks Press, 1994.

38. E.g. Block, Jennifer. *Pushed: The Painful Truth About Childbirth and Modern Maternity Care*. New York: Da Capo, 2008; Gaskin, Ina May. *Ina May's Guide to Childbirth*. New York: Bantam-Dell, 2003; Jordan, Brigitte. *Birth in Four Cultures*. Prospect Heights, IL: Waveland Press, 1993.

39. Davis-Floyd, Robbie. "The Rituals of American Hospital Birth." In *Conformity and Conflict: Readings in Cultural Anthropology*, edited by Eavid McCurdy, 323-40. New York: HarperCollins, 1994. (Also available at davis-floyd.com/the-rituals-of-american-hospital-birth)

40. Davis-Floyd, Robbie. *Birth as an American Rite of Passage*. Berkeley: University of California Press, 1992.

41. Davis-Floyd, Robbie. "The Rituals of American Hospital Birth." In *Conformity and Conflict: Readings in Cultural Anthropology*, edited by Eavid McCurdy, 323-40. New York: HarperCollins, 1994.

42. Ibid.

43. Bugg, George J, Farah Siddiqui, and Jim G Thornton. "Oxytocin Versus No Treatment or Delayed Treatment for Slow Progress in the First Stage of Spontaneous Labour." In *The Cochrane Library*, 2011. onlinelibrary.wiley.com/doi/10.1002/14651858.CD007123.pub2/abstract.

44. Jordan, Brigitte. *Birth in Four Cultures*. Prospect Heights, IL: Waveland Press, 1993.

45. Gaskin, Ina May. *Ina May's Guide to Childbirth*. New York: Bantam-Dell, 2003.

46. Davis-Floyd, Robbie, and Joseph Dumit. "From Technobirth to Cyborg Babies: Reflections on the Emergent Discourse of a Holistic Anthropologist." In *Cyborg Babies: From Techno-*

Sex to Techno-Tots, edited by Robbie Davis-Floyd and Joseph Dumit. New York: Routledge, 1998, pg. 260.

47. Henkart, Andrea Frank, ed. *Trust Your Body! Trust Your Baby! Childbirth Wisdom and Cesarean Prevention.* Westport, CT: Bergin & Garvey, 1995, pg. 52.

48. Davis-Floyd, Robbie, and Joseph Dumit. "From Technobirth to Cyborg Babies: Reflections on the Emergent Discourse of a Holistic Anthropologist." In *Cyborg Babies: From Techno-Sex to Techno-Tots*, edited by Robbie Davis-Floyd and Joseph Dumit. New York: Routledge, 1998, pg. 10.

49. Adams, Alice E. *Reproducing the Womb: Images of Childbirth in Science, Feminist Theory, and Literature.* Ithaca, NY: Cornell University Press, 1994, pg. 222.

50. Mauger, Benig. "Childbirth as Initiation and Transformation: The Wounded Mother." *Journal of Prenatal & Perinatal Psychology and Health* 11, no. 1 (1996): 17-30.

51. Davis-Floyd, Robbie, and Joseph Dumit. "From Technobirth to Cyborg Babies: Reflections on the Emergent Discourse of a Holistic Anthropologist." In *Cyborg Babies: From Techno-Sex to Techno-Tots*, edited by Robbie Davis-Floyd and Joseph Dumit. New York: Routledge, 1998, pg. 274.

52. England, Pam. *Birthing from Within.* Albuquerque, NM: Partera Press, 1998, pg. 151.

53. Gaskin, Ina May. *Ina May's Guide to Childbirth.* New York: Bantam-Dell, 2003, pg. 287. Gaskin outlines the facts and medical risk implications of the recent trend away from the traditional double-layer closure to a single-layer suturing following cesarean.

54. Ibid, pg. 152.

55. Gaskin, Ina May. *Ina May's Guide to Childbirth.* New York: Bantam-Dell, 2003.

56. Ibid, pg. 299.

57. Grady, Denise. "New Guidelines Seek to Reduce Repeat Caesareans." New York Times, www.nytimes.com/2010/07/22/health/22birth.html?pagewanted=print.

58. Gaskin, Ina May. *Ina May's Guide to Childbirth.* New York: Bantam-Dell, 2003, pg. 302-303.

59. Goer, Henci. *The Thinking Woman's Guide to a Better Birth.* New York: Perigee, 1999.

60. Kurth, Lisa, and Robert Haussmann. "Perinatal Pitocin as an Early Adhd Biomarker: Neurodevelopmental Risk?" *Journal of Attention Disorders* 15, no. 5 (2011).

61. Wahl, Roy U Rojas. "Could Oxytocin Administration During Labor Contribute to Autism and Related Behavioral Disorders?—a Look at the Literature." *Medical Hypotheses* 63, no. 3 (2004): 456-60.

62. Odent, Michel. "The Long Term Consequences of How We Are Born." *Journal of Prenatal and Perinatal Psychology and Health* 17, no. 2 (2002): 107-12.

63. Buckley, Sarah. *Gentle Birth, Gentle Mothering.* Berkeley, CA: Celestial Arts, 2009. An excellent research overview of cord clamping: Mercola, Joseph. "Why Do Obstetricians Still Rush to Clamp the Cord?" Mercola.com, articles.mercola.com/sites/articles/archive/2010/12/02/obstetricians-immediate-cord-clamping-routine.aspx.

64. Ibid, pg. 159.

65. Davis-Floyd, Robbie, and Joseph Dumit. "From Technobirth to Cyborg Babies: Reflections on the Emergent Discourse of a Holistic Anthropologist." In *Cyborg Babies: From Techno-Sex to Techno-Tots*, edited by Robbie Davis-Floyd and Joseph Dumit. New York: Routledge, 1998, pg. 262. The attentive reader will recall that Davis-Floyd's first birth was by C-section; this one was a midwife-attended home VBAC.

66. Kitzinger, Sheila. *The Experience of Childbirth.* New York: Viking Penguin, 1984, pg. 201.

67. Davis-Floyd, Robbie, and Joseph Dumit. "From Technobirth to Cyborg Babies: Reflections on the Emergent Discourse of a Holistic Anthropologist." In *Cyborg Babies: From Techno-Sex to Techno-Tots*, edited by Robbie Davis-Floyd and Joseph Dumit. New York: Routledge, 1998, pg. 264.

68. Odent, Michel. *The Caesarean*. London: Free Association Books, 2004, pg. 103-104.

69. Gettler, Lee T, Thomas W McDade, Alan B Feranil, and Christopher W Kuzawa. "Longitudinal Evidence That Fatherhood Decreases Testosterone in Human Males." *Proceedings of the National Academy of Sciences* 108, no. 39 (2011): 16194-99; and Abrams, Douglas Carlton. "The Making of a Modern Dad." *Psychology Today*, March/April 2002.

70. Personal communication, 2010.

71. Gaskin, Ina May. *Ina May's Guide to Childbirth*. New York: Bantam-Dell, 2003, pg. 191.

72. Houser, Patrick M. *The Fathers-to-Be Handbook*. London, UK: Creative Life Systems Ltd, 2007.

73. Alibrandi, Gina Maria. "Accept the Process: A Commentary on Childbirth Education." In *Trust Your Body! Trust Your Baby!*, edited by Andrea Frank Henkart. Westport, CT: Bergin & Garvey, 1995.

74. Gaskin, Ina May. *Ina May's Guide to Childbirth*. New York: Bantam-Dell, 2003.

STEP FIVE

1. Potos, Andrea. "Instructions for the New Mother." *Mothering*, 1998.

2. E.g. Maté, Gabor. *In the Realm of Hungry Ghosts: Close Encounters with Addiction*. Berkeley, CA: North Atlantic Books, 2010; Odent, Michel. *The Scientification of Love*. London: Free Association Books, 1999; Ornish, Dean. *Love & Survival: The Scientific Basis for the Healing Power of Intimacy*. New York: HarperCollins, 1997.

3. Davis-Floyd, Robbie, and Joseph Dumit, eds. *Cyborg Babies: From Techno-Sex to Techno-Tots*. New York: Routledge, 1998, pg. 6.

4. Davis-Floyd, Robbie. *Birth as an American Rite of Passage*. Berkeley: University of California Press, 1992.

5. Davis-Floyd, Robbie, and Joseph Dumit. "From Technobirth to Cyborg Babies: Reflections on the Emergent Discourse of a Holistic Anthropologist." In *Cyborg Babies: From Techno-Sex to Techno-Tots*, edited by Robbie Davis-Floyd and Joseph Dumit. New York: Routledge, 1998, pg. 260.

6. Bystrova, Ksenia et al. "Early Contact Versus Separation: Effects on Mother-Infant Interaction One Year Later." *Birth* 36, no. 2 (2009): 97-109.

7. Perry, Bruce, and Maia Szalvitz. *Born for Love: Why Empathy Is Essential—and Endangered*. New York: William Morrow, 2010, pg. 20.

8. Hrdy, Sarah Blaffer. *Mother Nature: Maternal Instincts and How They Shape the Human Species*. New York: Ballantine, 1999.

9. Ibid, pg. 399. I am grateful to the monkeys whose lives were spent in the pursuit of this revolutionary understanding, and it is my fervent hope that we can honor and learn from Harlow's and Hinde's landmark work, so that no more monkeys—or any other animals—need suffer this kind of scientific derangement.

10. Perry and Szalvitz. *Born for Love: Why Empathy Is Essential—and Endangered*, Chapter 6.

11. Hopson, Janet. "Fetal Psychology." *Psychology Today*, Sept. 1 1998.

12. Hofer, Myron A. "On the Nature and Consequences of Early Loss." *Psychosomatic Medicine* 58 (1996): 573. This excellent, highly readable article is available in its entirety at www.psychosomaticmedicine.org/cgi/reprint/58/6/570.pdf.

13. Morgan, Barak E, Alan R Horn, and Nils J Bergman. "Should Neonates Sleep Alone?" Biological Psychiatry 70, no. 9 (2011): 817-25.

14. McKenna, James J, and Thomas McDade. "Why Babies Should Never Sleep Alone: A Review of the Co-Sleeping Controversy in Relation to SIDS, Bedsharing and Breast Feeding." *Padediatric Respiratory Reviews* 6 (2005): 134-52. Available at www.naturalchild.org/james_mckenna/cosleeping.pdf.

15. Phillips, David P, Kimberly M Brewer, and Paul Wadensweiler. "Alcohol as a Risk Factor for Sudden Infant Death Syndrome (Sids)." In *Addiction*: John Wiley & Sons, 2010.

16. Lewis, Thomas et al., *A General Theory of Love*. New York: Random House, 2000, pg. 83.

17. E.g., Amini, Fariborz et al. "Affect, Attachment, Memory: Contributions toward Psychobiologic Integration." *Psychiatry* 59, no. 3 (1996): 213-39; Gareau, Mélanie G et al. "Neonatal Maternal Separation Causes Colonic Dysfunction in Rat Pups Including Impaired Host Resistance." *Pediatric Research* 59, no. 1 (2006): 83-88; Jimenez-Vasquez, P. A. et al. "Early Maternal Separation Alters Neuropeptide Y Concentrations in Selected Brain Regions in Adult Rats." *Brain Res Dev Brain Res* 131, no. 1-2 (2001): 149-52; Raine, A et al. "Birth Complications Combined with Early Maternal Rejection at Age 1 Year Predispose to Violent Crime at 18 Years." *Archives of General Psychiatry* 51 (1994): 984-88; Science Daily. "Prolonged Maternal Separation Increases Breast Cancer Risk in Neonatal Mice." Science Daily, www.sciencedaily.com/releases/2010/11/101108071906.htm; Kuhn, Cynthia M, and Saul M Schanberg. "Responses to Maternal Separation: Mechanisms and Mediators." *International Journal of Developmental Neuroscience* 16, no. 3-4 (1998): 261-70.

18. E.g. Levine, Peter. "When Biology Becomes Pathology." Paper presented at the From Neurons to Neighborhoods: The Effects of Emotional Trauma on the Way We Learn, Feel and Act, Mt. St. Mary's College, Los Angeles, March 2-3 2002; Van der Kolk, Bessel, and et al. *Traumatic Stress: The Effects of Overwhelming Experience on Mind, Body, and Society*. New York: Guildord Press, 1996.

19. E.g. Lewis, Thomas, Fari Amini, and Richard Lannon. *A General Theory of Love*. New York: Random House, 2000; Solomon, Marion F. *Narcissism and Intimacy*. New York: Norton, 1989.

20. Share, Lynda. *When Someone Speaks, It Gets Lighter: Dreams and the Reconstruction of Infant Trauma*. New Jersey: Analytic Press, 1994, pg. 60.

21. Prescott, James. "Affectional Bonding for the Prevention of Violent Behaviors: Neuro-Biological, Psychological and Religious/Spiritual Determinants." In *Violent Behavior Vol. I: Assessment and Intervention*, edited by L.J. Hertzberg et al., 110-42. New York: PMA Publications, 1990. Prescott served as Health Scientist Administrator of the Developmental Behavioral Biology Program at the National Institute of Child Health and Human Development at the NIH from 1966-1980. He was commissioned to do the most comprehensive study to date of the root causes of violence. What he turned up tanked his career because, as Joseph Chilton Pearce puts it, "it wasn't good for the gross national product." Prescott's suggested solutions to violence—keeping babies and mothers together; discouraging formula feeding; encouraging supportive/unconditional v. authoritarian parenting—wasn't good for the economy. Essentially his

research found that failed mother love in primates results in developmental brain disorders that lead to lifelong patterns of depression, violence and drug addiction. Prescott has continued driving home his message ever since, albeit as an outsider scientist.

22. Eberstadt, Mary. "Home Alone America." *Policy Review*, no. 107 (2001).

23. Hrdy, Sarah Blaffer. *Mother Nature: Maternal Instincts and How They Shape the Human Species*. New York: Ballantine, 1999.

24. Prescott, James. "How Culture Shapes the Developing Brain and the Future of Humanity." *Touch the Future*, Spring (2002): 15-18.

25. Ibid, pg. 17.

26. O'Donohue, John. *Beauty: The Invisible Embrace*. New York: Harper Perennial, 2005.

27. Ayres, A Jean. *Sensory Integration and the Child: Understanding Hidden Sensory Challenges*. Los Angeles: Western Psychological Services, 2005.

28. Kendall-Tackett, Kathleen. "Nighttime Breastfeeding and Maternal Mental Health." In *Science & Sensibility*: Lamaze International, 2010. When co-sleeping caught on in America in the 1970s, the rates of postpartum depression dropped dramatically within those groups practicing it.

29. Hrdy, Sarah Blaffer. *Mother Nature: Maternal Instincts and How They Shape the Human Species*. New York: Ballantine, 1999.

30. Petherick, Anna. "Development: Mother's Milk: A Rich Opportunity." *Nature* 468 (2010): S5-S7. This article reports that breastfed babies have fewer infections and may have fewer food allergies and less diarrhea. Breast milk also appears to actually affect gene expression in the stomach cells of infants—a finding whose implications aren't yet well understood but seem to further support the natural role of nursing in the postpartum year.

31. McCraty, Rollin et al., *Science of the Heart: Exploring the Role of the Heart in Human Performance*. Boulder Creek, CA: Institute of HeartMath, 2001.

32. Perry, Bruce. "Nature and Nurture of Brain Development: How Early Experience Shapes Child and Culture." In *From Neurons to Neighborhoods: The Neurobiology of Emotional Trauma*. Los Angeles, 2003.

33. Kendall-Tackett, Kathleen. "Nighttime Breastfeeding and Maternal Mental Health." In *Science & Sensibility*: Lamaze International, 2010.

34. Verrier, Nancy. *The Primal Wound: Understanding the Adopted Child*. Baltimore, MD: Gateway, 1993.

35. McGinn, Michael F. "Attachment and Separation: Obstacles for Adoptees." *Journal of Social Distress & the Homeless* 9, no. 4 (2000): 273-90.

36. Axness, Marcy. *What Is Written on the Heart - Primal Issues in Adoption*. Los Angeles: Adoption Insight, 1998.

37. Brodzinsky, David M. "Prevalence of Adoptees among Special Education Populations." *Journal of Learning Disabilities* 27, no. 8 (1991): 484-89.

38. Shelton, Deborah, and Bonnie Miller Rubin. "More Mental Disorders in Adopted Youth." *Los Angeles Times*, May 6 2008, A17.

39. Maté, Gabor. *In the Realm of Hungry Ghosts: Close Encounters with Addiction*. Berkeley, CA: North Atlantic Books, 2010.

40. Slap, G. "Adoption as a Risk Factor for Attempted Suicide During Adolescence." *Pediatrics* 108, no. 2 (2001): E30.

41. Abbott, Scott William. "When There's No Place Like Home: Heidegger, Hermeneutics, and the Narratives of Adopted Adolescents." *Dissertation Abstracts International: Section B: The Sciences & Engineering* 60, no. 9-B (2000): 4871.

42. Szejer, Myriam. *Talking to Babies: Psychoanalysis on a Maternity Ward.* Boston: Beacon Press, 2005.

43. Ibid, pg. 65.

44. Ibid, pg. 198-199.

45. Christakis, Dominic A. "The Effects of Infant Media Usage: What Do We Know and What Should We Learn?" *Acta Paediactrica* 98 (2009): 8-16. The researchers put so fine a point on the infant media debacle as to declare, "Parents hoping to raise baby Einsteins by using infant educational videos are actually creating baby Homer Simpsons." My contempt knows no bounds for an enterprise that leverages parents' insecurities and fears (*Will my child have what it takes to succeed in this ever more complicated world?*) into a frantic market for baby-improvement "infotainment" that flies in the face of everything science knows about what infants and young children need for healthy development. They even thumbed their nose at the American Pediatric Association's guideline that children under two shouldn't watch any television.

46. Stern, Daniel N. *Diary of a Baby.* New York: Basic Books, 1998, pg. 48.

47. Schore, Allan. *Affect Regulation and the Origin of the Self: The Neurobiology of Emotional Development.* Mahwah, NJ: Lawrence Erlbaum, 1999 (if you're the intrepid sort and want to read the original work of one of the founding godfathers of the field); Lewis, Thomas et al. *A General Theory of Love.* New York: Random House, 2000 (if you'd prefer a simpler explanation designed for lay people, and one of the most gorgeously written books ever on *any* subject, let alone the neurobiology of attachment!).

48. Solomon, Marion F. *Narcissism and Intimacy.* New York: Norton, 1989. Solomon contributes an excellent understanding to the distinguishing features of affect, emotion, and feeling—terms that are often used interchangeably in psychological literature. *Affect*s, of which there are a limited repertoire present from birth (or even before), are undefined global sensations related to experiences with bodily functions—physical comfort or pain deriving from nurturing and/or deprivation experiences between infant and caretaker. These are basic to the development of the core self during the early months of life. At first they are not psychological events but purely biological responses; however, they quickly become linked to encoded memory traces and become the building blocks of *emotions*, responses that incorporate patterns of seeing, hearing, smelling and touching. Emotions are formed during interactional experiences that include some awareness of self and other. *Feelings* combine emotions and affects with cognitive processes, which can begin when the infant is capable of symbolic thought—generally by around 18 to 24 months. (Pg. 82)

49. E.g. Amini, Fariborz, et al. "Affect, Attachment, Memory: Contributions toward Psychobiologic Integration." *Psychiatry* 59, no. 3 (1996): 213-39.

50. Schore, A. N. "Attachment and the Regulation of the Right Brain." *Attachment and Human Development* 2, no. 1 (2000): 23-47.

51. Lewis, Thomas et al. *A General Theory of Love.* New York: Random House, 2000.

52. Buck, R. "The Neuropsychology of Communication: Spontaneous and Symbolic Aspects." *Journal of Pragmatics* 22 (1994): 265-78, quoted in Schore, Allan N. "The Neurobiology of Attachment and Early Personality Organization." *Journal of Prenatal and Perinatal Psychology and Health* 16, no. 3 (2002): 249-63; italics added for emphasis.

53. Schore, Allan N. "The Neurobiology of Attachment and Early Personality Organization." *Journal of Prenatal and Perinatal Psychology and Health* 16, no. 3 (2002), pg. 258.

54. Goleman, Daniel. *Social Intelligence: The New Science of Human Relationships.* New York: Bantam/Dell, 2006, pg. 143.

55. Maté, Gabor. *Scattered: How Attention Deficit Disorder Originates and What You Can Do About It.* New York: Penguin, 1999.

56. Siegel, Daniel J., and Mary Hartzell. *Parenting from the inside Out: How a Deeper Self-Understanding Can Help You Raise Children Who Thrive*. New York: Jeremy Tarcher/Putnam, 2003.

57. Perry, Bruce, and Maia Szalvitz. *Born for Love: Why Empathy Is Essential—and Endangered*. New York: William Morrow, 2010, pg. 125.

58. Lewis, Thomas, Fari Amini, and Richard Lannon. *A General Theory of Love*. New York: Random House, 2000.

59. Friday, Nancy. *The Power of Beauty*. New York: Harper-Collins, 1996, pg. 133.

60. Breeding, John. *The Wildest Colts Make the Best Horses*. UK: Chipmunka Publishing, 2007.

61. Siegel, Daniel J. "Emotional Trauma and the Developing Mind." Paper presented at the From Neurons to Neighborhoods: The Effects of Emotional Trauma on the Way We Learn, Feel and Act, Mt. St. Mary's College, Dept. of Psychology, March 2-3 2002.

62. Axness, Marcy. "Malattachment and the Self Struggle." *Journal of Prenatal and Perinatal Psychology and Health* 19, no. 2 (2004): 131-47.

63. Perry, Bruce, and Maia Szalvitz. *Born for Love: Why Empathy Is Essential—and Endangered*. New York: William Morrow, 2010.

64. Schwartz, Jeffrey M, and Sharon Begley. *The Mind and the Brain: Neuroplasticity and the Power of Mental Force*. New York: HarperCollins, 2002.

65. Siegel, Daniel J., and Mary Hartzell. *Parenting from the inside Out: How a Deeper Self-Understanding Can Help You Raise Children Who Thrive*. New York: Jeremy Tarcher/Putnam, 2003.

66. Liedloff, Jean. "Who's in Control? The Unhappy Consequences of Being Child-Centered." In *Pathways to Family Wellness*. Philadelphia, PA: Int'l Chiropractic Pediatric Assn., 2005.

67. Ibid.

68. Pearce, Joseph Chilton. *The Biology of Transcendence: A Blueprint of the Human Spirit*. Rochester, VT: Inner Traditions, 2002.

69. Schore, Allan. *Affect Regulation and the Origin of the Self : The Neurobiology of Emotional Development*. Mahwah, NJ: Lawrence Erlbaum, 1999.

70. Leo, Pam. "Connection Parenting." connectionparenting.com.

71. Erikson, Erik H. *Childhood and Society*. New York: Norton Co., 1963. Erikson was prescient of our recent understanding of the importance of the *quality* of parental presence and attunement on the development of the social psyche.

72. Cooper, Glen et al. "Circle of Security." www.circleofsecurity.net.

73. Siegel, Daniel J., and Mary Hartzell. *Parenting from the inside Out: How a Deeper Self-Understanding Can Help You Raise Children Who Thrive*. New York: Jeremy Tarcher/Putnam, 2003, pg. 163.

74. Di Blasio, Paola, and Chiara Ionio. "Childbirth and Narratives: How Do Mothers Deal with Their Child's Birth?" *Journal of Prenatal and Perinatal Psychology and Health* 17, no. 2 (2002): 143-51.

75. Goleman, Daniel. *Social Intelligence: The New Science of Human Relationships*. New York: Bantam/Dell, 2006, pg. 11.

76. Ibid.

77. Panuthos, Claudia. *Transformation through Birth*. Westport, CT: Bergin & Garvey, 1984, pg. 132.

78. Jordan, Brigitte. *Birth in Four Cultures*. Prospect Heights, IL: Waveland Press, 1993.

79. Shields, Brooke. *Down Came the Rain*. New York: Hyperion, 2006.

80. Rettner, Rachael. "Perfectionists at Risk for Postpartum Depression." LiveScience.com, www.livescience.com/6696-perfectionists-risk-postpartum-depression.html.

81. Axness, Marcy. "A Mother's Call to Healing: Old Wounds Surface When Children Are Born." *Whole Life Times*, July 1995, 14-15.

82. Orthof, Claudia and Eleanor M Luzes. "Immediate Postpartum: Mother-Baby Bonding." In *XVI Encounter of Conscious Pregnancy and Natural Childbirth*, edited by Carla Maria Garcia Machado. Rio de Janeiro, 2006.

83. Hagen, Edward H. "Does Postpartum Depression Serve an Evolutionary Purpose?" In *Scientific American Mind*: Scientific American, 2009.

84. Mendizza, Michael, and Joseph Chilton Pearce. *Magical Parent, Magical Child: The Optimum Learning Relationship*. Nevada City, CA: In-Joy, 2002.

85. Robbins, John. *Reclaiming Our Health: Exploding the Medical Myth and Embracing the Source of True Healing*. Tiburon, CA: H.J. Kramer, 1996, pg. 42.

86. Lewis, Thomas et al. *A General Theory of Love*. New York: Random House, 2000, pg. 88.

87. Perry, Bruce, and Maia Szalvitz. *Born for Love: Why Empathy Is Essential—and Endangered*. New York: William Morrow, 2010.

88. Ibid, pg. 47.

89. Di Blasio, Paola, and Chiara Ionio. "Childbirth and Narratives: How Do Mothers Deal with Their Child's Birth?" *Journal of Prenatal and Perinatal Psychology and Health* 17, no. 2 (2002): 143-51.

90. Margulis, Jennifer. "What No One Tells You About Bonding with Baby." In *Mothering*. Santa Fe, NM: Mothering 2011. mothering.com/jennifermargulis/infancy/what-no-one-tells-you-about-bonding-with-baby.

91. Maté, Gabor. *Scattered: How Attention Deficit Disorder Originates and What You Can Do About It*. New York: Penguin, 1999.

92. Travis, John W. "Why Men Leave—a Hidden Epidemic." ww.compleatmother.com/articles2/why_men_leave.htm.

93. Salter, Joan. *The Incarnating Child*. Gloucestershire, U.K.: Hawthorne Press, 1987, pg. 25.

94. Karp, Harvey, and Nancy Mohrbacher. "More Debate on Swaddling." *International journal of Childbirth Education* 26, no. 3 (2011): 26-31.

95. Marsa, Linda. "Study: Baby Walker May Delay First Steps." *Los Angeles Times*, July 1 2002, S-3.

96. The New York Times. "The Dangers of Baby Walkers." New York Times, consults.blogs.nytimes.com/2010/02/22/the-dangers-of-baby-walkers.

97. Science Daily. "Letting Infants Watch Tv Can Do More Harm Than Good." Science Daily LLC, www.sciencedaily.com/releases/2009/01/090113074419.htm.

98. Pierre, Summer. "Reflections on a Year of Motherhood." In *Summer Pierre Headquarters*. New York, 2011, summerpierre.wordpress.com/2011/01/10/reflections-on-a-year-of-motherhood/.

STEP SIX

1. White, Burton L. *New First Three Years of Life: Completely Revised and Updated*. New York: Fireside, 1995, pg. 355.

2. Eberstadt, Mary. "Home Alone America." *Policy Review*, no. 107 (2001).

3. Ibid.

4. Dancy, Rahima Baldwin. *You Are Your Child's First Teacher*. Berkeley, CA: Celestial Arts, 2000, pg. 8.

5. Ibid, pg. 6.

6. Bartlett, Tom. "The Case for Play." The Chronicle of Higher Education, chronicle.com/article/The-Case-for-Play/126382.

7. Elkind, David. "The Disappearance of Play." In *Child Education Series*. Caltech University, Pasadena, CA, 2004.

8. Larsen, Kate. "There Are Ways to Give Kids a Good Head Start on Literacy." *The Sun*, July 17 2003.

9. Johnson, Susan. "Teaching Our Children to Read, Write & Spell." *Pathways to Family Wellness*, Spring 2010, 44-47. An excellent article explaining how early reading taxes the child's developing brain; can be found at icpa4kids.org/Wellness-Articles/teaching-our-children-to-write-read-a-spell.html.

10. Suggate, Sebastian P. "School Entry Age and Reading Achievement in the 2006 Programme for International Student Assessment (Pisa)." *International Journal of Educational Research* 48, no. 3 (2009): 151-61.

11. University of Otago. "Late Readers Close Learning Gap." Science Alert, www.sciencealert.com.au/news/20100401-20448.html.

12. Clarkson, Beth. "Early Poor Readers Remain Poor Readers." James Randi Educational Foundation forum, forums.randi.org/showthread.php?t=76797.

13. Bartlett, Tom. "The Case for Play." The Chronicle of Higher Education, chronicle.com/article/The-Case-for-Play/126382/.

14. Schore, Allan. *Affect Regulation and the Origin of the Self: The Neurobiology of Emotional Development*. Mahwah, NJ: Lawrence Erlbaum, 1999. We are indebted to Schore for his groundbreaking work that has enlightened so many. "Affect" is a word that refers to an infant's early emotional experiences, and also to primitive emotions we all continue to negotiate at all ages.

15. Johnson, Susan. "The Importance of Warmth." www.youandyourchildshealth.org/youandyourchildshealth/articles/the%20importance%20of%20warmth.html.

16. Ibid.

17. Johnson, Susan. "Fever." www.youandyourchildshealth.org/youandyourchildshealth/articles/fever.html. Written by a developmental pediatrician, all of the articles on this site are great resources. I especially appreciate Dr. Johnson's sense of humor: she writes about the first time she did lemon wraps for her son's high fever, "All I could think of while doing this was the headlines in the morning newspaper—'Son dies of a febrile seizure while mother, who is a pediatrician, applies lemon juice to his calves.' Well, the headlines didn't turn out like that. My son's fever immediately came down to 102 and the hallucinations stopped, all in 10 minutes."

18. Block, Melissa. "Healing Crisis: Don't Worry, Mom—I'm Just Growing!" *Mothering*, July/August 2003. (Also available at mothering.com/health/healing-crisis-dont-worry-mom-im-just-growing.)

19. Goleman, Daniel. *Social Intelligence: The New Science of Human Relationships*. New York: Bantam/Dell, 2006, pg. 154.

20. Lyddon, William J., and Alissa Sherry. "Developmental Personality Styles: An Attachment Theory Conceptualization of Personality Disorders." *Journal of Counseling & Development* 79, no. 4 (2001): 405-14. Many mental health experts express the opinion that labels such as

narcissistic or borderline personality disorder are "charged with pejorative meaning" and frequently used in the mental health professions as "little more than a sophisticated insult," writes Judith Herman (*Trauma and Recovery*. New York: Basic Books, 1997, pg. 123). In that spirit, and inspired by Ivey's more compassionate term "developmental personality style," cited in Lyddon and Sherry, over the conventional "personality disorder," I prefer the term "defensive personality style." This harmonizes well with Alice Miller's classic exploration of these styles, which she saw "less as an illness than as a tragedy" (Miller, Alice. *The Drama of the Gifted Child*. New York: Basic Books, 1981, pg. xvi). It articulates such personality constellations not as "disorders," or "flaws," but rather, unique ways a person has learned to adapt to and survive the pain of insecure or disorganized attachments and the rejection, abandonment, or abuse inherent in them.

21. Zahn-Waxler, Carolyn. "Becoming Compassionate: The Origins and Development of Empathic Concern." *Shift: At the Frontiers of Consciousness*, December 2006-February 2007 2007, 21-23.

22. Paul, Pamela. "Fearless Preschoolers Lack Empathy? ." *New York Times*, November 21 2010.

23. In *Born for Love: Why Empathy Is Essential—and Endangered*. New York: William Morrow, 2010, pg.112-119, authors Perry and Szalavitz offer a good explanation of the hyporesponsive stress system—lower resting heart rate, lower skin conductance response to stress (a primary measure taken by polygraph), and lower resting levels of cortisol—often found in "fearless" children, along with a thorough discussion of the implications of various parenting approaches for the development of empathy, for future aggression and violence, and even for the flourishing or foundering of entire societies and nations.

24. Ackerman, Jennifer. *Sex Sleep Eat Drink Dream: A Day in the Life of Your Body*. New York: Houghton Mifflin, 2007, pg. 8.

25. Liedloff, Jean. "Who's in Control? The Unhappy Consequences of Being Child-Centered." In *Pathways to Family Wellness*. Philadelphia, PA: Int'l Chiropractic Pediatric Assn., 2005. icpa4kids.org/Wellness-Articles/whos-in-control-the-unhappy-consequences-of-being-child-centered.html.

26. Mendizza, Michael, and Joseph Chilton Pearce. *Magical Parent, Magical Child: The Optimum Learning Relationship*. Nevada City, CA: In-Joy, 2002.

27. Grille, Robin. *Parenting for a Peaceful World*. NSW, Australia: Longueville, 2005.

28. Payne, Kim John, and Lisa M Ross. *Simplicity Parenting: Using the Extraordinary Power of Less to Raise Calmer, Happier, and More Secure Kids* New York: Ballantine, 2010.

29. Pearce, Joseph Chilton. "The Biology of Trancendence: Shaping Your Life in a Radically Changing World." Santa Barbara Graduate Institute, September 20-21 2002. In this talk, Joe recalled an article in *Forbes* magazine all about the new market for advertisers to fruitfully target—the four-to-seven year olds—whose overarching message was, "Stabilize your consumer market from the very beginning."

30. Kuhl, Patricia. "The Linguistic Genius of Babies." TEDxTalks, www.ted.com/talks/patricia_kuhl_the_linguistic_genius_of_babies.html.

31. Toole, Carol. "The First Four Years of Childhood." *Renewal: A Journal for Waldorf Education* 11, no. 1 (2002): 5-9.

32. Healy, Jane M. *Endangered Minds: Why Children Don't Think and What We Can Do About It*. New York: Touchstone, 1990.

33. Schmitt, Kelly L. "Children's Visual Attention to Formal Features of Television at Home." In *60th Bienniel meeting of the Society for Research in Child Development*. New Orleans,

LA, 1993. www.eric.ed.gov/ERICWebPortal/search/detailmini.jsp?_nfpb=true&_&ERICExt Search_SearchValue_0=ED362272&ERICExtSearch_SearchType_0=no&accno=ED362272.

34. Healy, Melissa. "Losing Focus." *Los Angeles Times*, May 25 2004, F1.

35. Lillard, Angeline S, and Jennifer Peterson. "The Immediate Impact of Different Types of Television on Young Children's Executive Function." *Pediatrics* 128, no. 4 (2011): 644-49.

36. Healy, Jane M. *Endangered Minds: Why Children Don't Think and What We Can Do About It*. New York: Touchstone, 1990.

37. Badenoch, Bonnie. "Mindfulness/Mindlessness." YouTube, www.youtube.com/watch?v=pbyTRSnwhsI. This state when the mind "lets go" relies on the newly recognized *default network* in the brain; notable discoveries, inventions, and works of creativity have arisen from this state.

38. Mendizza, Michael, and Joseph Chilton Pearce. *Magical Parent, Magical Child: The Optimum Learning Relationship*. Nevada City, CA: In-Joy, 2002, pg. 143.

39. Postman, Neil. *The Disappearance of Childhood*. New York: Vintage Books, 1994, pg. 90.

40. Payne, Kim John, and Lisa M Ross. *Simplicity Parenting: Using the Extraordinary Power of Less to Raise Calmer, Happier, and More Secure Kids* New York: Ballantine, 2010, pg. 8.

41. Payne, Kim John. "The Soul of Discpline." Highland Hall Waldorf School, Northridge, CA, February 2003.

42. Neufeld, Gordon, and Gabor Maté. *Hold on to Your Kids: Why Parents Need to Matter More Than Peers*. New York: Ballantine, 2006, pg. 215.

43. Personal communication, 2010.

44. Goodman, Brenda. "Self-Control in Childhood Brings Adult Success." WebMD, LLC, children.webmd.com/news/20110124/self-control-in-childhood-brings-adults-success.

45. Ibid.

46. Essex, Marilyn J, W Thomas Boyce, Michael S Kobor, et al. "Epigenetic Vestiges of Early Developmental Adversity: Childhood Stress Exposure and DNA Methylation in Adolescence." *Child Development*, no. DOI: 10.1111/j.1467-8624.2011.01641.x (2011).

47. Grille, Robin. *Parenting for a Peaceful World*. NSW, Australia: Longueville, 2005. See pg. 181-191 for a thorough discussion of the topic of corporal punishment.

48. Grille, Robin. *Parenting for a Peaceful World*. NSW, Australia: Longueville, 2005, pg. 187.

49. Ibid.

50. Brown, Brené. "TedxHouston." TEDxTalks, www.youtube.com/watch?v=X4Qm9cGRub0.

51. Grille, Robin. *Parenting for a Peaceful World*. NSW, Australia: Longueville, 2005.

52. Paul, Pamela. "Can Preschoolers Be Depressed?" New York Times, www.nytimes.com/2010/08/29/magazine/29preschool-t.html.

53. Grille, Robin. *Parenting for a Peaceful World*. NSW, Australia: Longueville, 2005, pg. 199.

54. Ibid, pg. 187.

55. Cohen, Lawrence. *Playful Parenting*. New York: Ballantine, 2001, pg. 235.

56. Goleman, Daniel. *Social Intelligence: The New Science of Human Relationships*. New York: Bantam/Dell, 2006; excellent discussion of safety as a prerequisite for playing on pg. 180.

57. Ibid, pg. 17.

58. Patterson, Barbara, and Pamela Bradley. *Beyond the Rainbow Bridge: Nurturing Our Children from Birth to Seven*. Amesbury, MA: Michaelmas Press, 2000. Many of the discipline in-

sights and ideas in this step are inspired by this lovely book, for which I'm grateful to Barbara and Pamela.

59. Neufeld, Gordon, and Gabor Maté. *Hold on to Your Kids: Why Parents Need to Matter More Than Peers.* New York: Ballantine, 2006, pg. 72.

60. Kohn, Alfie. *Punished by Rewards.* Boston: Houghton Mifflin, 1993, pg. 104.

61. Ibid, pg. 102-3, emphasis by the author.

62. Aldort, Naomi. "Getting out of the Way." *Mothering*, 1994, 38-43.

63. Richtel, Matt. "A Silicon Valley School That Doesn't Compute." New York Times, www .nytimes.com/2011/10/23/technology/at-waldorf-school-in-silicon-valley-technology-can-wait .html?_r=3&hp.

64. Poplawski, Thomas. "Etheric? Astral? Ego? An Esoteric View of the Human Being and Its Value in the Education of the Child." *Renewal: A Journal for Waldorf Education* 11, no. 1 (2002): 11-16.

65. Carey, Benedict. "Psychiatry and Preschoolers." *Los Angeles Times*, June 30 2003, F1.

66. Myers, David G. *Psychology* Ninth ed. New York: Worth, 2010, pg. 634.

67. Bailey, Becky. *Easy to Love, Difficult to Discipline.* New York: Quill, 2002, pg. 30-31.

68. Payne, Kim John. "The Soul of Discpline." Highland Hall Waldorf School, Northridge, CA, February 2003.

69. Steingraber, Sandra. "The Environmental Life of Children." In *Child Honoring: How to Turn This World Around*, edited by Raffi Cavoukian and Sharna Olfman, 107-15. Westport, CT: Praeger, 2006.

70. Poplawski, Thomas. "Etheric? Astral? Ego? An Esoteric View of the Human Being and Its Value in the Education of the Child." *Renewal: A Journal for Waldorf Education* 11, no. 1 (2002): 11-16.

71. Payne, Kim John, and Lisa M Ross. *Simplicity Parenting: Using the Extraordinary Power of Less to Raise Calmer, Happier, and More Secure Kids* New York: Ballantine, 2010, pg. 6.

72. Science Daily. "Depression Treatment: Mindfulness-Based Cognitive Therapy as Effective as Anti-Depressant Medication, Study Suggests." ScienceDaily, www.sciencedaily.com/ releases/2008/11/081130201928.htm.

73. Steingraber, Sandra. "The Environmental Life of Children." In *Child Honoring: How to Turn This World Around*, edited by Raffi Cavoukian and Sharna Olfman, 107-15. Westport, CT: Praeger, 2006.

74. Payne, Kim John. "The Soul of Discpline." Highland Hall Waldorf School, Northridge, CA, February 2003.

75. Ferrucci, Piero. *The Power of Kindness.* New York: Jeremy Tarcher/Penguin, 2006, pg. 10.

76. Grille, Robin. *Parenting for a Peaceful World.* NSW, Australia: Longueville, 2005, pg. xvii.

77. Elkind, David. *Miseducation: Preschoolers at Risk.* New York: Alfred Knopf/Borzoi, 1987, pg. 120.

78. McKinney, John. "Thoreau Was Right: Nature Hones the Mind." Miller-McCune, www .miller-mccune.com/health/thoreau-was-right-nature-hones-the-mind-26763/#.

79. Ferrucci, Piero. *The Power of Kindness.* New York: Jeremy Tarcher/Penguin, 2006, pg. 7.

80. Elkind, David. *Miseducation: Preschoolers at Risk.* New York: Alfred Knopf/Borzoi, 1987, pg. 161-183. (The page numbers will vary slightly in the more recent edition; the chapter is entitled "Making Healthy Educational Choices.")

81. Barnes, Henry. "An Introduction to Waldorf Education: Learning That Grows with the Learner." In *Waldorf Education: A Family Guide*, edited by Pamela Johnson Fenner and Karen L. Rivers. Amesbury, MA: Michaelmas Press, 1992.

82. Payne, Kim John, and Lisa M Ross. *Simplicity Parenting: Using the Extraordinary Power of Less to Raise Calmer, Happier, and More Secure Kids* New York: Ballantine, 2010.

83. Mercola, Joseph. "Sugar May Be Bad, but This Sweetener Is Far More Deadly." Mercola.com, articles.mercola.com/sites/articles/archive/2010/01/02/highfructose-corn-syrup-alters-human-metabolism.aspx.

84. Batmanghelidj, Fereydoon. *Your Body's Many Cries for Water*. 3rd ed: Global Health Solutions, 2008.

85. Gross, Terry. "Jon Stewart: The Most Trusted Name in Fake News." In *Fresh Air*: NPR, 2010. www.npr.org/templates/story/story.php?storyId=130321994.

STEP SEVEN

1. Barnes, Henry. "An Introduction to Waldorf Education: Learning That Grows with the Learner." In *Waldorf Education: A Family Guide*, edited by Pamela Johnson Fenner and Karen L. Rivers. Amesbury, MA: Michaelmas Press, 1992.

2. Perry, Bruce. "Nature and Nurture of Brain Development: How Early Experience Shapes Child and Culture." In *From Neurons to Neighborhoods: The Neurobiology of Emotional Trauma*. Los Angeles, 2003. Sometimes, when parents are coming to these principles when their child is already in the school-age years, what is needed is a bit of "catch-up"—implementation of earlier steps to, for example, fulfill the child's needs for more security, consistency, warmth, etc. Any developmental need that is not fulfilled during its rightful stage doesn't simply go away; it tends to persist lifelong and a person's attempts to meet those needs (which are usually unconscious) get expressed in maladaptive ways, such as in obsessive-compulsive behavior, manipulation, etc.

3. Quoted in Cobb, J.J. *Cybergrace: The Search for God in the Digital World*. New York: Crown, 1998, pg. 56.

4. McGlauflin, Helene. "Struggling with Screens: One Mother's Story." *Renewal: A Journal of Waldorf Education* 14, no. 2 (2005).

5. Murray, John P. "Television Violence and Its Impact on Children." In *The Kansas Journal of Law and Public Policy*: DocStoc.com, 1995. www.docstoc.com/docs/8390796/Television-Influence.

6. Tompkins, Aimee. "The Psychological Effects of Media Violence on Children." AllPsych Online, allpsych.com/journal/violentmedia.html.

7. The Kaiser Family Foundation. "Key Facts: Tv Violence." Washington, DC: The Kaiser Family Foundation, 2003.

8. Livingston, Karen. "Some Thoughts on Television." *Mariposa*, 1999.

9. Huesmann, L Rowell et al. "Intervening Variables in the Tv Violence-Aggression Relation: Evidence from Two Countries." *Developmental Psychology* 20, no. 5 (1984): 746-75.

10. Oppenheimer, Todd. *The Flickering Mind: Saving Education from the False Promise of Technology*. New York: Random House, 2003.

11. Oppenheimer, Todd. "Schooling the Imagination." *Atlantic Monthly*, June 1999.

12. Oppenheimer, Todd. *The Flickering Mind: Saving Education from the False Promise of Technology*. New York: Random House, 2003.

13. Sblendorio, Christopher. "Push-Button Entertainment and the Health of the Soul." *Renewal: A Journal for Waldorf Education*, 1991.

14. Brooks, Barbara. "Menarche." In *Encyclopedia of Children and Childhood in History and Society*: Gale Group, 2008. www.faqs.org/childhood/Me-Pa/Menarche.html.

15. Wierson, M et al. "Toward a New Understanding of Early Menarche; the Role of Environmental Stress in Pubertal Timing." In *Adolescence*, 913-24: PubMed.gov, 1993. www.ncbi.nlm.nih.gov/pubmed/8266844.

16. Postman, Neil. *The Disappearance of Childhood*. New York: Vintage Books, 1994, pg. 83-85.

17. Poplawski, Thomas. "Taming the Media Monster." *Renewal, A Journal for Waldorf Education* 10, no. 1 (2001).

18. Ibid.

19. Meyer, Rudolf. *The Wisdom of Fairy Tales*. Edinburgh, GB: Floris Books, 1988.

20. Coplen, Dotty. *Parenting for a Healthy Future*. Gloucestershire, UK: Hawthorn House, 1995.

21. Gatto, John Taylor. *The Underground History of American Education*. New York: Oxford Village Press, 2000. Gatto reveals the little-known fact that Mann and his wife visited Prussia in the summertime, when schools were out of session; Mann's positive assessments were based on conversations with vacationing schoolmasters, tours of empty classrooms and reading old reports.

22. Visser, Michiel. "Public Education Versus Liberty: The Pedigree of an Idea." Acton Institute, www.tysknews.com/Depts/Educate/education_versus_liberty.htm.

23. Hammond, Linda Darling. *The Right to Learn*. San Francisco: Jossey-Bass, 1997, pg. 40, emphasis mine.

24. Gatto, John Taylor. *The Underground History of American Education*. New York: Oxford Village Press, 2000.

25. Elkind, David. *The Hurried Child: Growing up Too Fast Too Soon*. Cambridge, MA: Perseus Publishing, 2001.

26. Ibid. With what we now know about early brain development and the fundamental role attachment plays in healthy wiring of the circuitry in a child's frontal lobes, the main thing these children were missing out on at home wasn't necessarily "academic preparedness" such as learning their letters and numbers, but simply time spent in relationship with an attuned, responsive, lovingly authoritative parent. Along with a rich environment of stories and play opportunities, the gains enjoyed by children in Head Start derive largely from the enrichment of having relationships with human adults who are interested and who have time to interact with them.

27. Visser, Michiel. "Public Education Versus Liberty: The Pedigree of an Idea." Acton Institute, www.tysknews.com/Depts/Educate/education_versus_liberty.htm.

28. Gatto, John Taylor. "American Education History Tour." Odysseus Group, www.johntaylorgatto.com/historytour/history5.htm.

29. Ibid, pg. 9.

30. Kohn, Alfie. "The 500-Pound Gorilla." www.alfiekohn.org/teaching/500pound.htm.

31. Dewey, John. *The Child and the Curriculum*. Chicago: University of Chicago Press, 1902, pg. 13.

32. Glasser, William. *Schools without Failure*. New York: Harper & Row, 1969.

33. Gatto, John Taylor. *Dumbing Us Down: The Hidden Curriculum of Compulsive Schooling*. New York: New Society Publishers, 2002, pg. 2.

34. Ibid, pg. 4.

35. Oppenheimer, Todd. "Schooling the Imagination." *Atlantic Monthly*, June 1999.

36. Ibid.

37. Dominus, Susan. "Play-Doh? Calculus? At the Manhattan Free School, Anything Goes." New York Times, www.nytimes.com/2010/10/05/nyregion/05bigcity.html?_r=1&hp=&page wanted=print.

38. Gerber, Charlotte. "Statistics on Homeschooling in the United States." lovetoknow, home-school.lovetoknow.com/Statistics_on_Homeschooling_in_the_United_States.

39. Postman, Neil. *Teaching as a Subversive Activity*. New York: Delacorte Press, 1969, pg. 81.

40. Ibid, pg. 62-65.

41. Jan Evans Bowman, personal communication, 2010.

42. Sblendorio, Christopher. "Push-Button Entertainment and the Health of the Soul." *Renewal: A Journal of Waldorf Education* (1991).

43. Mann, Christine. "Family Dinner Time Creates Lasting Benefits." suite101.com, www.suite101.com/content/family-dinner-time-builds-health-success-a69810.

44. Spiegel, Alix. "The Family Dinner Deconstructed." In *Morning Edition*: NPR, 2008. www.npr.org/templates/story/story.php?storyId=18753715.

45. Elkind, David. "The Disappearance of Play." In *Child Education Series*. Caltech University, Pasadena, CA, 2004.

46. Coakley, Jay. *Sports in Society: Issues and Controversies*. 10th ed. New York: McGraw-Hill, 2008.

47. Zopa, Sifu. "Teaching Martial Arts to Kids." Yun Hoi Chun Kuen, www.yunhoiwingchun.com/Articles/General/TeachingMartialArtstokids/tabid/93/Default.aspx.

48. Stepp, Laura Sessions. *Our Last Best Shot: Guiding Our Children through Early Adolescence*. New York: Riverhead Books, 2000, pg. 321.

49. Ibid, pg. 319.

50. Ibid, pg. 306.

51. Giedd, Jay. "Inside the Teenage Brain (Unedited *Frontline* Interview)." PBS, www.pbs.org/wgbh/pages/frontline/shows/teenbrain/interviews/giedd.html, 2002. We can thank the reprogramming of cerebellum circuitry at this phase of development for the fact that teens are so often clumsy, like the proverbial fast-growing puppy dog who hasn't quite caught up with its own size!

52. Ibid.

53. Pearce, Joseph Chilton. *The Biology of Transcendence: A Blueprint of the Human Spirit*. Rochester, VT: Inner Traditions, 2002, pg. 53.

54. Friday, Nancy. *The Power of Beauty*. New York: Harper-Collins, 1996, pg. 127.

55. Marks Psychiatry. "Sense of Fatalism Encourages Risky Behavior in Teens." Marks Psychiatry, markspsychiatry.com/sense-of-fatalism-encourages-risky-behavior-in-teens/. Some think this study, published in the journal *Pediatrics*, challenges the conventional perception that teens engage in risky behaviors because of their perception that they are invulnerable to harm; most likely—as in most either-or questions about causality—both are true in different cases and in complex interrelatedness.

56. Staley, Betty. *Between Form and Freedom*. Stroud, UK: Hawthorne Press, 1988, pg. 8.

57. Spinks, Sarah. "Inside the Teenage Brain." In *Frontline*, 2002. www.pbs.org/wgbh/pages/frontline/shows/teenbrain/etc/script.html.

58. Payne, Kim John. "The Soul of Discpline." Highland Hall Waldorf School, Northridge, CA, February 2003.

59. Prescott, James. "How Culture Shapes the Developing Brain and the Future of Humanity." *Touch the Future*, no. Spring (2002): 15-18.

60. Pearce, Joseph Chilton. *The Biology of Transcendence: A Blueprint of the Human Spirit.* Rochester, VT: Inner Traditions, 2002, pg. 49.

61. de Zengotita, Thomas. "The Numbing of the American Mind: Culture as Anesthetic." *Harper's*, April 2002, 33-40.

62. DiCarlo, Russell E., ed. *Towards a New World View: Conversations at the Leading Edge.* Erie, PA: Epic, 1996, pg. 164.

63. Lewis, Thomas et al. *A General Theory of Love.* New York: Random House, 2000.

64. Maté, Gabor. *In the Realm of Hungry Ghosts: Close Encounters with Addiction.* Berkeley, CA: North Atlantic Books, 2010.

65. Frank, Scott et al. "Hyper-Texting and Hyper-Networking: A New Health Risk Category for Teens?" In *American Public Health Association's 138th Annual Meeting & Expo: Social Justice.* Denver, CO: APHA, 2010.

66. Pearce, Joseph Chilton. *The Biology of Transcendence: A Blueprint of the Human Spirit.* Rochester, VT: Inner Traditions, 2002, pg. 51. Pearce highlights research suggesting that "the increase of intelligence at each stage of development is disproportionately greater than the increase exhibited in the previous stage, similar to the order of increase found in the Richter scale for measuring earthquakes. Thus the intelligence increase in the stage designed to open at late adolescence is an order of magnitude vastly beyond that of the previous stage, suggesting an intelligence in no way related to anything coming before. Adding up all experience and knowledge gained to that point gives no hint of the possibilities ready to unfold somewhere around age twenty-one."

67. Neufeld, Gordon, and Gabor Maté. *Hold on to Your Kids: Why Parents Need to Matter More Than Peers.* New York: Ballantine, 2006, pg. 98.

68. Ibid, pg. 131-132.

69. Ibid, pg. 102.

70. Ibid, pg. 103.

71. Ibid, pg. 103.

72. Ibid, pg. 262.

73. Poplawski, Thomas. "Paradise Lost: The Nine-Year Change " *Renewal: A Journal of Waldorf Education* 13, no. 1 (2004): 4-8.

74. Rosenberg, Marshall. *Nonviolent Communication.* Boulder, CO: Sounds True, 2004.

75. Walbridge, Jean. "On Trusting Your Adolescent." SelfGrowth.com, www.self growth.com/articles/On_Trusting_Your_Adolescent.html.

76. Payne, Kim John, and Lisa M Ross. *Simplicity Parenting: Using the Extraordinary Power of Less to Raise Calmer, Happier, and More Secure Kids* New York: Ballantine, 2010, pg. 34.

EPILOGUE

1. Eberstadt, Mary. "Home Alone America." *Policy Review*, no. 107 (2001).

2. NIH: Child Health and Human Development. "Child Care Linked to Assertive, Noncompliant, and Aggressive Behaviors; Vast Majority of Children within Normal Range." National Institutes of Health, www.nichd.nih.gov/news/releases/child_care.cfm.

3. Groch, Judith. "Daycare May Lessen Aggression in Children of Low-Education Mothers." University of Pennsylvania School of Medicine and MedPage Today, www.medpagetoday.com/Psychiatry/GeneralPsychiatry/7250.

4. NIH: Child Health and Human Development. "Child Care Linked to Assertive, Non-compliant, and Aggressive Behaviors; Vast Majority of Children within Normal Range." National Institutes of Health, www.nichd.nih.gov/news/releases/child_care.cfm.

5. Jong, Erica. "Mother Madness." The Wall Street Journal, online.wsj.com/article/SB10001424052748704462704575590603553674296.html.

6. Begley, Sharon. "Adventures in Good and Evil: The Evolutionary Roots of Morality." *Newsweek*, May 4 2009, 46-48.

7. Ibid, italics added for emphasis.

8. Chua, Amy. *Battle Hymn of the Tiger Mother*. New York: Penguin Press, 2011.

9. Lewis, Thomas, Fari Amini, and Richard Lannon. *A General Theory of Love*. New York: Random House, 2000, pg. 32.

10. Lipton, Bruce, and Steve Bhaerman. *Spontaneous Evolution*. Carlsbad, CA: Hay House, 2009, pg. 340.

11. Laszlo, Ervin. *Chaos Point: 2012 and Beyond*. Newburyport, MA: Hampton Roads, 2010.

12. Lipton, Bruce, and Steve Bhaerman. *Spontaneous Evolution*. Carlsbad, CA: Hay House, 2009, pg. 359.

13. Perry, Bruce, and Maia Szalvitz. *Born for Love: Why Empathy Is Essential—and Endangered*. New York: William Morrow, 2010, pg. 116.

14. Lewis, Thomas, Fari Amini, and Richard Lannon. *A General Theory of Love*. New York: Random House, 2000.Lewis, pg. 225-226.

15. Cavoukian, Raffi, and Sharna Olfman, eds. *Child Honoring: How to Turn This World Around*. Westport, CT: Praeger, 2006, pg. xix-xx.

16. Teilhard de Chardin, Pierre. *The Phenomenon of Man*. New York: Harper & Row, 1959/Perennial reprint 2002, 1959, pg. 255.

17. Postman, Neil. *The Disappearance of Childhood*. New York: Vintage Books, 1994, pg. 153.

INDEX

ABOUT THE AUTHOR

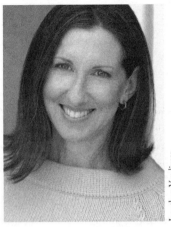

Jonathan Vandiveer

Her own life and discoveries as an adopted person and a mother led Marcy Axness to pursue a deeper understanding of how we become who we become, how early it begins, and how we can do it in a healthier, more joyful way. She is a popular international speaker on attachment, culture, and child and parent development. Featured in several documentary films, she is an expert in adoption, prenatal development and Waldorf education. She counsels parents and pre-parents in her private Quantum Parenting practice, applying, honing, and documenting the successful results of *Parenting for Peace* principles in real life. With her former husband of twenty-five years, she has raised a son, twenty-four, and a daughter, twenty-one, both of whom are engaging, thoughtful, flourishing young adults.

In her pre-motherhood life, Marcy won multiple awards and an Emmy nomination as a documentary writer and producer, covering emerging topics in health for CBS News, and has produced programming for Lifetime, Showtime, and The Disney Channel. She has a solid constituency built up over nearly twenty years of teaching, writing, counseling, and networking within multiple intersecting communities focused on progressive human insights, development, and evolution. Her combination of life experience, cultural acumen, and scholarly credibility uniquely equip her to chart this compelling, entertaining, and engaging human roadmap through attachment theory, developmental neurobiology, epigenetics, cell biology, prenatal psychology, child development, and consciousness research to illuminate a pathway of healing and wholeness for coming generations.

Marcy invites you to join her at www.ParentingForPeace.com.

Sentient Publications, LLC publishes books on cultural creativity, experimental education, transformative spirituality, holistic health, new science, ecology, and other topics, approached from an integral viewpoint. Our authors are intensely interested in exploring the nature of life from fresh perspectives, addressing life's great questions, and fostering the full expression of the human potential. Sentient Publications' books arise from the spirit of inquiry and the richness of the inherent dialogue between writer and reader.

Our Culture Tools series is designed to give social catalyzers and cultural entrepreneurs the essential information, technology, and inspiration to forge a sustainable, creative, and compassionate world.

We are very interested in hearing from our readers. To direct suggestions or comments to us, or to be added to our mailing list, please contact:

SENTIENT PUBLICATIONS, LLC

1113 Spruce Street
Boulder, CO 80302
303-443-2188
contact@sentientpublications.com
www.sentientpublications.com